Violence in the
Emergency Department

Patricia B. "Nikki" Allen, MBA, BS, RN, has spent her entire career in diverse areas of health care management. She has created a violence prevention plan including violence prevention tools to help the multiple Emergency Departments (EDs) with which she has been involved. Since then, Ms. Allen has become increasingly interested in addressing the explosive but underreported incidence of violence occurring in Emergency Departments across the United States. She has been a regular invited speaker about violence in the Emergency Department at the Leadership Conference of the Emergency Nurses Association (ENA). She is passionate about continuing her work in developing strategies to deal with violent individuals, to help protect ED patients, and to help physicians, nurses, and ED staff protect themselves from harm. Ms. Allen's other passions are her three grown children, her daughter-in-law, and her friends. One of her children is a health care professional in an environment that is high-risk for violence.

Violence in the Emergency Department

Tools and Strategies to Create a Violence-Free ED

PATRICIA B. ALLEN, MBA, BS, RN

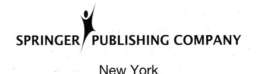

SPRINGER PUBLISHING COMPANY

New York

No part of this publication may be reproduced, stored in a retrieval system, or transmitted in any form or by any means, electronic, mechanical, photocopying, recording, or otherwise, without the prior permission of Springer Publishing Company, LLC, or authorization through payment of the appropriate fees to the Copyright Clearance Center, Inc., 222 Rosewood Drive, Danvers, MA 01923, 978-750-8400, fax 978-646-8600, info@copyright.com or on the web at www.copyright.com.

Springer Publishing Company, LLC
11 West 42nd Street
New York, NY 10036
www.springerpub.com

Acquisitions Editor: Margaret Zuccarini
Project Manager: Mark Frazier
Cover design: Mimi Flow
Composition: Apex CoVantage, LLC

Ebook ISBN: 978-0-8261-1060-2

09 10 11 12 13 / 5 4 3 2 1

The author and the publisher of this Work have made every effort to use sources believed to be reliable to provide information that is accurate and compatible with the standards generally accepted at the time of publication. Because medical science is continually advancing, our knowledge base continues to expand. Therefore, as new information becomes available, changes in procedures become necessary. We recommend that the reader always consult current research and specific institutional policies before performing any clinical procedure. The author and publisher shall not be liable for any special, consequential, or exemplary damages resulting, in whole or in part, from the readers' use of, or reliance on, the information contained in this book. The publisher has no responsibility for the persistence or accuracy of URLs for external or third-party Internet Web sites referred to in this publication and does not guarantee that any content on such Web sites is, or will remain, accurate or appropriate.

Library of Congress Cataloging-in-Publication Data

Allen, Patricia, MBA, R.N.
    Violence in the emergency department : tools & strategies to create a violence-free ED / by Patricia "Nikki" Allen.
        p. ; cm.
    Includes bibliographical references and index.
    ISBN 978-0-8261-1059-6 (alk. paper)
    1. Violence in hospitals—Prevention.   2. Hospitals—Emergency services—Safety measures.   I. Title.
    [DNLM: 1. Emergency Service, Hospital.   2. Violence—prevention & control.   3. Security Measures. WX 185 A428v 2009]
    R727.2.A45 2009
    362.18—dc22   2009009495

Printed in the United States of America by Victor Graphics

This book is dedicated to my beloved children, Amanda, Andrew, and Jennifer, and to my daughter-in-law, Ashley. I cherish you all very much. Thank you for being wonderful adults and amazing individuals!
Second, I dedicate this book to my friends Paul Clere, Wendy Fordyce, and Pam King, who enthusiastically supported my passion to help curb violence in U.S. EDs and pushed me toward my goal of writing this book.
I could not have finished the book without my devoted and detailed friend, Marilyn Wright. And to Margaret Zuccarini and Brian O'Connor, my ever-patient editors, thank you; you know what you did!
I dedicate this book to the Emergency Department nurses, directors, and physicians with whom I have had the pleasure to work and for whom I have the greatest respect and utmost admiration.
I further dedicate this book to my ENA speaking partner, Vicki Owens, who as the director of a large suburban ED has experienced violence in her own ED despite being ahead of the curve in protecting their ED environment against intrusion.
Finally, to my former boss, Suzanne Stone-Griffith, who saw a need for hospital Emergency Departments to be made aware of the dangers of violence and who addressed the need for prevention programs.

Contents

Preface

My goal in writing this book is to share the tremendous amount of information that I have amassed over several years of research and practice, and through the Emergency Nurses Association (ENA) forum that allowed me to speak about a subject that is of immense interest to me. During a literature review to update my current information, three themes recurred about violence in the Emergency Department.

First, our dedicated Emergency Department nurses, physicians, and staff are being threatened, spit on, harassed, kicked, punched, and seriously injured by patients and exposed to other types of violence on nearly an everyday basis. Some nurses believe that patient abuse is part of the job, while other nurses just seem reluctant to report abuse. Several resources attribute this trend to the fact that nurses apparently believe there is no logic in reporting any level of patient abuse because of they believe that violence will not be addressed. "We are out there on the front lines without guns, bulletproof vests and mace. We are out there trying to help. When did it become OK to hit or beat us?" (Harmacinski, 2003). Fellow nurses, it is simply not OK to be treated with abuse or violence—no matter what. Please immediately report any violence or abuse!

Second, violence is more than the type of violence that I refer to as walking-in-the-door violence. It can include the violence and abuse delivered by violent street gangs; perpetrators of violence; patients, including psychiatrically ill patients; families; friends; and strangers. I realized that street gangs and abuse to nurses by patients must certainly be discussed but that other forms of violence exist that may present themselves in the ED, such as domestic/intimate partner violence/abuse; teen dating violence/abuse; lateral/workplace violence; and elder violence/abuse. I felt it necessary to expand on the subject matter of *all* violence, although this book is not intended to be a complete resource for each type of violence against patients.

Third, there is scant information about the larger topic of ED violence. I have searched and researched newspaper archives, journals, Web sites, books, academic literature, and personal recollections to little avail. There is inadequate contemporary information in any written source about violence in U.S. EDs. Surprisingly, I found more information from the prior decade and a good bit of journalistic information from Britain, Canada, and Australia, some which is relevant to U.S. EDs and that I will share.

I know that violence has not gone away from the doors of our U.S. Emergency Departments. Quite the contrary; violence is occurring to a much greater extent, and the problem of violence is becoming more complex and difficult to address. I decided to write this book with the intent of sharing what I have learned and with the hope of impeding even one death or disability due to violence in U.S. Emergency Departments.

Violence in the Emergency Department is larger than just workplace violence. It envelopes every facet of violence and is affecting the safety and welfare of our nurses and health care providers and of our patients, who entrust us to care for them.

Patricia B. "Nikki" Allen, MBA, BS, RN

Introduction

Violence in the ED, while an incongruity, is a crisis for U.S. hospitals. Emergency Departments are places that people come to be cared for, and the perception—and the reality—is that no one should encounter danger in the ED.

However, violence in the ED is increasing and is responsible for death, job-ending physical assault, loss of work days, decreased job satisfaction, career change of talented and committed emergency medicine physicians and nurses, and change in the environment of emergency care in the United States and internationally. Violence in the ED may be partially responsible for the closing of hospitals and Emergency Departments across the U.S.

Emergency Departments of all sizes and demographics in the U.S. and in the world are becoming the victims of violence. The incidence and the extent of violence are rapidly escalating. Being a rural or a suburban medical center is no longer an automatic guarantee that violence will not occur. No Emergency Department is immune.

There are five types of individuals who threaten and/or instigate violence in U.S. Emergency Departments:

- The individual or family who becomes volatile and assaults the professional caregiver in the ED for diverse reasons, often due only to long waits to obtain emergency care
- Psychiatric patients, especially those who are not compliant with their medication regimen
- The gang member or other perpetrator who is seeking drugs or revenge or responds in his habitually violent way (Savelli, personal communication, 2008)
- The substance abuser who is seeking drugs or is acting out due to the effects of drugs or alcohol intoxication
- The angry individual who perceives himself as a victim and who seeks out specific individuals to assault or harm; this individual often has a past history of violent behavior

The reasons that these individuals or groups incite violence are many, complex, and varied: overcrowded ED waiting rooms, staffing shortages, untrained triage nurses, limited interpersonal communication, uninitiated ED staff, and the patient's perception of being forgotten in the waiting room are documented reasons for violent outbursts. Individuals who are patients in the Emergency Department may have a psychiatric illness or an acute personality disorder, and such patients are taken to the Emergency Department because there is no other place to go.

When individuals feel threatened (being sick or in pain) or out of control (waiting hour after hour for medical assistance), and perceive inactivity by the ED staff, a normally calm individual can often be incited to explosive anger.

There are several other notable types of violence whose victims may present as patients in the ED:

- The victim of domestic abuse, now commonly called intimate partner violence or IPV (both male and female)
- Victims of dating violence that has become rampant among teenagers and adolescents
- The coworker, the so-called lateral abuser, who victimizes a cohort in the workplace
- Elder abuse victims, a blight on the U.S. that exists in alarming numbers
- The child who is the victim of violence or abuse.

Street gangs present a powerful challenge for Emergency Departments. When a gang member is injured, it is characteristic for other members of his gang to follow the injured person to the ED and take up residence in the waiting room. The act of cutting off a shirt or taking off a hat or gang beads, which may be necessary for emergency treatment, is considered disrespectful to the gang and can provoke violence.

Identifying the potential risk for violence in *your* ED is the *critical first step* to prevention. Each hospital must recognize and address the potential for violence in its own Emergency Department with the ultimate goal of protecting the physicians, nurses, staff, and other patients who are customers of the hospital.

Hospitals need to anticipate that violence will occur and have a plan to prevent it. Each staff member, whether employed full-time, part-time, or PRN, needs to be trained in de-escalation tactics and to have the tools, support, and empowerment necessary to know how to act rapidly when a violent episode does erupt in the Emergency Department.[1]

Hospital leaders must recognize the risks that may be inherent within their hospitals, such as multiple access points into the Emergency Department and hospital, limited security personnel, unmanned video surveillance, untrained ED staff, and so forth and work toward correcting these deficiencies.

Limited data are published about violence in U.S. Emergency Departments often due to the conflict between the need to attract and retain patients in a hospitable way and the reality of caring for individuals who may have a violent lifestyle. Staff generally underreports violence because many staff perceives assaults or abuse by patients as part of the job. In a 2008 position statement, the Emergency Nurses Association (ENA) tells hospitals that "healthcare organizations have a responsibility to provide a safe and secure environment for their employees and the public. Emergency Nurses have the right to take appropriate measures to protect themselves and their patients from injury due to violent individuals" (ENA, 2008).

Violence prevention can become a core competency for a hospital Emergency Department if violence prevention is employed consistently, is successful, and is communicated to the community.

So, why isn't violence in the Emergency Department the new hot topic of the year, constantly on the mind of every red-blooded American, discussed around the water cooler or before football games? The reason is that no one outside of the business of health care—most especially those in hospital emergency services—is aware of the significant impact that violence in the Emergency Department is creating. Violence in the ED may be well-known and recognized among hospital administration. The problem of ED violence may be insufficiently admitted, perhaps due to the fact that hospital administrators must do everything possible to generate one more customer/paying patient to ensure their hospital's—and their own—longevity and success.

This book is a guide for Emergency Departments, hospitals, and for health care professionals involved in the care of patients in the Emergency Department. *Violence in the Emergency Department* is designed to help you become aware of the potential for violence and to identify risk in your Emergency Department. This book will help you take the critical first steps toward implementing a violence defense strategy and program to protect your hospital and your invaluable Emergency Department staff. Additionally, this book will assist you in creating a violence-free

ED and help create a core competency to enable your hospital to market *your* Emergency Department to patients as the safe place to come for emergency services.

Violence in the Emergency Department is also a primer for non–health care individuals who want and/or need to understand the complex nature of violence in U.S. Emergency Departments. It is my hope that this information will provide the insight and knowledge necessary to make crucial decisions for yourself and your family when emergency care is needed.

NOTE

1. PRN is a hospital staffing strategy and refers to staffing on an as-needed basis.

REFERENCES

Emergency Nurses Association (ENA) position statement: violence in emergency care settings. (September, 2008). Retrieved May 14, 2009, from www.ena.org

Harmacinski, J. (2003). *Emergency room violence growing concern for nurses.* Salem, Massachusetts: The Salem News.

The Emergence of Violence in Society and Health Care Settings

We used to wonder where war lived, what it was that made it so vile. And now we realize that we know where it lives, that it is inside ourselves.
—Albert Camus

1 The Sociology of American Violence

The past two decades in the United States have been met with an amazing amalgam of change: sophisticated technological change; change in transportation methods; change in how goods and services are manufactured, advertised, and delivered; and dramatic population and demographic change. Much of the change in the U.S. has been negative and toxic, threatening individuals and communities. I recall the innocent America of my youth and in contrasting the 1950s and 1960s to the escalating international and social tensions of today, I have questioned the onset of violence in contemporary society and I have attempted to identify even one source for the arrival and acceleration of violence into our previously untouched lives. How and when did violence begin to creep into our perfect American world?

The naiveté that many of us experienced in our youth often was created by the shield of a small-town existence. Around us—yet far away—the rumblings of social and racial tension was beginning. Civil rights, the Bay of Pigs, and Vietnam were introduced into every U.S. living room as radio and television broadcasting technology improved. Mothers canned and prepared food and clothing for bomb shelters and in school; we practiced shielding ourselves beneath our desks in the event that the *red alert* was sounded. Singers and songwriters captured the social change that the U.S. was experiencing, notably in the anthem dedicated to the students at Kent State University (Ohio) who died from violence, and tributes to Martin Luther King and Bobby and President John Kennedy, who were violently assassinated by U.S. citizens. The remoteness and inaccessibility of the rest of the world were disappearing as images of the political and social change in allied and in hostile countries became part of the fabric of everyday American life.

HOW DID VIOLENCE BEGIN?

It is a vast and difficult challenge to interpret the various theories and analyses of political, social, and economic thinkers and to decipher and assimilate one or several theories into a causal agent for the beginnings of violence as a social voice.

There are three key factors that may have been responsible for the formation and function of society and that may help to explain a foundation for violence in the late 18th-century U.S.

The first key factor, the structure of the economy, such as the presence of or lack of a democracy (Barrington Moore, n.d.), may be a significant factor in whether a society embraces—or rejects—violence as a way to express displeasure. Individuals who live in tyrannical societies, who do not have a vote in how their taxes are spent or in the making of governing rules, can become frustrated and angry. U.S. democracy has based its foundation on *by the people, for the people,* and as in other democratic governments individual citizens define the policies and laws. Autocracy, by its very nature, appears to fuel frustrated and violent action in the form of coups or demonstrations. The basis of democracy is to promote and encourage independent thinking and accomplishment, empowering people with jurisdiction over their own lives, resulting in less frustration and violent behavior.

The second key factor, the type of labor or employment system implemented by government, may be a cause. In Japan, employment became "internalized" (Mosk, 2008) in the 1940s through the legalization of labor unions. The government approval of unions resulted in one very important outcome: the loyalty of the workforce that was further strengthened by the offer of high wages and assured employment for both white-collar and blue-collar workers, promised to the workers in the best *and* in the worst of economic times. As a valuable byproduct, the Japanese workers became a very flexible workforce so that when technological opportunity presented itself, the workers were able to capitalize on the change that we recognize as the just-in-time inventory strategy (Bnet business dictionary, n.d.).[1] While there is no direct evidence that an employment system of this kind was a sustaining feature in creating loyalty and/or reducing worker dissatisfaction—and therefore in decreasing the potential for violence—it is an intuitive leap to assume that employees appreciated this intervention. In the U.S., there is no such mechanism to garner employee loyalty. The U.S. is, and has been, fraught with layoffs, downsizings, and right-sizings. These unemployed individuals are likely to feel disenfranchised and desperate—and far from loyal. All of this has contributed to growing employee *hostility* against the employer, which has, at times, culminated in workplace shootings and other forms of violence from angry and frustrated individuals.

The timing of industrialization of a society (Bendix, n.d.), occurring in the late-19th century in America, represents historical levels of technological advance (Dore, n.d.) that led to a flurry of entrepreneurial investment and great advances by inventors. In the U.S., both the investors and the entrepreneurs enjoyed great wealth. The Gilded Age in the U.S. was an explosion of growth and was thus labeled and intended to imply "outwardly showy but internally corrupt" (David, 1936, p. 12). This phrase sums up the circumstances of the U.S. at the end of the 19th century: the U.S. government was mired in corruption, and great prosperity and wealth was held by only a handful of people, while the remaining citizens were desperately poor and deprived.

We can assume that societal industrialization in other countries has had much the same impact as it had in the U.S., whereas violence in preindustrial societies may be less furious, less intense. The point in time that industrialization and mechanization occur may signal the beginning of change that creates the rationale for irrational behavior that is violence.

CLUES ABOUT VIOLENCE IN EARLY SOCIETY

A growing disregard for the worth of human values during the pinnacle of industrialization (David, 1936), when cities were growing and commerce was spreading westward, may have stimulated the rapid development of labor unions in the U.S. in 1886. The dramatic changes in *industrial technique* broadened the chasm between employer and employee. "Sweeping industrialization" and change and improvement in technology created the opportunity for the extensive exportation of goods (David, 1936, p. 4). Factory workers were underpaid, underappreciated, and exploited. One employer was said to have remarked to Samuel Gompers, "I regard my employees as I do a machine, to be used to my advantage, and when they are old and of no further use I cast them in the street" (David, 1936, p. 7).

The law of supply and demand affected the U.S. worker and his ability to earn a decent wage. Public and private investment in industrialization and mechanization was rampant, and since machines could do the work of the labor force faster and better, more machines and fewer workers were used. In 1886, Carroll Wright, the Commissioner of Labor, reported that machines had taken the place of one-half of the human workforce that heretofore had been irreplaceable 20 years prior. One account from a small arms manufacturing operation projected that the number of gun stocks that could be manufactured by one laborer using a machine was greater by a factor of 45–50 times than what could be accomplished by a cadre of workers in an entire day. It was estimated that this one operation alone had displaced "44–49" men (David, 1936, p. 5).

The workforce in the U.S. had grown very large because the "stream of cheap European labor entering the country" (David, 1936, p. 4). Competition and the thirst for wealth drove the business owners to pay their workers the smallest wage they could pay so as to pocket more money for themselves. This disparity in wealth "drove a powerful wedge between the workers and the owners" to a degree that had not been seen before" (David, 1936, p. 8). The workers—the *working poor*—were accused of being destitute because of "poor education; drink, laziness, [gambling] and improvidence" (David, 1936, p. 8) rather than as a result of the rapid expansion of mechanization that reduced the need for human manpower. "If one examines the economic and social condition of the United States working class during the 'eighties, one can understand why labor was restive and discontented" (David, 1936, p. 8). The limitless number of workers who were able and willing to accept insufficient wages fueled a growing economic hardship for a great many people, creating a vast number of poor workers and poverty-stricken families in the U.S. If one man refused to work long hours for a paltry wage, there were two or three other men standing in line who would gladly accept. It is no revelation that extreme discontent among the new working class was mounting to a dangerous level. The men had no control over their environment and had no ability to make change; they were forced to accept intolerable working conditions, deficient wages, and miserable living circumstances. In 1883, 10% of the population in U.S. cities lived below the poverty level, with the average worker's wages less than $1.00 a day (David, 1936).

The political system was corrupt, and the politicians flaunted the wealth, privilege, and social status that accompanied their election to office. The workers had much to complain about and accused the employers of being the "destroyers of human rights" (David, 1936, p. 12). The expanding division of social standing and economic assets is perhaps the beginning of the phrase the *haves and the have-nots,* referred to by social scientists as the "frustration-aggression mechanism" (Conflict Resolution Consortium, Staff, 1970, p. 10).

SOCIAL REVOLUTION

By 1881, the social revolutionary movement was growing in the U.S., but there was still only a modest interest in the principles of the movement or support through participation until a German man, Johan Most, arrived in the U.S. in 1882. Johan Most is credited with revving up the quasi-anarchists by providing a rational basis for social-revolutionary action in the U.S.

Most had spent an unhappy, humiliating childhood in Germany. He had a visible physical deformity that may have played a large part in his belief that he was to be relegated to the role of a "martyr for society" (David, 1936, p. 84). Interestingly, Johan Most was a victim of violence himself, having had an "unfortunate experience with a parish priest" during his youth (David, 1936, p. 85). As a young adult in Germany, Most was becoming more radical in his thought. He acquainted himself with Marxist thinking and action and was frequently criticized and questioned by law enforcement regarding his increasingly extremist socialistic views.[2] Before he was forced to leave Germany in 1878 under antisocialist law, he had managed to serve two terms in the Reichstag, the German Parliament. In London, following his ejection from Germany, he published a weekly socialist newsletter and became actively involved with Russian terrorists, writing in favor of the assassination of Tsar Alexander II. Through Most's publications, the public was confronted with the reality of Most as a violent man, which added to his critical notoriety. Most was a robust and fanatical proponent of violence, defending the "use of violence to achieve the necessary end" (*(Johan) Most Biographical Sketch,* n.d.).

Upon his arrival in the U.S., Most's anarchist views and his ability to speak with conviction and passion created idol-like curiosity and veneration wherever he visited. Johan Most believed that states (the U.S. and other countries) must be governed by a group of citizens, and he spoke against the structure of a government, rejecting the strength, protection, and involvement of any government in society. Most, in fact, did not believe in formal government and argued for methods to overthrow authority. Initially, Most was able to convince large numbers of U.S. citizens that through the use of force, government could be changed and made to succumb to the wishes of the people, encouraging governance by the people without the influence of an official government. Eventually the influence and power that Most had briefly enjoyed during his time in the U.S. was weakened as U.S. citizens grew increasingly disbelieving of Most and of his radical and unfamiliar ideas. Most died in the U.S. nearly 20 years after he had first arrived and had been welcomed and heralded as a visionary (David, 1936, p. 91). Most may have been successful in influencing his maxim of violence before falling out of favor.

THE EARLY 20TH CENTURY AND AMERICA'S GILDED AGE

By 1890, 11 million of the 12 million employed U.S. citizens were earning less than $1,200/year. The average annual wage was $380.00 (David, 1936, p. 13) as compared with a projected average wage for U.S. workers in 2009 of $52,909 (N.D., 2008). Cities offered citizens an opportunity to earn more money than could be earned in rural agricultural areas, which created a massive migration into the cities. Additionally, immigrants continued to arrive in the U.S. in unprecedented numbers. Both groups flowed into the city, hoping to make their fortunes.

An economist of the time is quoted as saying, "a widespread feeling of unrest and brooding revolution . . . violent strikes and riots wracked the nation through the turn of the Century. The middle class whispered fearfully of 'carnivals of revenge'" (*America in the Gilded Age*, 1999). The middle class of the day—the working poor—was the group of workers who were suffering abject poverty and horrendous living conditions in tenements in the cities. The *frustration-aggression mechanism* appears to be recognized by social scientists during this era as an important keystone in the rise of violence (Conflict Resolution Consortium, Staff, 1970, p. 10).

The Gilded Age of the U.S. brought about the formation of a social structure in large urban cities after the U.S. Civil War. The Gilded Age was characterized by a bifurcation of interests representing a change from the middle-of-the-road sociopolitical viewpoint that had been the prevailing position for most U.S. citizens until the early part of the 20th century. This developing dichotomy of positions was apparent in the surfacing of a class structure producing a high-society faction that became interested in demonstrating the good life with irrepressible displays of wealth, including elaborate houses and excessive material possessions, and an opposing segment representing the lowest of the low society— beggars, thieves, and murderers who lived in hovels often down the street from the opulent, extravagant homes and buildings owned by the other half (*America in the Gilded Age*, 1999). The situation created by this social positioning during the Gilded Age may have been the impetus for the social theorists' discussions—an attempt to put a name to the changes that were occurring. An increase in frustration, anger, and aggression resulted in violence as a means to collectively express displeasure at the disparity of social circumstances.

The early beginnings of change—a division in the group's social interests—was apparent from the political splinter groups that formed on either side of the central political opinion and were based on the driving interests within each group. The group that was right of center (the former, central political position) was gravely concerned about the new, developing culture and the "waning of patrician society and standards," whereas the group left of center strongly favored correcting "mass poverty and inequality" (Monti, 1999, p. 33). Both groups had a zeal for the evolving social and industrial capitalism of the U.S., each hoping to cash in on fortunes of their own, but the groups were dissimilar in their approach to solving the problems of cities (Monti, 1999, p. 33).

Andrew Carnegie, an immigrant from Scotland, is one of the U.S.'s most illustrious, yet most malevolent, entrepreneurs. He is known as the originator of the sweatshop, in which workers labored many hours a day in dangerous and inadequate buildings, making minute wages. The sweatshops were organized to support his business interests in New York City. In Pennsylvania, Carnegie monopolized the steel industry of the nation. Aside from being known as one of the U.S.'s most important innovators of the Gilded Age, Andrew Carnegie is also known for his ability to engage a "ruthless determination to thwart his rivals by fair means or foul" (Cashman, 1984). Much public anger toward Carnegie resulted eventually in his decision to donate large amounts of the money he had earned. Even today, his generous philanthropy is well-known and well-regarded.

The Gilded Age was tumultuous, creating massive wealth for a few and extraordinary poverty for many. Men, it seems, were out for themselves, a frame of mind captured from the earlier century. A quote from Mark Twain sums up the tenor of the Gilded Age: "what is the chief end of man?—to get rich. In what way? Dishonestly if we can; honestly if we must" (*America in the Gilded Age*, 1999).

Nothing in this historical view or the observation of developing political stylists in cities in the early days of the U.S. points to or explains definitively how violence developed. However, the abject poverty of the working poor coupled with the documented maltreatment by appalling employers can unequivocally explain how frustration and anger can grow and lead to violent emotion and action. The discrepancies in wealth and new opportunities to learn and participate in radical thought and action led to formation of early—and violent—working-class social revolutions within the U.S. The "classic view of the escalation of violence," says Cheryl Jorgensen-Earp, is "that movements reach a point of frustration" when bargaining or attempts at resolution no longer work; that is when violence occurs (Jorgensen-Earp, 2008, p. 5).

Late in the 19th century and early in the 20th century in the U.S., the development of labor unions played an important role in mobilizing the dissatisfaction of the workers. U.S. industrial workers joined together as collective bargaining units in an attempt to improve wages and to decrease the length of the workday. Aggression may have been the members' only recourse as a means to express frustration and resentment at their inability to control the work environment, and violence emerged as a demonstration of the workers' unhappiness.

Jorgensen-Earp in her book *In the Wake of Violence* suggests that "despite the potentially negative weight that it brings to a movement, violence in social protest is more common than generally thought" (Jorgensen-Earp, 2008, p. 18). Jorgensen-Earp tells us that in 1973, William Gamson "spoke of US social protest as 'liberally speckled with violent episodes' and estimates (in 1973) that 25% of all social movements had 'violence somewhere in their history'" (Jorgensen-Earp, 2008, p. 18).[3]

Paradoxically, while the formations of labor unions may be at the root of collective social activity in the U.S., professional nursing unions have become a growing staple of U.S. health care delivery systems, primarily in hospitals. Professional nurse unions have become a method for nurses to protect their staffing positions and their licenses. Nurses, too—through their unions—have *fought* for fewer hours, improved pay, worker rights (for example, to lower nurse-to-patient ratios), and as a means to thwart management mistreatment. Professional nurse unions are a tool for compensation negotiation and collective lobbying for the political and legal rights and representation of nurses. The following pages of this book explore another perspective of the protection of nurses' rights—protection from violence in the Emergency Departments in the contemporary U.S.

To absolutely identify and define the reason(s) for a beginning or an upsurge of violence in the U.S. from the beginning of recorded history would require an entire social discourse on U.S. and international social history and philosophical thought. For the purposes of this book, the brief overview that I have provided presents clues about how frustration leads to anger and drives the impetus for individuals to join together, forming collectives of action in an attempt to resolve some of their distressing work and social circumstances, both in the early part of the U.S. 20th century and today.

THE HISTORY AND SOCIOLOGY OF AGGRESSION AND VIOLENCE

Theorists and philosophers who provide an account for the beginning of social aggression and violence in the U.S. have provided much insight into the beginnings and timeline of the emergence of violence in contemporary U.S. society. There is much written information to support theories demonstrating the impact of cultural and societal expectations on the way an individual evolves, the experiences that he has or does not have, the environment in which he lives, and the role models who influence him (Bendix, n.d., p. 1; Katznelson & Zolberg, n.d., p. 12; Staff, 1970, p. 9). The combination of these forces aggregate to shape a potential for *individual* pacifism or for violence.

Cultural factors of a society contribute to what is acceptable behavior and what is not acceptable behavior. We learn ethics and moral values from our parents, teachers, and social peers. The expectations of behavior are formed early and are supported or changed throughout the formative years. Expectations about right and wrong may change depending on the path an individual chooses. For example, if one individual selects a career path that encourages a daily visit to a tavern or bar with his buddies after work or one is employed in an environment that does not prohibit the use of profanity (a form of aggression), the individual will likely have a different view of the world than does the individual who works in an office environment that commands a completely different set of values and expectations (Moffatt, 2002). Dr. Gregory Moffatt in his book, *A Violent Heart*, believes that if he relocated a white-collar businessman, who had expectations of proper behavior in his daily office environment, into a prison situation, the businessman would "very quickly take on a more aggressive personality" (Moffatt, 2002, p. 3).

The thinkers of the day in the early 20th century must have been confronted with trying to understand the issues that were responsible for the collective aggression that had been occurring in the cities during the Gilded Age and in the prior century. A group of Yale psychologists in the 1930s led by John Dollard first described a rationale for group aggression and violence. They called this theory the *frustration-aggression mechanism*. In summary, this theory says that:

> the primary source of the human capacity for violence appears to be the frustration-aggression mechanism. Frustration does not necessarily lead to violence, and violence for some men is motivated by expectations of gain. The anger induced by frustration, however, is a motivating force that disposes men to aggression, irrespective of its instrumentalities. If frustrations are sufficiently prolonged or sharply felt, aggression is quite likely, if not certain, to occur. To conclude that the relationship is not relevant to individual or collective violence is akin to the assertion that the law of gravitation is irrelevant to the theory of flight because not everything that goes up falls back to earth in accord with the basic gravitational principle. The frustration-aggression mechanism is in this sense analogous to the law of gravity: men who are frustrated have an innate disposition to do violence to its source in proportion to the intensity of their frustrations. (Miller, 1941)

Collective aggression or group violence appears to develop not from angry individuals in concert but instead from the group *as a collective,* which decides to act in violent ways. Earl Conteh-Morgan, in his 2004 book titled *Collective Political Violence: An Introduction to the Theories and Cases of Violent Conflicts*, talks about a concept of aggression. Conteh-Morgan argues that the frustration-aggression model does not take *deprivation* into account as a determining factor in the cause of aggression. Deprivation could certainly have been a motivating factor to incite aggression and violence for the have-nots in the 19th- and 20th-century U.S. (Conteh-Morgan, 2004).

Researchers disagree about the definition of aggression. Some believe that aggression is the purposeful causing of pain, while others view aggression simply as unacceptable social behavior, perhaps as simple as a rude remark. Conteh-Morgan says, "For most people an action is aggressive in nature if the perpetrator had a socially *un*justified motive" (Conteh-Morgan, 2004, p. 70, emphasis added); in other words, aggressive acts are not considered aggression if the act is socially justified. But what is considered socially justifiable?

It appears that the acceptance or rejection of aggression as a social norm directly correlates to the level of advancement or economic largesse that a society enjoys: aggression is unacceptable in developed societies, whereas less-advanced societies accept aggression. Conteh-Morgan states that the 1960s in the U.S. saw much political change and social upheaval, which drove political scientists, sociologists, and psychologists to rethink, redefine, and reintroduce collective political aggression or violence as linked—once again—to the frustration-aggression model. The U.S. in the 1960s was caught up in revolution against the Vietnam War, against the government, and against the laws prohibiting marijuana, and the youth of the U.S.—excited to make changes and to put their mark on history—were ready for a fight. It seems that I was not totally incorrect in my 1960s assumption that big change was happening.

J. C. Davies suggests that the principle cause of revolution is the "reaction to a short-term economic downturn following a prolonged period of objective economic and social development" (Davies, 1962, p. 5). Conteh-Morgan labels Davies' assessment *shattered dreams;* when shattered dreams are coupled with the fear of losing everything that an individual has already attained the result can be a revolution (Conteh-Morgan, 2004, p. 71). The goal of aggression or revolution, Conteh-Morgan purports, is "self-enhancement by the group of protesters who perceive themselves to be threatened, challenged or devalued" (Conteh-Morgan, 2004, p. 71).

The way that a specific culture—with its traditions, religious influences, and majority laws and values—helps form our own personal views can differ based on the history and lifestyle of that culture. A perfect illustration of the influence that culture has in the formation of individual values, expectations, and actions—and deprivation—is the modern culture of Iraq and its people. For many years, the Iraqis have lived in a dictator-run country where they have had to witness their quasi-elected leader living a much richer lifestyle that the ordinary Iraqi citizen lives. Iraqis must budget their daytime responsibilities around the hours that they know electricity will be available and live in constant fear for their safety, things that people in the U.S., on the whole, have rarely had to worry about. In Iraq, there is a distinct environment of civil tension among the many ethnicities, cultures, and religiously diverse groups. Iraqis' perception of acceptable behavior may be skewed with unusual expectations of what appropriate and acceptable behavior looks like. In the U.S., there is no question as to what is the appropriate behavior of its citizens. The culture that Iraq has—and the expectations that Iraqis have of other Iraqis—is very different from American's expectations of other Americans.

It is important to know that a theory is simply that: someone's interpretation of why something is occurring. Understanding the entire spectrum of sociological theory and succumbing to the exploration of the social scientists' and philosophers' evidence in support of their theories with the extensive pro/con arguments that could be made, would take us completely off track in determining a timeframe and possible rationale for aggression and violence in the U.S.

These explanations are solely an overview of some of the important views of the day. This discussion is based on the assumption that one reason for group aggression, revolution, or violence may be partially explained by the frustration-aggression mechanism, and the timeframe for its origin may be the middle to late 1930s in the U.S. Dr. Moffatt (2002) believes that "theories concerning the causes of aggressive behavior can be grouped into three major categories—biological, sociological and psychological" (p. 4). It is from this framework that I present my research regarding the larger subject of violence.

THE BIOLOGY OF AGGRESSION AND VIOLENCE

Biologically speaking, individuals may inherently carry a violence gene. Dr. Gregory Moffatt (2002) suggests that individuals may have an aggressive nature due to genetics that drive or shape personality, producing "pre-programmed" (p. 5) tendencies toward aggression or violence. Similarly, just as tendencies toward alcoholism or other inherited diseases are built into our genetic individuality, violence, or aggression may also be genetic. Dr. Moffatt (2002, pp. 7–8) points out that the hypothalamus of the brain is a critical organ, and that this minute organ may function to direct an individual's violence potential. The following passage best supports the function of the hypothalamus in the control or jurisdiction of behavior and of rage:

> The tiny hypothalamus serves as the Health Maintenance Organization of the body, regulating its homeostasis, or stable state of equilibrium. The

hypothalamus also generates behaviors involved in eating, drinking, general arousal, rage, aggression, embarrassment, [and] escape from danger, pleasure and copulation. It does an amazing number of housekeeping chores for such a small piece of tissue. Its lateral and anterior parts seem to support activation of the parasympathetic nervous system: drop in blood pressure; slowing of pulse; and regulation of digestion, defecation, assimilation, and reproduction in such a way as to contribute on the whole to rest and recovery. The medial hypothalamus and the posterior hypothalamus regulate activation and acceleration of pulse and breathing rates, high blood pressure, arousal, fear and anger. The stimulation of specific groups of cells in these areas can elicit pure behaviors. For example, rats placed in an experimental situation where they can press a lever to stimulate a pleasure center will do so to the exclusion of eating and drinking. Stimulation of another area can produce rage. (Kore Liow, 2001)

A brief discussion of testosterone, a male sex hormone (androgen) and anabolic steroid, may help explain why males are generally more aggressive than females. Testosterone is secreted by the male testes, the endocrine system, and to some degree by specific neurons in the brain. Female testosterone is secreted by the ovaries and the endocrine system and also by the neurons in the brain, the same as males. The key difference is that the level of female testosterone secretion is a relative microquantity when compared with males, as males produce 20 times more testosterone than females do. Testosterone and other hormones are also responsible for the equilibrium of body functions, for libido, for regulation of levels of water, glucose, and electrolytes, and for stimulation of growth. Importantly for this discussion, testosterone functions to help an individual manage stress, especially in the face of changing physical circumstances (Mitchell, 1998).

The fact that males far outnumber females as perpetrators of violence is not disputed (Fonagy, 1999; Ridley, 2005). It certainly seems possible that the huge differential in the amount of testosterone produced by males may lie at the foundation of a heightened level of aggression among males. The elevated natural production of testosterone or taking additional supraphysiologic doses of steroids has been linked to aggressive behavior. Interestingly, hypogonadism, or the production of unusually *low* quantities of testosterone, also is associated with aggressive behavior. The use of alcohol, amphetamines, and phencyclidines have also been shown to increase agitation and may intensify violent behavior (Mitchell, 1998).

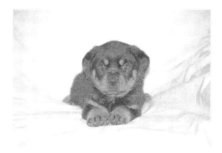

Figure 1.1 Through socialization, both man and animal can be docile and aggression-free. Photo courtesy of Vladimir Petrovic (www.bullenfeld.com).

Anyone who owns a rottweiler puppy (see Figure 1.1) can attest to the fact that providing plenty of love and training, and with the proper socialization, the rottweiler's innate sense of aggression will never develop. The puppy will never know that he was bred for aggression. The same may be true for all animals who learn from their human cohabitants about love, respect, and caring. While there doesn't appear to be scientific research to support the theory about the rottweiler, it does appear to be true. The case of the rottweiler, an animal known for violence and aggression, is an example of the influence that culture and socialization can have on both humans and animals.

As for humans, Moffat (2002) suggests that the male physiology may be responsible for a higher tendency toward aggression due to testosterone, although the presence of normal amounts of testosterone, in and of itself, cannot and should not be labeled the culprit of violence.

THE PSYCHOLOGY OF AGGRESSION AND VIOLENCE

The inability to cope, anger, sleeping problems, or posttraumatic stress syndrome, all considered psychological disorders, can create aggression and violence, possibly triggered by the release of high levels of cortisol—the so-called stress hormone—from the adrenal gland (Scott, 2008). Significant psychiatric or mental disorders of psychosis, schizophrenia, and other serious illnesses can create aggressive and violent behavior as a manifestation of the disease state. Disordered thinking that is a hallmark of many mental illnesses can cause a misunderstanding of words or a misinterpretation of the behavior of others. The disordered thinking that is commonplace in psychiatric illness may be especially pronounced if the disorder is severe and not managed by pharmacologic means.

Mental deficiencies, dementia, Alzheimer's disease, or mental retardation can inhibit appropriate social skills and/or coping, which may result in frustration and the potential for aggression and/or violence (Moffatt, 2002; Scott, 2008).

As with the frustration produced by psychiatric disease states, the frustration generated from a lack of control of one's environment—or situational inequity—the feeling or awareness of not being able to control may be characterized as a form of relative deprivation. In simple terms, relative deprivation comes into play when an individual is deprived of what the individual feels is appropriately due to him or her. Although relative deprivation is typically applied to collective violence, there is some evidence that the extent of frustration and anger can generate violence in society (Moffat, 2002, p. 72).[4] This type of situational frustration could be the cause of violent outbursts or aggression caused by patients who sit waiting for hours in the Emergency Department to see a provider. The situation is out of their control and as stress builds, so does the potential for the development of aggression, even in the absence of a psychological or psychiatric disease state.

Violence in movies, video games, television, music, advertisements, and athletics and the greater than normal exposure to these media sources create a high likelihood for the development of increased aggressive responses because the message of violence that is communicated becomes an accepted norm, over time.

SOME THEORETICAL VIEWS OF VIOLENCE

Professor Gregory Moffatt introduces Jack Katz's explanation of violent action as the outcome of humiliation. Katz, who is a professor of sociology at UCLA, interprets the act of violent behavior as a skewed emotion created by the perpetrator who believes that his act of violence is justified and that he was in some way provoked and driven to committing violence.[5] In a simplistic explanation, the provocateur undergoes a process in which he experiences humiliation that transforms to rage *if* the individual is not able to reject the emotion created from humiliation. The individual, in dismissing or suppressing the emotion of humiliation may not even recognize it as humiliation. But, if the individual is humiliated, recognizes that he has been humiliated, and allows the emotion of humiliation to surface, he will likely become enraged. Enraged individuals are the individuals who attack violently and without notice, perhaps as in the case of the student killer at Virginia Tech (Moffatt, 2002, p. 23).

Each individual has a preconceived notion of what violence is and what violence looks like, determined by experiences with violence and the unique factors that have contributed to his social and genetic makeup. Katz offers an explanation of how criminal violence may occur within an individual and may also provide the basis for the occurrence of *delayed aggression* as in workplace violence. In most cases of workplace violence, latent emotions erupt suddenly, causing an individual to impulsively return to a former workplace in search of an unfair boss or a cruel and impudent ex-girlfriend, and then to kill. Motivation is the reason that incites a perpetrator or perpetrators to act and provides one clear rationale and explanation for violent behavior (Moffatt, 2002, p. 23). The entire range of factors that join together to make up the emotional being of an individual are responsible for the ways that people act, react, and generally behave. A situation or circumstance that incites motivation, creates momentum, or changes equilibrium can incite one to react violently.

The changes in the range of emotions from humiliation to rage are used by Katz to describe criminal acts of homicide. But the mechanism of emotional change combined with motivation may be one explanation for the triggering of violence and violent acts.

Most individuals who have healthy psyches also have the ability to normally process unpleasant experiences or impassioned emotion, such as humiliation, and are capable of turning the emotion inward, absorbing the experience, and redirecting it in a socially acceptable way.

Leon Festinger, a renowned social scientist, theorized that one of the forces that shapes human behavior is *cognitive dissonance* (Festinger, 1957). Loosely interpreted, cognitive dissonance could be taken to mean conscience, or as Festinger explains, a lack of balance between beliefs and actions. Festinger hypothesizes that individuals will actively work to remove the dissonance, or the psychological discomfort one is experiencing, since the dissonance conflicts with what the individual truly believes. Festinger theorizes that acting in a dissonant way, or against what the individual believes, can only be accomplished by the individual changing his basic belief or opinion—his cognition or understanding of what is true. One way that basic beliefs are changed is through the *social support* of one's new thinking. In applying the theory freely to collective violence, it may be possible that the social network of disgruntled workers in the early 20th century recognized and believed that violence—as a solution to the horrendous social conditions—was wrong. But, as Festinger explains, if the magnitude of the conditions or elements to which the individuals were subjected was great, the workers were highly motivated to correct and improve the conditions. This new paradigm—or new thinking—may have been reinforced by others in the group thus providing adequate social support resulting in a change in opinions and beliefs about violence.

From a summary of Ted Gurr's book *Why Men Rebel,* Gurr hypothesizes that the "primary source of the human capacity for violence lies within the *frustration-aggression mechanism,*" introduced in an earlier section. Gurr believes that frustration alone does not trigger violence, but if the frustration is protracted, as was the case in the late 19th and early 20th centuries in the U.S., violence can result (Conflict Resolution Consortium, Staff, 1970). Another of Gurr's explanations for internalized frustration and conflict, *relative deprivation,* may help explain the onset or development of individual violence that resulted early in the U.S.'s industrial age, motivated by the disparity between the great wealth of the business owners and the great poverty of the workers. According to Gurr, relative deprivation is the state of mind of an individual based on an understanding of what he thinks he deserves and what he thinks he will get. If the gap between the two is large, aggression, violence, or rebellion can ensue. Gurr believes that the frustration-aggression mechanism is an individual trait, while relative deprivation is an indicator of violent thought and action within a group of individuals and is best explained as *collective* aggression or violence.

"Aggressive behavior develops over time," reports distinguished psychologist Dr. Carl Goldberg. In a review of the book *Speaking With the Devil: A Dialogue With Evil,* Dr. Gregory Moffatt explains that Goldberg believes individuals progress through "six stages in the process of becoming thoughtless, emotionless, and mean" (Moffatt, 2002, p. 23). Goldberg defines the six stages as shame, contempt, rationalization, justification, the inability or unwillingness to self-examine, and magical thinking (Moffatt, 2002, p. 23).

Magical thinking is a type of thinking, according to Goldberg, in which the individual has convinced himself that he is perfect. The process of magical thinking "involves obtaining power over the source of life by creating 'a moral and emotional distance between the perpetrator and victim' " (Goldberg, 1996, p. 155). Magical thinking is a "form of grandiosity in which the person believes that others have failed to recognize his unique qualities and the person or other people must be forced to see. Self-examination is impossible because it is believed to be unwarranted" (Goldberg, 1996, p. 157).

Dr. Goldberg (1996) is convinced that evil is not a product of mental illness nor is it the influence of the devil; instead, he says that people learn by doing (p. 10), similar to the supposition that I have presented. According to Dr. Goldberg (1996, p. 6), people make choices between good and evil all of the time and that the response to these many decisions "shape our moral—or immoral—choices now and in the future" (p. 10). Furthermore, Goldberg asserts that a "malevolent personality" emerges when the wrong choices—harmful choices—are made that give credence to the individual's decision to commit bad and evil acts (Goldberg, 1996, p. 15).

THE IMPACT OF 9/11

The occurrence of violence in society, particularly in our contemporary society, can be summed up in one phrase: September 11. The U.S. was unprepared for what happened on September 11, and the events that occurred that day have changed U.S. society and its perceptions of violence and evil. This section will focus on the short-term impact of September 11 on the U.S.'s viewpoint of the accepted, understood, and trusted way of life that U.S. citizens enjoy and how the violence of September 11 tainted the U.S.

The violence that occurred on September 11 was conveyed by an outside force: foreign nationals who violated the U.S.'s ideals and accustomed sense of security.

Until that day in September 2001, the possibility that anything of this magnitude or horror could occur in the U.S. was unimaginable in the current environment of the U.S as the most powerful, and secure, nation on earth. New York had been turned into a war zone, with images and descriptions of Armageddon. Two thousand seven hundred and twenty-six innocent lives were lost on September 11 ("Deaths in World Trade Center Terrorist Attacks," 2002), and life as it was known would never be the same again, especially for the victims' families and the survivors of the massive attack.

Following the events of September 11, the U.S. did not know who or what to trust. Citizens were determined to recapture the pre–September 11 landscape that supported and enhanced our basic and time-honored tenet of freedom, especially freedom from violence. The

U.S. had worked hard for its freedom and for its culture of safety, protection, and for its expansive efforts toward nonviolence, and we were not willing to give it up.

The first human instinct one has when attacked is to attack back, and a great many U.S. citizens experienced this emotion on September 11. Being defensive to the point of attacking back may be an unfamiliar emotion to many; but the response that was elicited after the September 11 violent assault should be recognized as an expected reaction. The U.S. was built on the integration of many immigrants from diverse countries along with its own U.S.-born citizens, and the heterogeneity of the U.S. is one of the many elements that creates exciting and distinctive communities and cultures in our towns and cities. After September 11, the cultures that we enjoyed and with which we were interconnected in our everyday lives suddenly became frightening intruders, not to be totally trusted. Some fear of the anonymous purposes of our neighbors had merit: the motto of *better safe than sorry* was a basis for a significant change in the way a majority of native U.S. citizens viewed neighbors and merchants who were not U.S.-born.

Rajeev Bhargava in his chapter, "Ordinary Feelings, Extraordinary Events" from the book *Understanding September 11* sums it up well: "It is extremely abnormal if self-respecting persons do not experience righteous anger, even hatred, toward those who have wronged them" (Barghava, 2002, p. 328).

Since that frightening time several years ago, the U.S. has adjusted to the new rules that were adopted for protection from invisible enemies and to quash any opportunity for another September 11. Most Arabs are not dissident or extreme radicals and most Afghanis or Pakistanis do not have bombs hidden in their apartments or car trunks. We have also learned, though, that some are and some do. But there are also native-born U.S. citizens who have very evil intentions and work tirelessly to put the U.S. in harm's way.

Several years following September 11, the New York Advisory Committee and the U.S. Commission on Civil Rights issued the findings of the commission. The report focused on civil rights and racial profiling regarding the groups of citizens and noncitizens of U.S., the racial groups who were blamed for the infiltration and insurgence into the U.S. on September 11. This commission study was not designed to examine the national security controls or the U.S. Department of Homeland Security policies and procedures that had been put into place to protect the U.S. from another unknown and unrecognizable force. This report was about one thing: the violence and the hate that was the impetus that would shape a segment of U.S. citizens' thoughts and beliefs for years to come (Hanley & Berry, 2003).The commission found that the current policies and practices of various law enforcement agencies in New York City, particularly within communities occupied by Muslim, Arab, and South Asian residents, were reacting with methods that violated U.S. civil rights and liberties. The harsh practices were in response to an interpretation that all Middle Eastern nationals—whether citizens or legal visitors—were violent activists who had the ability and the desire to harm the United States as had been done several years prior, by alleged similar racial and or ethnic individuals. The commission believed that there are several nonproductive outcomes from harsh acts of racial profiling, including, the distrust of law enforcement authorities, hindrance of crime reporting, and lessening of the cooperation between police officials and Middle Eastern and other communities. The commission believes it is essential to "identify and thwart future terrorists" (Hanley & Berry, 2003, p. 1) and recognizes that a spirit of collaboration, trust, and understanding would go far to protect all New York City residents from further terrorist incursion. The agreement to proctor the interactions of these communities of citizens with law enforcement was dubbed the Handschu Agreement.[6]

We have one united goal—to prevent further terror and violence in the U.S. But all citizens and law enforcement professionals need to proceed with a spirit of fairness. Violence took on an entirely new significance on September 11 that would leave the U.S. and U.S. citizens forever changed. We have more reasons than ever to combat all forms of violence with a vengeance that will serve to alter and expel the ever-growing presence of violence in our culture as an accepted way of life in the U.S.

CASE STUDY

This case study is from Dr. Gregory Moffatt's book, A Violent Heart. *Dr. Moffatt's rendition and explanations throughout the story and the story itself are surprising communiqués of human nature and violence.*

(Continued)

At Yale University in 1963, Stanley Milgram did a fascinating study that portrayed how far people would go, even harming another human being, if they felt justified in their actions. In Milgram's study, subjects were told that they were a part of a research project studying the effects of punishment on learning. The subjects were supposedly given an electrical shock if they did not learn a set of facts properly. In this study, one group of subjects, known as "teachers" would read pairs of words over an intercom to another group, known as "learners" in an adjacent room. The "learners" would be shocked if they recalled the pairs [of words] incorrectly. In actuality, the subjects who were allegedly receiving the electrical shocks were cohorts with Milgram in the study. The terminology for this type of research participant is called a *confederate in research*. Milgram's confederates were never actually (electrically) shocked. The real purpose of the study was to see to what extent the "teachers" would obey Milgram and continue administering electrical shocks to the learners. Milgram had predicted that most subjects would refuse to harm other people, but what he found was quite the opposite.

The panel of 30 switches supposedly ranged from 15 to 450 volts of electricity, with each successive switch representing a more powerful shock. The higher voltages were clearly marked with danger warnings. In the adjacent room, the confederate would make sounds as if he or she was really being shocked when the "teacher" administered the punishment. As the study progressed, the confederate would complain about the pain, ask to be allowed to quit the study, and eventually would stop responding altogether, as if unconscious.

Some of Milgram's subjects refused to continue the experiment when they believed that they were hurting the "learner." However, most of the subjects continued to administer shocks even when the "learner" stopped responding. An astounding 65% of the subjects administered shocks all the way through the 450 volt level. Most of Milgram's subjects were visibly uncomfortable with the study. Some of them argued with him, complaining that the study was unethical, and yet they continued to participate. In follow-up interviews, with the subjects, Milgram asked them to explain why, despite their discomfort with the study, they continued to administer shocks. The most common answer was that they believed he knew what he was doing, so they continued. In other words, they justified their behavior and obeyed Milgram simply because he was in a position of authority. (Moffatt, 2002, p. 10)

NOTES

1. Just-in-time (JIT) is a strategy originated in the Japanese auto manufacturing industry; JIT is an inventory strategy that improves return on investment (ROI) by reducing on-hand inventory and instead initiating a process to have the inventory that is needed, just in time for its use in a process. JIT reduces inventory and carrying costs.

2. *Marxism* is defined as the political and economic philosophy of Karl Marx and Friedrich Engels, in which the concept of class struggle plays a central role in understanding society's allegedly inevitable development from bourgeois oppression under capitalism to a socialist and ultimately classless society.

3. William A. Gamson is a professor of sociology at Boston College, Boston, Massachusetts, where he is also the codirector of the Media Research and Action Project. Gamson, the author of many books on political science and social movements, can be reached at his Web site http://www2.bc.edu/~gamson/Homepage(Frames).html.

4. The term *situational inequity* is linked to many interpretations, from racial inequity to story writing. For the purposes of this book situational inequity refers to the frustration or dissatisfaction of inequity or deprivation.

5. Dr. Katz is the author of a collection of sociology-themed books and articles, among them *Seduction of Crime: Moral and Sensual Attraction in Doing Evil*, published in 1988, and *How Emotions Work*, published in 1999. Dr. Katz's Web site is http://www.sscnet.ucla.edu/soc/faculty/katz/.

6. The Handschu Agreement was originally established in 1971 following intensive police surveillance of certain political activists in New York City. The agreement is a "set of guidelines to regulate police behavior in New York City with regard to political activity" (Hanley & Berry, 2003, p. 1).

REFERENCES

America in the Gilded Age. (1999). Retrieved August 26, 2008, from http://www.pbs.org/wghb/amex/carnegie/gildedage.html

Average Wages in the U.S. (2008, January 14). Retrieved April 5, 2009, from www.politicalcalulations.blogspot.com

Barrington Moore, J. (n.d.). *The social origins of dictatorship and democracy.* Retrieved July 21, 2008, from http://ssr1.uchicago.edu/PRELIMS/Change/chmisc2.htm

Bendix, R. (n.d.). *Tradition and modernity reconsidered.* Retrieved July 21, 2008, http://ssr1.uchicago.edu/PRELIMS/Change/chmisc1.html

Bhargava, R. E. (2002). *Ordinary feelings, extraordinary events: Moral compliexity in 9/11.* P. P. Craig Calhoun (Ed.). Brooklyn, NY: Social Science Research Council.

Bnet business dictionary. (n.d.). Retrieved April 6, 2009, from http://dictionary.bnet.com/definition/just-in-time.html?tag=content;col11

Cashman, S. (1984). *America in the gilded age: From the death of Lincoln to the rise of Theodore Roosevelt.* New York: New York University Press.

Conflict Resolution Consortium, Staff. (1970). *Book summary of* Why men rebel *by Ted Gurr.* Beyond Intactability Project. Retrieved July 24, 2008, from www.beyondintractability.org/booksummary/10680

Conteh-Morgan, E. (2004). *Collective political violence: An introduction to the theories and cases of violent conflicts.* New York: Routledge.

David, H. (1936). *The history of the Haymarket Affair: A study in the American social-revolutionary and labor movements.* New York: Russell and Russell.

Davies, J. C. (1962, February). Toward a theory of revolution. *American Sociological Review, 27*(1), 5–6, 8.

Deaths in World Trade Center terrorist attacks. (2002). *MMWR, 51,* 16–18. Retrieved April 6, 2009, from www.cdc.gov/mmwr/preview/mmwrhtml/mm51spa6.htm

Dore, R. (n.d.). *British factory—Japanese factory.* Retrieved July 21, 2008, from http://ssr1.uchicago.edu/PRELIMS/Change/chmisc1.html

Festinger, L. (1957). *A theory of cognitive dissonance.* Palo Alto, CA: Stanford University Press.

Fonagy, P. (1999). *Male perpetrators of violence against women: An attachment theroy perspective.* Dallas Society for Psychoanalytic Psychology. Retrieved April 5, 2009, from www.dsp.com/papers/fonagy5.htm

Goldberg, C. (1996). *Speaking with the devil: A dialogue with evil.* New York: Penguin Book Group.

Hanley, M., & Berry, M. F. (2003). *Civil rights implications of post-Setpemember 11: Law enforcement practices in New York.* The New York Advisory Committee, Michael Hanley, Chairman. New York: United States Commission on Civil Rights.

(Johan) Most biographical sketch. (n.d.). Anarchist Archives. Retrieved August 12, 2008, from http://dwardmac.pitzer.edu/ANARCHIST_ARCHIVES/bright/most/biosketch.html

Jorgensen-Earp, C. R. (2008). *In the wake of violence: Image and social reform.* East Lansing: Michigan State University Press.

Katznelson, I., & Zolberg, A. (n.d.). *Working class formations.* Social Change. Retrieved July 21, 2008, from http://ssr1.uchicago.edu/PRELIMS/Change/chmisc2.html

Kore Liow, M. (2001). *Information about HH: The role of the hypothalamus.* Retrieved August 24, 2008, from http://www.geocities.com/hhugs2001/roleofhyp.htm

Miller, N. (1941). The frustration aggression hypothesis. *Psychological Review, 27*(1), 337–342.

Mitchell, N. (1998). *The slab.* Retrieved August 22, 2008, from http://www.abc.net.au/science/slab/testost/story.htm

Moffatt, G. K. (2002). *A violent heart: Understanding aggressive individuals.* Westport, CT: Greenwood Publishing Group.

Monti, D. J. (1999). *The American city: A social and cultural history.* New York: Blackwell Publishers.

Mosk, C. (2004, January 18). Japan, Industrialization and Economic Growth. (R. Whaples, Ed.). Retrieved August 1, 2008, from http://eh.net/encyclopedia/article/mosk.japan.final

Ridley, R. L., (2005). *Domestic violence survivors at work: how perpetrators impact employment.* Retrieved April 5, 2009, from http://www.maine.gov/labor/labor_stats/publications/dvreports/survivorstudy.pdf

Scott, E. M. (2008). *Control and stress: How to stay healthy.* Retrieved August 24, 2008, from http://stress.about.com/od/stresshealth/a/cortisol.htm

The Evolution of Health Care Delivery: Setting the Stage for Violence in the ED

THE HIGH PRICE OF HEALTH CARE

The past 8 years in the United States have been disturbing and in many ways irrational. The decade prior had been one of substantial growth and the continued assurance of the U.S. leadership position in the world, affording its citizens the good life and opportunities to innovate. However, in the past 8 years, the U.S. has been challenged, starting from a position of a strong financial and economic environment to one of instability due in part to our societal losses from 9/11 and the increasing investment in a war that seems to many U.S. citizens to be never ending. Recently, the correction of the housing market has added to the instability of U.S. residents—many of whom have lost their homes—and the immense downturns in the financial markets. Health care costs are skyrocketing, and typical, working citizens often cannot afford the exorbitant costs of health care insurance designed to defray huge outlays of capital in the event of a medical emergency. The high cost of health care, the gradual erosion of access to providers, the closure of hospitals and Emergency Departments, the increasing numbers of uninsured, and the mounting expense of providing health care to all citizens have been among the greatest challenges we have faced. Traditionally, U.S. citizens have had the assurance and expectation of indefinite access to quality and affordable health care, allegedly the best care in the world. But no health care is excellent if its citizens cannot afford it.

Health care spending in the U.S. in 2007 was a phenomenal $2.3 trillion dollars, an average cost of $6,697 per person. It is "16% (sixteen percent) of the nation's GDP and growing at unsustainable rates" (Jost, 2007, p. 8). By 2013 the expenditure is projected to be as high as $3.36 trillion (see Table 2.1). The U.S. spends more money on health care than on food, housing, or transportation, and the U.S. has more health care expenditures than any other country (Jost, 2007). "Lehman Brothers' equity research predicts that bad debt and charity care expenses for the for-profit healthcare industry will rise 15–17% in 2008 for a total expense of $14.6 billion in unfunded care" (Wilson, 2008). Between 2000 and 2004, the cost of health care increased at an average annual rate of 7.9% (Jost, 2007).

The rationale and theories used to explain the rising costs of health care, and maybe even some of the solutions to halt the growth, could fill an entire collection of encyclopedias. For the purposes of this book, the focus is to explore potential reasons for an increase in violence in U.S. society today and how that violence is expressed in our hospital emergency departments. Several of the triggers for the high costs of health care in the U.S. will be explored in an attempt to uncover reasons for escalating health care costs that may create frustration and anger and perhaps be an underpinning for a more violent society.

Health care in the U.S. is very expensive. There are many reasons for the year over year increases, including: research ($27.6 billion in

Table 2.1

HEALTH CARE EXPENDITURES

	2000	2005	2013 (PROJECTED)
% of GDP spent on health care	13.8	16.0	18.4
Health care expenditures	1.98 trillion[a]	$2.3 trillion	$3.36 trillion

[a]This figure is estimated.

2003; Jost, 2007, p. 2), innovation, the cost of delivering services, the immense expense required to develop technology, and the reporting of potential solutions to the many divisions of health care and its stakeholders. Some additional reasons for the high price of health care in the U.S. are:

1. The U.S. pays for the health care costs of the uninsured (safety net programs, bad debt, charity care).
2. A decrease in federal funding and reimbursement for public programs has resulted in more uninsured persons and a general increase in taxes.
3. The individual's share of the cost of insurance coverage has increased and affordable health care coverage options have decreased.
4. Health care services are expensive (Jost, 2007, p. 2).

Regina Herzlinger, in her book, *Consumer-Driven Healthcare* (2004), agrees that the sick are the greatest consumers of health care services and are the reason for the largest share of health care expenditures. She reports that in 1928, the top 5% of users of health care accounted for 52% of all expenditures and that this percentage remained the same through 1996. Herzlinger, and others, believe that improved health care leads to reduced costs, and Herzlinger suggests "three obvious strategies" (Herzlinger, 2004, p. 119) to approach and control the ever-increasing costs:

- "Integrate the many diverse sources of care around organizations focused on their needs.
- Support patients' ability to promote their health status and to care for themselves.
- Ensure the use of technological advances in treating chronic illness" (Herzlinger, 2004, p. 119).

Herzlinger further states that the best way to control health care costs is to focus on improving care for the sick, and she suggests that a consumer-driven insurance approach would involve consumers in all facets of their own care, such as health promotion, specific policies to cover costs, personalized medicine, and expanded use of the electronic health record (EHR). This overarching strategy can "motivate and reward the providers who develop it" (Herzlinger, 2004).

Electronic Health Record

The U.S. has not yet developed an EHR, a fully integrated health record system capable of connecting the spectrum of health care providers. Many independent vendors have developed electronic systems, and a number of health care providers use technology solutions, which is the beginning of a fully integrated system to be used by all facets of health care delivery: hospitals, physicians, clinics, and even patients.

The absence of an electronic means to coordinate, store, and share patient data accounts for excessive amounts of time (cost) that must be invested to find the right pieces of information for a particular patient or procedure or the time and expense required to copy and mail a multiple-page patient record so that the consulting physician has pertinent data. The availability of the capacity to store and retrieve individual health records electronically would advance the opportunity to deliver improved health care by slashing the investment of time currently required to retrieve needed health care records and the expense of recreating paper documents. Research focused at finding the right information technology system, the cost to purchase and integrate the systems, and the training involved for all users and stakeholders of the system will be vast. We are not there yet.

CASE STUDY

ELECTRONIC DOCUMENTATION LOWERS ED WAITS AND REDUCES POTENTIAL FOR VIOLENCE

King's Daughters Medical Center in Kentucky was able to reduce its Emergency Department length of stay (LOS) from 220 minutes to 118 minutes as part of its Emergency Department Performance Improvement project by adopting four strategies. The most important strategy was the adoption of an electronic documentation system that allowed ED nurses and physicians to electronically capture a large amount of patient information, so called charting that used to be relegated to paper charts. The electronic documentation system that was implemented by the King's Daughters ED used wheeled computers so that nurses and physicians could

(Continued)

*roll laptops to any location, facilitating nurses' or physicians'
ability to capture patient information wherever they happen to
be. The streamlining of data entry freed up documentation time
so that nurses and physicians focus more efficiently on delivering
patient care.*

*A second key strategy to the success of reducing the LOS was
the addition of flow coordinators, employees whose only (but very
critical) job was to improve communication among all Emergency
Department staff by tracking patients' location within the ED environment and aiding patients' efficient flow through the ED. At
busy times, the flow coordinator managed both ED patient and
visitor traffic.*

*A third strategy involved identifying peak traffic times and
planning for flex schedules of some of the ED nurse practitioners
and nursing technicians, thus accommodating peak patient arrival
times at the Emergency Department.*

*Last, to help patients understand that EDs are for serious ill-
ness and injuries and not for primary care, the King's Daughters
ED now requires a deposit of $200.00 as a co-pay upon arrival from
patients with non-emergency conditions* (Case Study: KY Hospital
ED Cuts Patient Wait Times With EMR, 2008).

RESEARCH

The U.S. is the health care research capital of the world, supported by
investments from the federal government. In 2003, the government invested $27.6 million in research, and, undeniably, that amount is much
greater today. Immense amounts of medical technology is created and
"adopted quickly and pervasively" in the U.S., more than in any other
country (Jost, 2007, p. 15). All health care research, including pharmaceutical research and marketing, is expensive. Most researchers have
multiple, advanced degrees that command high salaries. Research facilities must develop and use technologically innovative and cutting-edge
equipment and methods to achieve the rapid turnaround rates that are
expected and necessary for the research to pay off. One of the major reasons that medical centers are considered to be superior and are ranked

first class is due to the research capabilities. Such research activities provide medical centers with the opportunity to create or discover the next great medication or to potentially find a cure for a disease.

QUALITY HEALTH CARE

A popular adage has been that the U.S. has the best health care in the world. For the U.S. to have the best health care in the world, we must be willing to pay for it. U.S. citizens perhaps wish to explain away the growing costs of health care with the easy assumption that we are paying for the best. But the high cost of health care does not equate to high-quality health care.

Health care quality assures us that all systems are operational and efficient, but most of us would agree that this is not often the case. Quality of care is an old nomenclature used to define the "degree to which health care services increase the likelihood of desired health outcomes" (Institute of Medicine, 2008). The goal of quality is that the operations and efficient delivery of health care services will, or should, improve the end result. Quality measures are yardsticks or guidelines that are used to determine the end result and include access to care, outcomes, patient experience, process, and structure. Most of us, as health care professionals, chose to be in the health care business primarily to influence and improve the lives of others. Health care provider services are driven by the need and want to perform quality services so as to achieve optimal results for the patients. Often the inefficiencies of health care systems (hospitals, clinics, physician offices) bog down quality measures that have been established to achieve optimal results, or quality of care. Two of the important tenets of quality of care are *access to care* and *patient experience*. The lack of access or the inability to locate and receive the type of care that is needed has been affected by managed care and by cost. All of us can relate to the managed care barrier that we have experienced by having to call the administrator of our insurance plan to get their approval before scheduling a routine exam or procedure. Recently, family practice and primary care physician offices began employing individuals whose only job is to communicate with insurance companies and patients, and to provide letters of consent for specific services or procedures, helping the health care consumer work through the web of approvals required to obtain health care services (see Exhibit 2.1).

Exhibit 2.1

QUALITY MEASURES

Access—an access measure assesses the patient's attainment of timely and appropriate health care. Barriers to access may include inability to pay for health care, difficulty traveling to health care facilities, unavailability of health care facilities, lack of a "medical home," cultural and health beliefs that prevent recognition of the need for and benefits of health care, and disparities in responding to persons seeking health care.

Outcome—an outcome of care is a health state of a patient resulting from health care. An outcome measure can be used to assess quality of care to the extent that health care services influence the likelihood of desired health outcomes. Outcome-based measures of quality reflect the cumulative impact of multiple processes of care. Outcome measures may suggest specific areas of care that may require quality improvement, but further investigation is typically necessary to determine the specific structures or processes that should be changed.

Patient Experience—a patient experience measure aggregates reports of patients about their observations of and participation in health care. These measures provide the patient perspective on quality of care.

Process—a process measure assesses a health care service provided to, or on behalf of, a patient. Process measures are often used to assess adherence to recommendations for clinical practice based on evidence or consensus. To a greater extent than outcome measures, process measures can identify specific areas of care that may require improvement.

Structure—a structure measure is a feature of a health care organization or clinician relevant to its capacity to provide health care. Structure data describe the capability of organizations or professionals rather than care provided to, or results achieved for, specific patients or groups of patients. For example, nurse/patient ratio is a structure-based measure because it does not describe care given to specific patients or specific groups of patients.

From NQMC resources—http://www.qualitymeasures.ahrq.gov/resources/measure_use.aspx.

TENET 1: ACCESS TO EFFICIENT CARE

Any of us, as a patient at a health care clinic, realizes that efficiency is not paramount in many of their daily operations; we are nearly always required to wait, often well past the appointment time, and then we are asked to come back for a second visit to discuss the results of X-rays or laboratory tests for which we had to wait to have completed. The investment of time and money to follow the *process* of the health care provider is extraordinarily frustrating. It is rare that physician appointments can be accomplished within a short period of time; health care consumers often have to take time off work to accomplish even routine health care appointments.

TENET 2: THE OPTIMAL PATIENT EXPERIENCE

What is the optimal patient experience? Ideas about what defines a patient experience have changed over time. In the past, patients and their physicians had a strictly, albeit friendly, business relationship: the physician provided a service to the patient and the patient agreed to pay for the service. The more current philosophy of customer care encompasses the needs of the patient and the family and goes beyond having updated glossy periodicals in the physician's office waiting room. The total customer experience provides a superior and emotional connection with the patient in addition to efficient delivery of a health care service. At long last, health care providers have recognized that the patient, first and foremost, is our customer and has a *choice* in the health care services he selects. The quality of our current health care system has been seriously deficient in providing customer-centric care or experiences in ways that include comfort care (refreshments, special services), explanations of medications or procedures, aspects of disease management such as for diabetes or other chronic conditions, rollout beds in pediatric inpatient rooms, gourmet meals for the new postpartum mom and dad, communication of reasons that the patient has to wait 3 more hours until he can see the ED physician. Any small customer service enhancements and improvement will factor into a positive or negative total patient experience. Health care services are very competitive, and physicians and hospitals know that they must rethink the way that they are doing things, to improve the patient experience. Physicians and other health care providers must now be concerned about the patient encounter as other businesses are. By offering the best service, the best cost, and unique amenities, physicians and other health care providers will have greater success in attracting new customers and keeping their current patients happy and satisfied.

MANAGED CARE

Managed care, as we know it today, has been around since the 1970s as an attempt of the Nixon administration to begin a reform of health care.

The health care system was experiencing problems of "cost containment, coverage for the uninsured; access for the poor and minorities; consumer rights; and efficient delivery systems" (A *Brief History of Managed Care*, 1998, p. 2). The Nixon administration introduced a health care strategy to develop health maintenance organizations (HMOs) in an attempt to slow down the exorbitant growth of health care expenditures. This strategy was the brainchild of Dr. Paul Ellwood, who designed the HMO and coined the term (A *Brief History of Managed Care*, 1998, p. 3). Ellwood believed that the "traditional fee-for-service" (arrangements to pay physicians for services) was responsible for the growing cost chasm and that fee-for-service arrangements needed to change for reform to be successful (A *Brief History of Managed Care*, 1998, p. 3).

Managed care was initiated to control the cost of health care. According to Harold Luft, a well-regarded managed care expert, "HMO's (Health Maintenance Organizations) have not accomplished what their proponents had promised: changing clinical practice processes and improving quality of care relative to the existing system" (Herzlinger, 2004, p. 50).

Aetna has been accused of being "the only major company to force doctors to participate in low-paying HMO plans if they wanted to [participate] in higher-paying ones" (Herzlinger, 2004, p. 49).

If patients and patient advocates had taken the insurance companies to task initially, when problems were first encountered, it is possible that the cost of care and the delay in care associated with the extraordinary administration of managed care might have been avoided, reducing patient stress and physical pain. Unfortunately, physicians were the most accessible party to blame and this may be why malpractice lawsuits in the U.S. have increased in the past 20 years.

The *Wall Street Journal* sums up the effect of managed care succinctly when describing, in Herzlinger's *Consumer-Driven Healthcare*, one physician's experience with Aetna: "Aetna acts like we're liars" (Herzlinger, 2004, p. 49). Managed care and its "just say no" policies of the 1990s have been "conceded to be [a] failure [since] healthcare costs are once again rising at double-digit rates" (Herzlinger, 2004, p. 49).

Managed care, too, may be responsible for the integration of hospitals, an industry and system-salvaging strategy to share expenses by consolidating services and taking advantage of economies of scale. By 1972, the change in the political environment spurred interest in the consolidation of services in the "traditional, not-for-profit hospital sector" (Herzlinger, 2004, p. 651). Thomas F. Frist, Jr., one of the creators of the giant Hospital Corporation of America (HCA), believed that integration of hospitals and other health care services could be accomplished through "affiliation; management contracts; and purchasing consortia" (Herzlinger, 2004, p. 651). Managed care was in its infancy but was having an impact on the reduction of the revenue and payment methods that had been typically enjoyed up to that time.

In the 1990s the health care delivery model was beginning to shift from inpatient to outpatient services in order to deliver less expensive and higher quality services. Suddenly, hospitals were experiencing unused capacity (Herzlinger, 2004, p. 652), and many creative attempts to work within new payment and delivery systems were unsuccessful. Simply, the opportunities for more affordable outpatient services eclipsed the rising and prohibitive cost for inpatient care. The smaller specialty hospitals believed that a solution to help them gain market share and to potentially find alternative uses for the empty hospital beds was to create a partnership or affiliate arrangement by joining with existing hospitals or systems. The entities thought that such an arrangement would be mutually beneficial; however, most integration proved to be disastrous, often because of alleged fraud of Medicare and Medicaid payments. Dr. Frist remarked that "the inscriptions on the tombstones read SNFs, home health care, disease niche providers, risk-taking products (HMOs), and physician practice management (PPM) groups" (Herzlinger, 2004, p. 652). Today hospitals are struggling to survive not because of unused capacity, but because hospitals cannot financially sustain themselves with beds filled with patients who have no health insurance or have the limited ability to pay for the costs incurred during a hospital stay (Goldstein, 2009).

In today's health care environment, Frist says that hospital providers are under "unprecedented" pressure to reduce costs and increase quality (Herzlinger, 2004, p. 652). The drivers of the necessity to lower cost and improve the efficiency of health care delivery come from the changes in physician reimbursement from Medicaid, further growth of managed care, and monumental increases in the number of uninsured patients. The plan is to create a back-to-basics approach, to *cut costs,* and to make the health care services that providers are supplying "measurably" better in quality (Herzlinger, 2004, p. 652).

With the multitude of payers and the magnitude of cost-sharing strategies, managed care has become very complex and requires a detailed and focused study to intimately understand all facets of how managed care works. Suffice it to say that managed care has been around for

30 years and there isn't any sign that managed care will go away because of health care system reform, or some other reason, in the foreseeable future. Some say that managed care has been the salvation of the U.S.'s rising health care expenditures because insurance companies can arbitrarily refuse coverage; others say that managed care has taken health care decision making out of the hands of physicians. Certainly, both are true. Managed care could be evolving into health care services rationing, the cornerstone of other countries' national health plans.

THE UNINSURED

The sheer number of uninsured individuals in the U.S. is a primary reason for the high price of health care in the U.S. In 2006, according to the Current Population Survey (CPS) the number of U.S. citizens not covered by health insurance was 47 million (Smith, 2008, pp. 79–81). The number of uninsured citizens is predicted to grow to 56 million by 2013 and the uninsured population is growing "rapidly among the poor" (Jost, 2007, p. 3). Interestingly, the greatest increases of newly uninsured individuals were among working, middle-class adults. Most uninsured individuals live in the South, and the highest numbers of individuals and families covered by health care insurance reside in the Midwest. In 2007, the average cost for health insurance for a family was $12,000 per year (Jost, 2007, p. 80).

Individuals without health insurance are at risk for detrimental health condition outcomes, financial catastrophes leading to bankruptcies, financial challenges for providers, and the marginal likelihood that those who have no insurance will schedule and/or receive necessary diagnostic or restorative procedures. The higher cost of health care equates to lower access for care (Jost, 2007, p. 131). One-third of working-age adults in the U.S. are either paying off accrued medical debt or have had medical bill problems in the past few years. Medical debt is one of the most important contributors of bankruptcy in the United States (Jost, 2007, p. xiii). Surprisingly most bankruptcies caused by medical debt have been among insured individuals. In one year alone, 1.8 million individuals claimed bankruptcy due to their inability to pay medical bills (Jost, 2007, p. 131). Individuals and families face extraordinary stress and embarrassment when they find themselves unable to pay medical expenses and frequently must choose between deferring necessary medical care or having to bear the cost of an expensive procedure or medication.

MEDICARE, MEDICAID, AND THE STATE CHILDREN'S HEALTH INSURANCE PROGRAM

Understanding public health care funding and the ways that providers are paid is very complex. Forty-five percent of all health care expenditures in the U.S. are funded by public dollars and programs, primarily through Medicare and Medicaid. Experts in the field of economics and health care finance remind us that the basic problem with public funding of health care is that the value of the health care received is greater than the cost; however, the people who are receiving the health care, benefiting from the value of the service, are not the ones paying the cost (Jost, 2007). To illustrate, the State Children's Health Insurance Program (SCHIP) that provides health care *insurance,* or paid health care services for children (and some parents) in all states, provides health care services to those who do not pay for it. The most recent data, representing figures from 2005, disclose that 5 million children are covered by SCHIP programs (Centers for Disease Control [CDC], 2007). A snapshot of a high SCHIP utilization rate may reflect the proportion of uninsured children and families in certain states. California, a large state with a large population, has 816,406 children enrolled in its SCHIP program. New Jersey has a concentrated number of residents in a small state and has 115,222 children covered by SCHIP. Part of the explanation for low enrollment may be the typical bureaucratic process that creates extensive barriers to enrollment and care through its cumbersome requirements when applying for program(s), "frequent and onerous redeterminations" (Jost, 2007, p. 131), or the scarcity of 1-800 numbers to explain the details or encourage enrollment. (It is well known that a no-support strategy/methodology functions to discourage participation.) There is of course, no way to know for sure why citizens do not take advantage of an entitlement health care program for children.

SCHIP and Medicaid are not paid for solely by the individuals who use and benefit from the health care services. The general population of the U.S. who works every day and pays for their own health insurance also pays a portion of the health care costs for those who cannot afford to do so. The costs of providing social insurance or for covering the cost of uninsured children and families shifts the cost of funding these government-mandated programs to individuals employed in the U.S. The costs to administer the programs and the cost of the expenditures for the health care services they provide keep rising. U.S. citizens are paying a sizable portion of the money they earn to subsidize fellow citizens. Together with archaic solutions, the results of the inefficient use of funds and outdated methods used to evaluate the impact of funding and utilization can create frustration for U.S. taxpayers.

The rate at which health care services are reimbursed is low. Thirty percent of the total bill is reimbursed to hospitals and Emergency Departments for the care they provide recipients of Medicaid. Recent data reveals that 82 of the 100 people who visited Emergency Departments in 2006 were covered by either Medicaid or SCHIP (Nawar, Niska, & Xu, 2006).

Uninsured patients are creating a financial crisis for Emergency Departments. It is no surprise that the higher proportion of SCHIP utilization occurs in states that have the highest number of uninsured families. Of course, there is always the outlier statistic that clouds analysis. For example, New Jersey has a high proportion of uninsured families. This high percentage of uninsured families may point to a reason for the high closure rate of hospitals and Emergency Departments in states like New Jersey, as will be discussed later in the book. It stands to reason that if hospitals are receiving only 30% of the expenses for uninsured individuals and the state has dramatically cut its charity care funding for hospitals, hospitals are going to struggle financially, which will lead to closures due to the financial inability to sustain operations. Legal immigrants who arrived in the U.S. after 1997 are not eligible for public funding of health care. The federal government primarily funds the program as a state entitlement allowing each state to have 70% of the federal match rate (for Medicaid programs). The fund provides greater than $40 billion (through 2005) for hospitalizations, physician visits, check-ups, and specific services for children whose families have incomes that are too high to qualify for Medicaid but could not get or afford traditional health care insurance. These SCHIP programs are the safety net for children of the United States (Centers for Medicare and Medicaid, 2008).

A review of the sources from which public funding for Medicare and Medicaid are derived clearly points to the potential for serious funding difficulties in the years to come. Increasingly, employers are not providing health care insurance for their employees, creating additional household encumbrances and potentially a greater number of uninsured U.S. citizens. Medicare is the federally mandated social insurance program for U.S. citizens over the age of 65 that was initiated by President Lyndon Johnson in 1965 (Centers for Medicare and Medicaid, 2008). Medicare Part A pays for institutional care and inpatient services in hospitals for the Medicare population and receives funding from all employees who pay a portion of the cost in payroll taxes to support the Medicare benefits. Medicare Part B pays for physician and other professional services, and Medicare Part D supports a pharmaceutical benefit.

Medicare Part A and Part D and a fraction of the Medicaid program are funded by federal taxes. The remainder of the expense for Medicaid, the public health care program for the poor, is provided by state taxes. There is no question that the tax burden to fund these programs will continue to increase and affect the bottom line of every working U.S. citizen. The only alternative to increasing the tax rate over time and as costs increase is for the federal government to dramatically cut health care benefits to this population (Jost, 2007). Baby Boomers in particular have paid numerous tax dollars into the Medicare program during their many years of employment and have anticipated their right to the Medicare entitlement. Due to the immense draw down of the funds supporting the program, Medicare does not cover the expense of all health care services that U.S. seniors may need. To bridge the gaps in coverage, senior U.S. citizens have had to purchase additional, or supplemental, policies.

As much as $700 billion, over 30% of our health care dollar expenditure, was spent on the administration of insurance plans and benefits. The costs to administer one insurance payer are expensive, but administrative costs for multiple payers create complexity, inefficiency, and duplicate costs. All insurance providers, both public and private, incur high administrative costs that are passed on to the insurance consumer to pay for accounting, billing, and claims processing staffs. Private insurance companies incur the same expenses but have additional costs for advertising, sales, lobbying, underwriting, and profit. The Canadian and other national health care systems have a one-payer system and are able to manage and control their administrative costs, spending less than 16% of their total expense for administration of the program (Pitts, Niska, Xu, & Burt, 2007). The greater the numbers of payers, the more complex the rules, the less efficient the system, and the more it costs.

PHYSICIAN COST FOR MALPRACTICE INSURANCE

Malpractice insurance is costing physicians, hospitals, and other providers of health care millions of dollars annually in insurance premiums. Malpractice insurance is liability insurance purchased by physicians and others to protect personal or institutional assets against litigation that may ensue because of a patient's bad outcome or for other perceived failures, such as the failure to obtain a specific test. Malpractice insurance for physicians and hospitals is a complex array of legal ramifications and questions including fiduciary responsibility, client–physician (or hospital) relationship, and standard of care. For our purposes, malpractice insurance is a cost and a necessary protection for the health care provider. Malpractice liability insurance is regulated by states. The premium rates that physicians or hospitals pay for coverage are based on several factors including their risk (what they do, in terms of providing health care services) and the potential profit the physician or hospital is seeking. In other words, if the physician is in a specialty in which costs for equipment are large and the cost to perform the procedure is high, malpractice premium rates will be high. Physicians and hospitals pay a large percentage of their income to protect themselves from errors that are caused by them or caused by circumstances outside their control. A recent trend, and one that may be affecting the declining cost of malpractice insurance is that hospitals, who may be a part of a large self-insurance pool, have been including physicians in the pool or purchasing malpractice insurance for the physicians to encourage their alignment with the hospitals (*Texas May Change Medical Malpractice Law*, 2008).

Multiple sources report that health care spending could be reigned in if our government would reform malpractice (N.D., 2009; Pho, 2009). There is encouraging evidence that changes in the malpractice insurance environment may be on the horizon. In 2003, Texas capped non-economic damages in medical liability cases to $250,000 for physicians. Since then, liability rates for malpractice insurance have dropped by 24%, and Texas is benefiting from the influx of physicians into the state. Since 2003, applications for medical licensure in Texas have risen 58%, from 2,561 to 4,041. Other states, including Georgia and Colorado, have not been as progressive and have recently overturned the cap on malpractice payouts (*Texas May Change Medical Malpractice Law*, 2008).

THE BOTTOM LINE

There are many reasons for the high cost of health care in the U.S., but the primary reason that U.S. health care is expensive is due to one thing: health care goods and services are more expensive in the United

States. Timothy Jost, in his book *Health Care at Risk: A Critique of the Consumer-Driven Movement* (2000, p. 11), points out that the "most important cause of excess health care costs" in the U.S. are:

- Physician salaries are higher in the U.S. than in any other country; U.S. physicians enjoy salaries that are two times higher than those in Canada and Germany and are four times higher than salaries in Japan.
- U.S. citizens pay higher costs for goods and services than do citizens of other countries.
- Drugs cost more in the U.S. since there is no regulation on drug prices or on drug company profits (Jost, 2007).

The combination of cost and the extended period to obtain or access needed health care services can be a basis for frustration and anger, especially if the frustration is protracted. The potential for violence to occur may be rare, but rising health care costs and the lack of quality, efficiently delivered health care services in a genuine customer care environment may support a basis for anger and violence.

CASE STUDY

ED SUPER-USERS

George is a super-user of Camden, New Jersey's Emergency Departments. Super-users, a newly coined term, utilize the Emergency Department with "astonishing frequency and at an astonishing cost to [the] health system" (Addis, 2008, p. 1) for primary health care needs. George admits to being a patient at a Camden ED at least 30, and maybe 40, times this past year. His symptoms range from chest pain to shortness of breath and hypertension.

Super-users, a term that is borrowed from the population of nurses who are specially trained as a resource for new nurse users of an electronic documentation system, cost Emergency Departments, like those in Camden, $9.2 million annually (Addis, 2008, p. 2). One percent of Camden's Emergency Department user popu-

(Continued)

lations are super-users like George. Over a 5-year period, in the city's three EDs, the super-users logged 39,000 visits.

A family physician in Camden, Dr. Jeff Brenner, has decided to confront the problem of ED overutilization by super-users and other patients. Dr. Brenner says that "no one benefits when people over-use the Emergency Department; not the hospitals, not the tax-payers and not the patients" (Addis, 2008, p. 2).

The evidence showed that one of the super-user patients cost the city $3.5 million over a 5-year period. Dr. Brenner computed that for the same amount of money that hospitals were spending to care for the super-users in Emergency Departments, he could "hire 50 physicians and provide a concierge-level of medical care, or [employ] 100 nurse practitioners who could provide one-on-one care for 10 patients each" (Addis, 2008, p. 2).

Most of the super-user patients are legitimately ill, but they do not have emergent, life-threatening conditions. Most have chronic conditions that may or may not respond with more-appropriate, more-frequent, and more cost-effective primary care visits. Most of the super-users are "homeless; get beaten up; get hit by cars; hit their heads." "Some do not speak English" (Addis, 2008, p. 3). Dr. Brenner says that so-called treat 'em and street 'em philosophy of emergency care is costly and ineffective. But, for these super-users, there is no other place to go but to the Emergency Department when they are ill.

Dr. Brenner believed that he had a better method. Armed with a sizeable grant from the Robert Wood Johnson Foundation, Dr. Brenner built a "medical home without walls" (Addis, 2008, p. 3), designated the Camden Coalition of Healthcare Providers. The group includes a nurse practitioner, a community health worker and a social worker who visit homes, shelters, and other locations, including the streets to find the ED super-users before they need medical care and end up in the Emergency Department. The team signs up the super-users and encourages them to practice health improvement tasks such as checking their blood sugar. One of the ED super-users said that he was taking better care of himself and commented that "it makes a difference when people show you that they really care" (Addis, 2008, p. 4).

(Continued)

A similar program, established in San Francisco 10 years ago, helps program participants find housing, drug and alcohol rehab, and government assistance. Dr. Okin, the program creator and director, says that every "$1.00 [that is] put into the program saves $1.44 in hospital costs" (Addis, 2008, p. 4).

Okin believes that targeting this 1% of ED users, the super-users, will not solve all of the Emergency Department overcrowding problems but will make a "substantial difference" (Addis, 2008, p. 4).

In Camden, any reduction in the numbers of patients visiting Emergency Departments will make an impact. The ED at Cooper University Hospital was built for an ED visit population of 22,000 visits annually, yet it had 53,000 visits in 2007 (Addis, 2008).

How Do Health Care Cost Increases Affect Our Personal Bottom Line?

The classic distribution adage applies here: 20% of all patients account for 80% of the spending. Most of the emergency room visits are for infants 12 months and younger and for chronically ill patients with multiple comorbidities. In 2006, 3.5 million infants under the age of 12 months, or 84.5 visits per 100 infants, visited the Emergency Department. The second highest group utilizing ED services was among the elderly, 75 years of age and above, who had 10.2 million visits, representing 60.2 visits per 100 persons 75 years of age or older (Pitts et al., 2007). (The data does not specifically state that the elderly group had the greatest chronic illness or comorbidities, but this is a reasonable assumption.)

It seems that the Emergency Department can't get a break. In 2006, one of the largest health care insurers in the state of Ohio cut physician reimbursement by 50%. The cuts affected all physicians, including Emergency Department physicians. In the same year, Tennessee removed 100,000 people from its TennCare rolls.[1] Both of these cuts were designed to reduce state health care expenditures. The cut in reimbursement and the Medicaid participant reduction by Ohio and Tennessee placed the burden directly on the shoulders of the ED—in Tennessee—to cover any emergency cost for 100,000 of its citizens who visit the Emergency Department.

In Tennessee, 100,000 additional people without health care insurance would not be able to visit their primary care physician because they could not pay for the care. If a medical emergency arose or a health care situation became more serious, uninsured individuals would have no other option than to visit the ED, leaving the Emergency Department to cover the majority of the expense for the visit. In Ohio, hospitals had the unfortunate dilemma of paying the physicians for the shortfall in their reimbursement to prevent the risk of losing the physician services contract ("Reimbursement Cuts," 2007).

In the U.S. today, 47 million men, women, and children do not have health care insurance. Who absorbs the costs for illness or injury incurred by this group of people? The hospitals do, particularly the Emergency Department (Brownlee, 2008).

CASE STUDY

"MORE AMERICANS DELAY HEALTH CARE: COST CONCERNS DRIVE EVEN THE INSURED TO FORGO TREATMENT" (RUBENSTEIN, 2008)

Sarah Rubenstein writes in the Wall Street Journal's *June 26, 2008, column "Health," that even insured individuals in the U.S. are "delaying or forgoing" (p. D2) medical care because of a concern about cost. The information is derived from the recent report produced by the Center for Studying Health System Change.*

A 2007 survey of 18,000 people admitted that they had delayed or ignored necessary medical treatment in the previous year; this figure was 14% higher than the survey results from 2003 (Rubenstein, 2008, p. D2).

Sixty-nine percent of the respondents replied that the reason that they had delayed or ignored necessary medical care was because of cost concerns. Peter Cunningham, the chief author of the report, stated that as health care costs increase, more of those costs are "shifting to people and families" (Rubenstein, 2008, p. D2). Deductibles, often chosen at high levels in the interest of saving a few bucks, and out of pocket expenses are more costly and cause elder and other consumers to withhold care rather than pay exorbitant costs. Patients have "reached a tipping point relative to the affordability of health care," says Cunningham (Rubenstein, 2008, p. D2).

(Continued)

The largest group of health care consumers who elected to withhold care was uninsured U.S. citizens, at 38%. Seventeen percent of insured consumers admit that they too chose to withhold health care necessities.

Karen Ignagni, who heads the U.S. insurance trade group America's Health Insurance Plans, lists three key issues for change that make health care more affordable:

- *Decrease the variability in quality of care.*
- *Reduce and control the high cost of surgery and imaging.*
- *Cull and coordinate the number of specialty drugs.*

Ignagni encourages the insurance industry and the policy makers to construct solutions to effect improved cost structures of health insurance.

Rubenstein tells of Mr. Peter Koerner, aged 65, who owns a small business in Pennsylvania but who does not have health insurance. When Koerner accidentally "sliced off half of his thumb" (Rubenstein, 2008, p. D2), his local Emergency Department suggested that he receive care in a distant trauma center that would require him to be flown in by helicopter. Koerner refused since he realized that the cost would be high and he did not want to be "responsible for that kind of a price tag" (Rubenstein, 2008, p. D2) for the flight alone. Mr. Koerner elected to pay the costs out of pocket. The bill added up to over $5,000 for the band-aid *surgery he received in his community (Rubenstein, 2008, p. D2).*

CASE STUDY: WHITE PAPER

EMERGENCY DEPARTMENTS AS A SAFETY NET

Safety Net Hospital Emergency Departments: Creating Safety Valves for Nonurgent Care

The following study illustrates the problem and costs of Emergency Department care for nonurgent health care needs. Emergency

(Continued)

Departments were designed to treat life-threatening illness and in-
juries, but in recent years, with the demise of many EDs and hospi-
tals, nurse staffing shortages, lack of primary care physicians, and
uninsured patients, Emergency Departments are becoming the de
facto safety net for many people.

This study, conducted by the Institute for Health System
Change (HSC) in 2007, evaluates 12 communities to interview
health care leaders about the health care commerce in their mar-
ket, the changes that have occurred in the past 2 years, and how
those changes have affected the community. The cities and areas
represented in the study are: Boston; Cleveland; Greenville, South
Carolina; Indianapolis; Lansing, Michigan; Little Rock, Arkansas;
Miami; (northern) New Jersey; Orange County, California; Phoe-
nix; Seattle; and Syracuse, New York.

The report derives information from CEOs, Emergency De-
partment directors (at the main safety net hospital in each commu-
nity), directors of community health centers, health departments,
Medicaid agencies, and consumer advocates based on interviews
with 453 individuals. While the HSC report examines only a small
sample size (12 communities), it represents what is happening
across the nation.

Hospital emergency departments (EDs) are caring for more
patients, including those with nonurgent needs that could be
treated in alternative, more cost-effective settings, such as a clinic
or physician's office. According to findings from the Center for
Studying Health System Change's 2007 report, site visits to 12 representative metropolitan communities, many emergency departments at safety net hospitals (the public and not-for-profit hospitals
that serve large numbers of low-income, uninsured and Medicaid
patients) are attempting to meet patients' nonurgent needs more
efficiently. Safety net EDs are working to redirect nonurgent patients to their hospitals' outpatient clinics or to community health
centers and clinics, with varied results. Efforts to develop additional primary, specialty and dental care in community settings,
along with promoting the use of these providers, could stem the
use of emergency departments for nonurgent care, while increasing access to care, enhancing quality and lowering and managing
costs.

Busy Emergency Departments See More Nonurgent Patients

Emergency department visits are rising, especially for patients with non-urgent conditions. Such conditions could include cold and flu symptoms, minor cuts and sprains, rashes, dental problems, and prescription refills. The National Hospital Ambulatory Medical Care Survey (NHAMCS) found that total ED visits classified as nonurgent, meaning the patient should be treated in 2 to 24 hours, increased from approximately 10% of ED visits in 1997 to 14% of visits in 2005, with uninsured patients experiencing a slightly higher increase.

1. People with private insurance accounted for most of the overall increase in ED visits. However, low-income uninsured and Medicaid patients rely more on Emergency Departments than do people with Medicare or private coverage.
2. Low-income, uninsured, and underinsured patients often turn to EDs for care because they lack timely access to outpatient care in other settings. The growing reluctance of physicians and dentists to serve Medicaid and uninsured patients, along with shortages of primary care physicians and certain specialists, such as psychiatrists, in some communities, make obtaining clinic or physician appointments increasingly difficult, according to findings from HSC's site visits (in 2007) to 12 metropolitan communities. Community health centers have expanded access to care in underserved areas but still struggle to respond to growing demand for primary care.
3. Many safety net hospitals face capacity constraints, and waits for appointments can be several months. As one Boston ED director said, "We see people coming back to the ED two to three times because they can't get an appointment with a specialist" (Wilson, 2008).

   • Emergency departments are expedient sources of care because they are open 24 hours a day, cannot turn patients away without screening them, and many are located in urban areas accessible by public transportation. At an ED in Lansing, a representative of a Medicaid health plan asked Medicaid enrollees why they chose the ED over their primary care providers. Key reasons included difficulty obtaining appointments with network providers and lack of affordable transportation to other providers. Moreover, some ED directors and other observers suggested that safety net EDs have accommodated low-income patients and have thus become the preferred provider of choice for some.

- There are concerns about use of the ED for nonurgent care. EDs are often crowded with patients waiting to be admitted to the hospital. People with nonurgent needs may contribute to increased wait times for all patients, including those with emergent needs, which can adversely affect patient outcomes.

4. In addition, ED capacity is costly given the range of stand-ready services and equipment that EDs must maintain, and studies have found the costs of providing nonurgent care may be higher in emergency departments than in other settings.

5. Interviews with ED directors at the main safety net hospitals in the 12 HSC communities spotlighted ways EDs are attempting to better manage the amount of nonurgent care they provide and improve access for people in the communities they serve.

REDIRECTING NONURGENT PATIENTS

Safety net hospitals are expanding Emergency Departments to accommodate increased numbers of patients overall and attract more well-insured patients, but this is a costly response to caring for patients with nonurgent needs. While some hospitals are trying to provide nonurgent care more efficiently, such as using a fast-track approach where mid-level practitioners provide care in a setting separate from the ED. Such strategies may attract even more nonurgent patients. For example, an Orange County hospital that created a small area in its ED for a physician to quickly treat patients with minor conditions has noted an increase in patient volume and more people traveling from longer distances.

Rather than attempting to serve more nonurgent patients, many safety net EDs are helping patients establish so-called medical homes that provide preventive and primary care for both episodic medical needs and chronic conditions, with coordination of follow-up visits and tests. Such providers, which include hospital outpatient clinics, community health centers, and individual primary care practitioners, may provide less costly care, reduce reliance on the ED for nonurgent conditions, and diminish the likelihood of a nonurgent problem going untreated and becoming more severe.

Some safety net hospitals are adding primary care capacity and working more closely with hospital specialty clinics to treat more patients needing follow-up care. For example, an Orange County hospital recently built an internal medicine clinic to serve uninsured patients, a Boston hospital added more family medicine clinics, and an Indianapolis hospital added a clinic for Spanish-speaking patients. In Miami, where a quarter of the population is uninsured, a safety net hospital restructured its clinics to make them more efficient and enable more patients to be seen, with a visit going from being an all-day experience to average waits of 75–90 minutes. That hospital also has added school-based clinics and mobile vans to deliver care in the community without the overhead costs of full-scale clinic facilities.

The federal Emergency Medical Treatment and Labor Act (EMTALA) requires that all patients who present in the Emergency Department for care must be screened. So, to encourage the use of outpatient clinics and community health centers, and to re-educate patients about the appropriate use of Emergency Departments, some EDs will screen patients to determine if the individual does not have an urgent or emergency condition and will then refer the patient to a lower-level, nonurgent level of care not typically provided by Emergency Departments.

To help these patients with nonurgent conditions identify other providers and schedule appointments, a Miami ED has added a nurse practitioner to discriminate between emergency and nonemergency conditions. Those patients who can be treated in an outpatient clinic setting are aided in making appointments with primary care or dental clinics on the same day or within three days, depending on appointment availability and urgency of the patient's condition. Over the course of 18 months, the ED staff referred an average of 50 patients a day to clinics—almost double what they initially expected and approximately 15% of the total ED volume. The hospital also placed posters around the hospital and clinics in an ongoing effort to educate patients about the types of conditions that are more appropriately treated in a clinic than in the Emergency Department.

Another approach used in some communities is to dedicate specific ED staff to work with patients prior to arrival, in some cases targeting patients with frequent ED visits, by adding nurses to serve as patient advocates. Nurse advocates help patients establish a medical home in the community by linking them to private physicians, free clinics, and community health centers for ongoing primary care. The advocate also focuses on patients with frequent ED visits to ensure that they obtain appointments with their care providers. In this way, routine problems do not turn into emergent problems. Similarly, a Seattle ED identifies patients—many with mental health conditions—who have 14 or more visits in 1 year and creates a patient care plan for these patients. Those patients who do not have a medical home or primary care physician are referred to the hospital's clinics or community health centers.

Other communities identify potential referrals if a patient is treated in the ED for a nonurgent condition. Personnel in the Emergency Department work to inform the patient about other care options to keep their condition from escalating into a more serious problem and requiring a return visit. As a Boston ED director remarked, "Once we see a patient, it's very important that there is good access to primary care, so patients don't come back [to the ED] many times because their diabetes or blood pressure is out of control" (Wilson, 2008).

COMMUNITY CLINIC LINKAGES

Involvement of community health centers and other primary care clinics is important to safety net hospital efforts to control the amount of nonurgent care provided in Emergency Departments, particularly for hospitals without their own clinics. The national associations representing community health centers and Medicaid health plans encourage efforts to provide a continuum of care through a medical home to mitigate the need for patients to turn to EDs for nonurgent care. Health center directors are largely supportive of such efforts to take on more patients diverted from the ED, and some have adopted same-day scheduling or walk-in appointments to enable patients to be treated more quickly.

Recognizing that community clinics can take pressure off of EDs, a number of safety net hospitals, in communities such as Seattle, Phoenix, and Miami, are collaborating with health centers. For example, one hospital is in discussions with an area health center to help the center extend hours to evenings and weekends to see more patients diverted from the ED or those who otherwise would have gone to the ED. However, without sufficient assistance to community health centers in the form of direct funding or the potential to generate additional revenue from treating more insured patients, taking on more patients could create a financial strain for health centers. One health center director noted a previous arrangement with a for-profit hospital where the ED sent the health center uninsured patients but few insured patients.

In a number of communities, health information technology enables scheduling appointments with other providers and/or sharing a patient's clinical information between the EDs and other providers. In Boston, Cleveland, Indianapolis, and Lansing, some clinics and physician offices can connect to the electronic medical record system in EDs to schedule appointments and better track a patient's condition and previous tests and treatments, although many systems provide read-only access and cannot transfer information back and forth. In Greenville, safety net providers and community organizations have developed an electronic referral system to transfer clinical and insurance information from the ED to the community clinics. Eventually this system is intended to facilitate referrals from the clinics to the hospital's clinics as well.

States, as part of Medicaid and other insurance coverage reforms, also are interested in encouraging the use of primary care providers instead of Emergency Departments. The Massachusetts universal coverage reform legislation included funding for Medicaid health plans to establish strategies to divert nonurgent patients away from EDs. These funds have helped community health centers expand operations to offer appointments outside normal business hours. And Florida funds health centers to help cover the costs of treating uninsured patients, with some of the funding directed toward initiatives that encourage the use of health centers over EDs for nonurgent care.

ONGOING CHALLENGES

Safety net hospitals' efforts to limit ED use for nonurgent conditions face a number of challenges. The amount of primary care available through clinics and health centers varies by community, and overall demand for care typically exceeds supply. Even as primary care capacity for low-income people has expanded across some communities in recent years, ED directors reported significant waits for appointments at health centers and clinics, particularly for new patients and for those current patients needing specialty care.

Also, the challenge of redirecting patients is more complex than expanding health center and hospital clinic capacity. Some health centers' extended hours have not been utilized as predicted: a health center in

Miami started a pediatric clinic on Saturdays but discontinued it because too few patients presented for care, and a health center in Boston noted similar concerns about new Sunday hours. The reasons for low demand are not always clear, but community respondents pointed to limited transportation and child care, and they suggested it takes time to inform people about health center and clinic options and encourage them to use those providers. Some low-income people still consider the ED their medical home. The director of a community clinic in Greenville lamented that people—especially those who are uninsured and have been offered attractive alternatives for care—seem to go to the Emergency Department. Additionally, adding staff to redirect patients to outpatient settings and investing in health information technology stretches safety net providers' limited funds.

Furthermore, expanding access to primary care through community health centers and clinics often does not address the need for specialty, mental health, dental care, and prescription drugs, so many EDs continue to treat those needs on site. EDs often rely on specialists employed by the hospital or who are paid a stipend to serve on call to treat nonurgent patients while they are still in the ED. Thus, it often happens that a doctor who wouldn't see a patient on the outside consults for the same patient in the ED.

IMPLICATIONS

Emergency Departments provide important access for people whose conditions do not require immediate treatment but who cannot access a community provider in a timely manner. However, EDs are not designed to treat ongoing, chronic needs, and wait times to receive care can be long. Strategies and policies that help direct patients to other outpatient settings could increase access, enhance quality, and contain costs if there are community providers willing and able to treat more low-income people. Findings across the 12 HSC communities suggest that a combination of approaches could help stem ED use for nonurgent care, including expansion of community health centers, community clinics, and hospital clinics and strategies to improve their accessibility. Alignment of hours of operation and available services among existing providers could increase people's care options at lower costs. Since transportation is a significant barrier for some, bringing services to low-income neighborhoods through mobile vans and school-based services could improve access in a cost-effective way. Furthermore, incentives to improve communication and coordination among community providers and ED staff could facilitate referrals so that care is provided in the most appropriate setting. Development of information technology among health care providers could improve communication among providers and ultimately reduce costs.

To prompt private practitioners to treat more low-income people, incentives such as enhanced Medicaid reimbursement appear essential. With the growth of Medicaid managed care, there is an increasing onus on Medicaid health plans to establish adequate networks of practitioners willing to treat Medicaid enrollees, but this too is impeded by the fact that low payment rates to health plans lead to low payment rates to physicians. Funded through the Deficit Reduction Act (DRA) of 2005, the Centers for Medicare and Medicaid Services recently awarded $50 million over 2 years to 20 state Medicaid programs to help develop capacity and programs to encourage primary care use over ED use.

Moreover, low-income people need to be informed about alternatives to the ED. Previous research shows that most uninsured people are unaware of providers that offer relatively low-cost care in their communities. Media campaigns and other outreach efforts could help raise awareness of health centers and hospital clinics, as well as the services offered and hours of operation.

Incentives, such as transportation vouchers and ensuring that patients pay less out of pocket for non-ED providers than they would in the ED, could also encourage people to use other providers. The DRA allows state Medicaid programs to permit EDs to charge copayments for nonurgent treatment, "but the impact on ED use and whether needed care is obtained has yet to be determined" (Felland, 2008).

NOTE

1. TennCare is the 1994 Tennessee Medicaid program.

REFERENCES

Addis, N. (2008, July 13). Super-users are swamping the ED. *Star-Ledger* (Camden, NJ).
A brief history of managed care. (1998). Retrieved July 24, 2008, from http://www.thci.org/downloads/briefhist.pdf
Brownlee, S. (2008, July/August). Why does health care cost so much? *AARP,* 51–55.
Case study: KY hospital ED cuts patient wait times with EMR. (2008). Retrieved September 2, 2008, from http://www.fiercehealth.com/story/case-study-Ky-hospital-ed-cuts-patientwaittimes-emr/2008/09/02

Centers for Disease Control (CDC). (2007, July 11). *The cost of violence in the United States.* Retrieved May 18, 2008, from http://www.cdc.gov/print.do?url-http%3A//www.cdc.gov/ncipc/factsheets/CostOf Violence

Centers for Medicare and Medicaid. (2008). Retrieved August 24, 2008, from http://www.cms.hhs.gov

Felland, L. H. (2008, May). *Safety-net hospital emergency departments: Creating safety valves for non-urgent care.* Retrieved August 15, 2008, from http://www.hschange.com/CONTENT/983/?PRINT=1

Goldstein, J. (2009, April 13). *Plans to close Northeastern Hospital stirs anger* (F. H. Dan Bowman, Producer). Retrieved April 13, 2009, from https://mail.google.com/mail/?account_id=pba9999%40gmail.com#inbox/120a14127c28188f

Herzlinger, R. (2004). *Consumer-driven healthcare: Implications for providers, payers and policymakers.* San Francisco: Jossey Bass.

Institute of Medicine (2008). *Definition of quality and quality measures.* Retrieved July 24, 2008, from http://www.qualitymeasures.ahrq.gov/resources/measure_selection.aspx

Jost, T. (2007). *Health care at risk: A critique of the consumer-driven movement.* Durham, NC: Duke University Press.

Nawar, E., Niska, R., & Xu, J. (2006). National hospital ambulatory medical care survey: Emergency department. *Advance data from vital and healthcare statistics, 7.* Hyattsville, MD: National Center for Health Statistics.

Pho, K. M. (2009, March 17). *Will reforming the malpractice system be a deal breaker for health reform?* Retrieved April 6, 2009, from http://www.kevinmd.com/blog/2009/03/will-reforming-malpractice-system-be.html

Pitts, S., Niska, R., Xu, J., & Burt, C. (2007). National hospital ambulatory medical care survey: Emergency department. *Advance data from vital and healthcare statistics, 386.* Hyattsville, MD: National Center for Health Statistics.

"Reimbursement cuts, payment delays threaten ED bottom lines." (2007, March). *ED Management.*

Rubenstein, S. (2008, June 6). More Americans delay health care: Cost concerns drive even the insured to forego treatment. *The Wall Street Journal,* p. D2.

Smith, D. J. (2008). The uninsured in the U.S. healthcare system. *The Journal of Healthcare Management, 52*(2), 79–81.

Texas may change medical malpractice law. (2008, September 2). Retrieved September 2, 2008, from www.fiercehealthcare.com/story/tx-may-change-medical-malpractice-law/2008-09-02

Why consider strategy to reform medical malpractice? Retrieved April 6, 2009, from http://www.mass.gov/Ihqcc/docs/meetings/2009_04_01_HCQCC_malpractice.pdf

Wilson, C. (2008). *Emergency room visits rise as primary care access drops.* Retrieved July 24, 2008, from http://www.insidearm.comgo/arm-news/emergency-room-visits-rise-as-primary-care-access-drops

3   Why Are EDs Targets for Violence?

The word on the street is that Emergency Departments (EDs) keep a lot of drugs. Drug seekers and gang members know this. They also know that it is easy to walk into an open-access Emergency Department and demand drugs, even if it takes the use of firepower to get what they want. By law and by their very inherent nature, Emergency Departments must deal with everyone and anyone who presents themselves for care, which makes the ED staff excessively exposed to violent individuals (Holleran, 2006).

During a 14-year period in Los Angeles, 14.7% of all trauma victims brought to an LA Emergency Department were found to have a concealed lethal weapon (*Emergency Department Violence*, n.d.). This statistic is at least 10 years old, and plausibly the number is much higher today.

Hospital security concerns, especially in the ED, have grown since the 9/11 assault on the United States. The rules of the game changed that day. In the days that followed 9/11, our once free and unfettered cities became heavy with terrorist experts who emptied subways and buildings at the sight of an unaccompanied box or bag and who disallowed a dram-sized container of mouthwash on commercial jets.

In like manner, even quiet suburban hospitals and small-town health care facilities, once an oasis for the ill or injured of a community, are confronted with complex crime and security issues (Harris, 2006), not so much due to copycat criminals, but more directly caused by a growth in the violent nature of the world in which we live. *Bioterrorism* was not a word that our first-graders needed to know 10 years ago.

Emergency Departments are faced with having to accept whoever walks though the door per the Emergency Medical Treatment and Labor Act (EMTALA), and the ED must rely on whatever level of security its particular hospital has chosen to implement.[1] Some Emergency Departments have walls of bullet-proof glass, lockdown capabilities, and staff who are trained in de-escalation techniques, while others are fortunate to have a part-time security guard on Saturday night.

ED OVERCROWDING AND THE INCREASE OF ED VIOLENCE

It is generally accepted that the increase in the numbers of patients visiting Emergency Departments is partially accountable for the increase in violence in the ED. With a growing number of emergency visits comes an increase in the wait time for patients to be attended to by a medical professional. A 2007 report, representing data from 1992 to 2004 and prepared by the Centers for Disease Control and Prevention (CDC), reveals that ED visits have increased by 20% (Rollins, 2007a), and another source has confirmed a 26% increase in ED visits (Zigmond, 2006) reported from a similar timeframe. Coping with an extraordinary surge in Emergency Department visits is challenging enough, but 20% increased ED visits in the face of 9% closures of Emergency Departments in the U.S. from 1995 to 2005 is a critical and dangerous trend (Nawar, Niska, & Xu, 2007, p. 2).

One of the major problems that EDs face today is patient crowding. *Patient crowding* is the term used to describe the immense numbers of patients who are waiting for medical care or for an inpatient bed and must wait or be boarded in the ED. Aside from the sheer numbers of patients and the space constraints, impatient and angry patients can potentially create violent situations resulting from frustration of waiting in the ED waiting room for up to 6 hours. Psychiatric and or mentally ill patients also come to the Emergency Department. This group of patients, in particular, is at risk to incite a violent episode. This population is competing with the large number of injured or ill emergency patients who frequently have to be diverted away from the Emergency Department to other facilities because the ED is over capacity and cannot accommodate one more patient. Also, psychiatric patients have more limited options, often because they cannot be admitted to the inpatient services they need as a result of closures of a large number of inpatient and outpatient psychiatric resources because of limited reimbursements for mental health care.

In a 2007 survey of 1,500 Emergency Department physicians, more than 1,200 physicians (greater than 80%) responded that there were serious crowding conditions in their EDs. Forty-seven percent of the physicians report that patients have suffered as a result of the crowded environment, and 13% identified a patient death as a direct result of crowding (*Docs Note Rise in Emergency Department Crowding*, 2007).

Patients and families who are waiting long hours in the waiting room of the ED can become angry and agitated because of pain, fear, or the perception of being passed over or ignored by the ED staff. Donna Mason, former director of the Vanderbilt University Medical Center adult ED (Nashville, TN), tells us that "crowding and boarding always tend to bring out the worst in people. When people have waited for hours to be seen or to get an inpatient bed, they grow impatient. Their anger is often directed to the nurse who spends the most time with the patients and their families" (Rollins, 2007b).

One statistic taken from a 2005 article in the *Annals of Emergency Medicine* states that the threat of violence is only going to increase as psychiatric and substance abuse services become less available and the length of stay (in emergency waiting and treatment rooms) gets worse (Kowalenko, 2005).[2]

CASE STUDY

Psychiatric patients, who need inpatient care, are waiting long hours in the Emergency Department before they can be admitted for treatment. Eighty percent of hospitals report that mentally ill patients wait for at least 4 hours or more before being admitted, and often the only available inpatient psychiatric treatment bed is a significant distance away. Ten percent of the hospitals report that patients frequently waited in the ED for more than 24 hours before an inpatient resource could be found.

(Continued)

The American College of Emergency Physicians (ACEP) conducted a survey in 2008 to determine the extent of psychiatric patients who are forced to stay for hours in a general (nonpsychiatric) emergency department while awaiting admission or transfer to a rare inpatient psychiatric bed (Appleby, 2008). Of the 328 Emergency Departments surveyed, fewer than 50% have inpatient psychiatric units. Since 2000, U.S. community hospitals have lost 12% of all inpatient beds for the treatment of psychiatric illnesses. One report confirms that 61% of U.S. hospitals do not have specialized, psychiatric staff caring for mentally ill patients in the Emergency Department. An overall loss of government funding has resulted not only in the decrease in the numbers of available psychiatric resources but also in decreased funding for the education of advanced-prepared mental health professionals such as psychologists and psychiatrists. As a result, many hospitals may have been forced to close their inpatient psychiatric units because of "inadequate payments from government and insurers; unpaid costs for the uninsured; and too few psychiatrists willing to work in hospitals," says James Bentley of the American Hospital Association (Appleby, 2008).

Patients with psychiatric illness can create serious problems for Emergency Departments, which often do not have the nursing or physician expertise to deal with a psychiatric illness. Psychiatric patients respond better to a special, therapeutic environment that is generally quiet and controlled. Emergency Departments are not quiet and are not controlled. EDs are the loudest and most chaotic departments in all of the hospital and do not offer the best environment for patients who are struggling to maintain control in the face of psychosis or dementia. Nurses and physicians who are not trained in how to respond to psychiatric patients in the most helpful way can sometimes become the target of violence as patients lash out in frustration.

TOO MANY PATIENTS!

U.S. hospitals are challenged by an increasing number of ED visits, often because EDs are considered the new front door to hospitals. This is where the problem of excessive capacity issues begins. Increased ED visits lead to a lengthy process for the patient simply because it takes longer for the medical professionals to see and treat the excessive and growing number of patients. Excessive crowding initiates a protracted process, which includes extended wait times, as a result of a backlog of patients in the ED waiting rooms and treatment areas. It is well-documented that the average wait time in U.S. emergency rooms is 4–6 hours (Reavy, 2001). Extreme numbers of patients, triggering long wait times, can lead to higher patient frustration levels and, eventually, increased potential for ED violence.

Crowding and boarding also contribute to Emergency Department concerns because both can result in compromised care of the patient. Crowding occurs when disproportionate numbers of patients arrive for care at U.S. Emergency Departments and boarding is the process of keeping patients in the ED who are destined for inpatient admission until a bed in the hospital becomes available. All of these conditions, including the sizable number of acute and nonacute patients, often results in a domino effect on staff performance and facility and equipment overcapacity. Daily, this circumstance leads to chaos and amplified patient and family frustration, ultimately leading to a higher potential for violence.

Until very recently, emergency room crowding, boarding, and the use of resources in the emergency room was perceived by the rest of the hospital as a specific ED problem contained within a silo. That is, most hospitals viewed the problem as strictly an ED problem rather than as a systemic, hospital-wide problem that needed to be resolved by the entire hospital. Hospitals that have taken the broader view of ED crowding as a system problem appear to be making more progressive strides toward alleviating the crowding issues in the ED than are others.

UNINSURED PATIENTS

The CDC reported in June of 2007 that ED visits to U.S. Emergency Departments rose to an all-time high of "115.3 million visits in 2005," (Nawar, Niska, & Xu, 2007) which is equivalent to 36.6 visits per 100 people and 5 million more visits in 2005 as compared with 2004 (Lubell, 2007). Reported in August of 2008, the number of Emergency Department visits for 2006 rose to 119.2 million, nearly 1 visit for every 2 people in America (40.5 visits for every 100 people) (Pitts, Niska, Xu, & Burt, 2008).

This is a dangerous trend for all of the aforementioned reasons. To understand the scope of the problem, it is helpful to know the reasons for these increasing ED visits. Some of the well-documented reasons include:

- A decrease in Medicare and Medicaid physician reimbursement and an overall increase in the number of uninsured patients have combined to drive physicians to send patients to the ED for treatment rather than treat them in the office environment. Physicians are faced with a new model of care to compensate for lower reimbursement. Physicians must see more patients per hour to increase their opportunity for profitability. To balance both books and caseloads, physicians may opt to send their more time-intensive patients to the ED for care.
- The uninsured patient presents a dichotomy of dilemmas for EDs in the U.S. It is generally accepted that many uninsured patients elect to use the emergency room as their primary care provider. Backing up this assertion is a 2004 Robert Wood Johnson/American College of Emergency Physicians survey of emergency room physicians, who believe that 30% of patients seen in the emergency room are uninsured (ACEP Foundation, 2004).

Uninsured patients present four disparate problems:

1. The unintended consequence of providing care to low-acuity, nonemergency, or primary care patients in the ED increases the reimbursement and waiting room crowding issues for EDs as they exacerbate the clog in the ED flow (Silberner, 2006).
2. Uninsured patients generally do not have a primary care provider and often wait until a medical problem is demanding immediate attention before seeking medical assistance. More serious illnesses consume a greater share of time and resources for the Emergency Department and staff. Sixty-seven percent of emergency room physicians polled in 2004 agreed that uninsured patients are sicker and have more serious conditions than those who have health insurance (ACEP Foundation, 2004).

   a. Medicine and surgery specialists and subspecialists are becoming less available to the patients who present to the ED for care. When an uninsured patient does not pay for his or her Emergency Department visit, often the specialist does not get paid. As budgets get trimmed to balance the unpaid expenses, hospitals and EDs cannot afford the on-call expense that specialists must charge to make their services available and to pay the extra malpractice insurance these specialists must hold to provide services to the ED.

b. Emergency Departments lose money when patients cannot pay for services. Ultimately, negative cash flow creates an unbalanced ED budget and a threat to the hospital's bottom line. Although every hospital plans for unreimbursed care in the annual budget, for-profit hospitals and not-for-profit hospitals cannot provide totally unpaid care forever. Uninsured care may account for the increasing number of Emergency Department closures over the past decade. According to the CDC, 381 (9%) Emergency Departments in the U.S. have closed in the past 12 years; 2008 statistics reveal that 425 EDs and 703 hospitals closed between 1993 and 2003, including the closing of 198,000 staffed inpatient beds (Pitts et al., 2008).

c. The expansion of immigration, notably of undocumented (illegal) immigrants, is of serious concern to EDs and hospitals, primarily in the four states where currently more than one-half of all uninsured resident immigrants live: California, Texas, Florida, and New York. The reasonable assumption is that these four states in particular will continue to have difficulties supporting U.S. citizens who have no health insurance but need emergency medical care in addition to supporting undocumented, uninsured immigrants (*Study: Uninsured Population Grows With Immigration*, 2008).

3. The so-called aging of America increases the demand for emergency services. The majority of older patients have numerous and complex health care problems and medications and, as a result, require more time in the ED. Joel Seligman, CEO of North Westchester County Hospital, New York, remembers that in the past, individuals could probably see their family physician as a work-in appointment on any given day. Today, however, overbooked physicians may elect to send an older person with a problem to the emergency room.

4. Hospitals, unable to sustain operating viability because of inadequate reimbursement, are closing at an alarming rate. "Today [2002] there are 900 fewer hospitals than there were in 1980" (*Cracks in the Foundation*, 2002, p. 6). Illinois reports the closure

of 50 hospitals in their state alone between 1980 and 2005, and California confirms the closing of 23 general acute care hospitals between 1995 and 2000. Also significant, 40 mental health facilities nationally have closed since 1993, according to the Department of Justice. When one hospital closes, other local EDs must accommodate the overflow of sick patients, increasing not only the numbers of patients but the stresses on the local ED and hospital. Hospitals are succumbing to fiscal instability, which is cited as the number one reason for hospital closures. Fewer hospitals and Emergency Departments funnel a larger number of patients to fewer medical care resources.

NURSING SHORTAGE

There is a sustained lack of registered nurses (RNs), which is forecast to escalate through the year 2020. Fewer nurses automatically create an inefficient use of time and resources for patient processing and care in the ED. Currently in the U.S., there are 100,000 vacant positions in U.S. hospitals for RNs. This number is predicted to increase to 434,000 in the U.S. and to 800,000 worldwide by 2020 (*Nursing Shortage Growing Worldwide,* 2007). The nursing shortage is directly responsible for inefficiency issues in a majority of U.S. EDs and indirectly contributes to crowding issues in the EDs because a lack of inpatient personnel often requires the closure of inpatient beds, causing the downstream effect of more patients waiting in already-crowded EDs.

HIGHER PATIENT ACUITY

Patients are sicker. When patient acuity is great, it takes more time, materials, and human resources to care for the patient.[3] Chronically ill patients often have multiple comorbidities that require a cadre of specialists and medications to manage and treat the complexity of physiologic system interactions. Based on the 2005 and 2006 CDC data, the number of patients who visited EDs and were triaged in triage levels I and II, the two highest categories of patient acuity, reflecting an increase in ED high-acuity patient visits: 2005 triage levels I and II = 17,640,900 patients; 2006 triage level I and II = 18,052,800 patients (Nawar et al., 2007; Pitts et al., 2008).

PHYSICIAN SHORTAGE

The shortage of physicians in all specialties, including ED physicians and primary care physicians (PCPs), currently is calculated to be 20% or more ("ED Workforce Appears Stretched to Its Limits," 2006). This shortage creates a twofold impact on the ED: there are fewer ED physicians to care for the multitude of high acuity patients and fewer PCPs in the community in which to route the lower acuity, nonemergency, patients. As a result, requests and referrals for specialty and primary care appointments often are scheduled months in the future. If the patient becomes acute during this interval, there is only one thing for the patient to do: Go to the Emergency Department. Compounding this predicament is the scarcity of emergency on-call specialists who might be needed to evaluate and treat specific disorders.

The reimbursement crisis, which began in 2006 and has ballooned as high as a 50% rate cut for physician fees, is making it difficult for hospitals and EDs to attract and retain talented ED physicians.

INSURANCE REIMBURSEMENT

In addition to rate cuts, payers (insurance companies) are bundling services so that the fee (rate) that might have been paid to a physician for one procedure may now encompass three procedures for the same fee.

A delay in payment or the frank denial of payments to EDs and to physicians for certain things, such as EKGs, observation of patients, or after-hours care, can create a financial crisis for many EDs. Hospitals may need to eliminate ED personnel positions to compensate for fewer hours that are being reimbursed by insurance companies.

An example of this is that Medi-Cal, California's Medicaid program, has implemented legislation to cut 10% from the fee-for-service provider reimbursement to "address California's significant structural budget deficit," which became effective July 1, 2008 (*Statement of Proposal*, 2008).

The heightened scarcity of PCPs may be creating unanticipated consequences for the ED. According to a study presented in September 2007 at the Fourth Mediterranean Emergency Medicine Conference in Italy (Weber, 2008), a survey revealed that the rise in ED visits between 1996 and 2003 is not solely due to ED utilization by the uninsured or poor. A large number of insured patients are also using the ED for care since many PCPs are unable to provide timely access in their offices.

PSYCHIATRIC PATIENTS, SUICIDAL PATIENTS, AND PATIENTS WITH UNDIAGNOSED DEPRESSION

The deinstitutionalizing of the mentally ill person in the 1980s and 1990s has created a massive deficit of inpatient psychiatric resources so that patients who are experiencing a psychiatric crisis have no place to go except the ED. Frantic daily caregivers are forced to ask EDs to assist in the care of their out-of-control parents, spouses, or children (*Hospital Closures*, 2007).

Patients may be unaware of their own behavior in certain states of illness or injury and may respond inappropriately. Depression can lead to thoughts of suicide and hopelessness. A severely depressed patient is capable of reacting violently, paralleling his state of mind. In a critical state of unhinged thinking, the depressed or psychologically ill individual may be unconcerned about the consequence of injury or death that he may instigate.

Many cities in the U.S., such as Las Vegas and Charleston, South Carolina, have very limited psychiatric inpatient beds or facilities to care for mentally ill patients. There is a grave misunderstanding of the impact that psychiatric patients are having on U.S. EDs. If a hospital does not have an inpatient psychiatric service, a patient waiting for psychiatric admission often waits in the ED for an extended period of time until a qualified professional can evaluate and admit the patient or locate a secondary referral source. Rarely is a patient who presents to the ED and who is in need of mental health support capable of being discharged home to his own care or to the care of an untrained relative. The risks for both the patient and the caregiver are simply too high. The only alternative is to hold the patient in the ED pending the availability of a hospital bed, either in that hospital or in another hospital facility. It is not uncommon for hospital employees to drive patients across the state so the patient can be admitted to a facility with an available psychiatric bed.

Timeframes for ED psychiatric patient holds can vary depending on the availability of psychiatric resources in the local market. If no psychiatric resources are immediately available, an ED may inherit a psychiatric patient for up to one week or longer. Envision how difficult it would be to manage and appropriately care both for critically ill and injured patients and for patients who are awaiting acute psychiatric evaluation and may present a serious violence risk to ED personnel.

PATIENTS WITH SUSPECTED SUBSTANCE ABUSE

Individuals who are abusing alcohol, illicit drugs, prescription medication, or other substances can have a violent state of mind. Individuals under the influence of physically altering substances contribute directly to violent episodes in the Emergency Department.

The state of Georgia has seven state psychiatric hospitals. In Georgia's state psychiatric system, 115 patients died from neglect, abuse, or poor medical care between 2002 and 2007, and there were 200 confirmed cases of patient abuse. In 2007, 21 patients died under "suspicious circumstances" (Judd, 2008).

Currently in the U.S. there is a demonstrated lack of inpatient psychiatric beds. The Treatment Advocacy Center conducted a study to evaluate the bed trend in the U.S. between 2002 and 2005. The current numbers of inpatient psychiatric beds were compared with the available beds in 1955. Several examples of the decrease of inpatient psychiatric beds available today as a percentage of the inpatient psychiatric beds that were available in 1955 are listed here:

New York—4.6%

California—6.1%

Tennessee—8.0%

Illinois—3.5%

There are 10 U.S. states that presently have a critical shortage of inpatient psychiatric beds, defined as 12 or fewer beds per 100,000 individuals. The 10 states are: Nevada, Arizona, Arkansas, Iowa, Vermont, Ohio, South Carolina, Oklahoma, Idaho, and Alaska. Since 2003, 40 psychiatric hospitals have closed yet during the same timeframe, there have been 400 new prisons opened (Torrey, 2003; see Table 3.1).

Patients who present for care in the ED must be seen and evaluated, yet ED personnel often are confronted with the challenge of managing patients with a history of violence without even knowing it. Typically, there is no information about patients arriving in the ED who have

Table 3.1

PSYCHIATRIC INPATIENT BEDS

STATE	NUMBER OF BEDS/ 100,000 POPULATION (1955)	NUMBER OF BEDS (2005–2006)	MINIMUM NUMBER OF BEDS NEEDED (2005–2006)	NUMBER OF BEDS TO BE ADDED TO MEET MINIMUM STANDARD	2004–2005 BEDS AS A % OF 1955 BEDS
Idaho	200.5	157	683	526	5.6
Alaska	N/A	74	322	248	N/A
Oklahoma	396.6	386	1,754	1,368	3.0
South Carolina	264.7	443	2,109	1,666	4
Ohio	319.7	1,210	5,762	4,552	3.3
Michigan	301.2	1,006	5,030	4,024	3.3
Vermont	342.3	55	306	251	2.6
Iowa	198.2	239	1,494	1,255	4.1
Arkansas	284.3	184	1,415	1,231	2.4
Arizona	172.4	338	2,817	2,479	3.4
Nevada	195.6	119	1,190	1,071	2.6

known prior violent activity records. Prior diagnosis of certain medical and/or psychiatric illnesses or conditions could help the ED staff predict a potential for violence and take appropriate precautions to protect themselves if patient records were readily available containing information about:

1. A past history of violent behavior
2. Substance abuse (alcohol and/or drugs)
3. Severe psychiatric illness and/or acute psychosis
4. Not taking medication (psychiatric medication) (Jackson & Flinn, 1994)
5. Traumatic brain injury
6. Antisocial personality disorder

Additionally, because of the decreasing availability of psychiatric resources, the use of EDs for medical clearance before individuals are jailed is on the increase, which contributes to the potential for violent patient behavior in the ED (Holleran, 2006).

CASE STUDY

VIOLENCE AGAINST NURSES IN MASSACHUSETTS

Nurses are the primary caregivers of patients and are the most vulnerable to patient violence. Until recently, the problems of workplace injury concerned back injuries or work-related asthma, according to Evelyn Bain, head of Massachusetts Nurses' Association (MNA) Occupational Health and Safety Office. MNA is a nurses' union. Now she receives reports of nurses being "punched, strangled, sexually assaulted and stuck with contaminated needles."

An Emergency Department nurse who is an 18-year veteran of the ED admits that getting attacked and abused is not what she signed up for. An angry patient grabbed the nurse and dug in her nails, threatening to find and kill the nurse's children. The same nurse had an encounter with an intoxicated, HIV-positive patient, and the nurse ended up being covered in blood. She is no longer working as a nurse.

CASE STUDY DISCUSSION

"Emergency rooms seem to be the hot spot for violent assaults, but general practice nurses or specialty nurses in other hospital units are not immune." Over 50% of the MNA, a union whose members practice in many disciplines and not just in the ED, report patient violence (Lothian, 2007). Emergency Department psychiatric nurses particularly are at risk. Often, violent patients will devise weapons from any object they can find. One particular example is a patient who created a switchblade from a harmonica and tried to

(Continued)

harm the nurse. In a separate incident, the nurse had to physically "fight off an aggressive, violent male patient." The nurse reports that attacks of similar circumstances have become "almost routine" (Lothian, 2007).

In an analysis by the MNA nursing union, the cause of the increase in patient violence toward nurses is attributed to "budget cuts, resulting in a shortage of nurses." Hospital officials at the Massachusetts Hospital Association (MHA) disagree that a lack of appropriate staffing is the cause of increasing numbers of violent patient attacks. The MHA Senior Vice President for Clinical Affairs believes that asking for higher levels of nurse staffing is a "knee-jerk reaction" (Lothian, 2007).

Those who have witnessed and experience patient violence would vehemently disagree with this belief. It is posited that if the nurse executives were experiencing the ED patient care environment, including the type of violence that ED nurses encounter every day, they would change their minds. Such firsthand experience of patient violence is not easily endured. When nurse executives find it easy to dismiss not only the serious nature of such ED personnel experiences but also do not investigate current published research or statistics relating to possible causes for the increase of such violence, they might find it easy to dismiss. In her remarks, the MHA vice president does go on to qualify her remarks and admits that improved security and de-escalation training for all nurses is a better approach since society is becoming more violent. The MNA is encouraging nurses to press charges, whereas in the past "nurses were discouraged from taking action against violent patients" because they were told that "unruly and sometimes violent patients were part of the job" (Lothian, 2007).

CASE STUDY

This case study highlights the serious problem of increasing numbers of mentally ill or psychiatrically unstable patients coming to Emergency Departments, often because there is no other place to

(Continued)

go, and how this circumstance creates a critical burden on the health care system and on patients and their families. Inpatient psychiatric facilities and community services for less acute or serious behavioral or mental health issues have closed, leaving communities struggling to provide care for patients who need treatment and monitoring.

A new psychiatric Emergency Department model in Louisiana is making a positive impact on the community and the state. A psychiatric ED, an adjunct and extension of the current ED at University Medical Center, Pineville, Louisiana, was created in response to the overwhelming needs of the local hospitals and of the mentally needy to fill the gap created by the disruption and depletion of the health care services in Louisiana after Hurricane Katrina. The model allows for patients who are mentally or behaviorally unstable to move to a therapeutic, quiet stabilization area that accommodates their needs. Additionally, the unit helps to decrease the sheer volume of patients in the ED. According to Mary Broussard, Director of Nursing at University Medical Center, the "addition of psychiatric patients to the acute ED environment limited our ability to effectively care for either group" (Sills, 2008, p. 2). This model program, referred to as MHERE, will be expanded into other hospitals in the state. Although the acronym MHERE is not defined, it refers to the specific mental health emergency room extension that has been created at University Medical Center in Pineville, Louisiana.

The new concept of psychiatric ED treated 696 patients between January and June 2008. Fifty-six percent of those patients were transferred to inpatient psychiatric facilities or UMC's inpatient psychiatric unit. Nurses, counselors, and social workers provide comprehensive care to the patients. Security personnel are placed within the middle of the unit, which includes tracking videos visible from each of the treatment rooms (Sills, 2008).

CASE STUDY

In two states, North Carolina and Florida, several hospitals have added separate space within the ED for the emergency care of

(Continued)

patients with psychiatric conditions. Forsyth Medical Center in Greensboro, North Carolina, has been able to reduce its through-put time for all patients by 9% on average. The ED renovation in 2004 incorporated a new area that is staffed by one psychiatric nurse on every shift. The psychiatric nurse is supported by a team of behavioral health care specialists, called the Access Team, who are available depending on the volume of patients requiring psy-chiatric evaluation.

The ED director, as part of the planning process for the new ED, evaluated the type of patients who were visiting the ED. This evaluation revealed an increase in the number of psychiat-ric patient visits, an important statistic that suggested the need for a new strategy to help manage these patients. The ED plan-ning team also recognized that assessment and initial treatment of the psychiatric patients took a longer period of time, and utilized more human resources, than did the medical-surgical emergency patients. As with most ED expansions, the new area drew more psychiatric patients to the ED, and psychiatric ED patient vis-its were up nearly 8% from the same period during the previous year ("Psych ED Helps Speed Throughput Time by 9%," 2006).

In Florida, a hospital in a resort area has provided a separate area for psychiatric patients in its ED for some time. The entire space for the ED is very small and narrow, so it is a challenge for the ED to have separate functions within the small space. In addi-tion to the detached reception and processing area, the hospital has a therapeutic inpatient unit to accommodate psychiatric patients in crisis.

UNREIMBURSED CARE

States provide some level of charity care funding for their hospitals to help cover the expenditures that hospitals acquire when treating unin-sured patients. Based on the amount of funding that is received from the state coffer, hospitals budget for the projected losses they will incur for treating the uninsured, or charity care. Charity care funds do not usually cover the total costs that hospitals have for uninsured or charity care, funding generally between 20%–70% of the actual costs.

In New York and New Jersey, cities are reeling from abrupt budget cuts for uninsured care, while consistently maintaining a surplus of patients requiring unfunded care in the ED. New York is one of four states that have the nation's largest population of uninsured patients, and New Jersey has a documented 1.3 million uninsured inhabitants (Zieger, 2008), which is 23% of all New Jersey residents (*NJ Hospitals Going Under as State Bailout Cash Ends*, 2008).

The budget cuts in New Jersey will reportedly top $110 million this year. With nearly one-half of all New Jersey hospitals currently operating in the red, these budget cuts will contribute to a potentially dangerous financial shortfall for most hospitals that provide even a small measure of charity care. In short order, the only remaining strategy will be hospital closure, since ED and hospital budgets will not be able to sustain continued losses from uninsured patients coupled with no incoming state revenue to subsidize the difference.

One New Jersey hospital, Muhlenberg Regional Medical Center, in Plainfield, one of the hospitals preparing for closure, has been in operation for over 130 years and provides care for an ethnically diverse community. The population of Plainfield likely has many residents who do not have health insurance. Muhlenberg Regional Medical Center lost over $16.5 million in 2007 and projects a loss of $18 million in 2008. Another New Jersey hospital, Barnert Hospital, in Patterson, a 256-bed acute care community hospital, declared bankruptcy and closed its doors in recent months. Many other New Jersey hospitals likely will be subject to the same prospects this year and in years to come.

The loss of hospitals and EDs can affect many things, including producing a glut of patients who then become dependent on the remaining hospitals and EDs for emergency and primary care. More patients and fewer resources create an intensified opportunity for violence to occur.

THAT PATIENT IS OUR CUSTOMER

The concept of customer service and hospitality is only now becoming a strategy for hospitals and Emergency Departments. Prior to the naissance of for-profit health care, hospitals did not have a need to vie for patient visits or loyalty. Health care was affordable and services were provided by locally available hospitals and physicians. *Hospitality* was relegated to the hotel, restaurant, and service industries.

Before mid-1970, there was typically only one hospital within a defined town or region so that all patients in need of health care services went to the one local hospital that supplied the health care needs, from birth to death, of the entire family. Hospitality was inherent to the local market, the neighborhood, since everyone knew everyone else. There was no need for a hospital to promote and sell its health care services, and it was deemed unethical for physicians to advertise.

In our contemporary for-profit hospital environment, hospitals publicize their services to compete with the many local hospitals that often provide the same or similar services. Other neighboring hospitals frequently offer competitive services for a lower price or with the promise of time savings through more efficient delivery. Physicians have marketing budgets and are no longer resistant to advertising via television or other marketing channels to promote their services. In fact, physicians are considered savvy when they create an advertising edge by touting their prestigious pedigrees, credentials and board certifications, or by offering a same as cash financing benefit to help patients afford their services.

This need to compete creates serious conflicts for hospitals. Because hospitals are vying for the next paying patient, they do not want the media to broadcast the occurrence of a violent episode in their ED waiting room. Such media broadcasts might frighten a potential customer, the patient of the facility, who would not wish to become the unwitting victim of ED violence.

A *hospitality* strategy can persuade patients/customers, especially those within a hospital's catchment area, to use the locally available services offered by EDs and hospitals. The overall objective of hospitality for a hospital is to generate new business by impressing the patient with a high level of therapies and equipment and customer service that will encourage patients to come back time after time. Often it is said that if an individual is pleased with service he has received, he will tell one person, but if he is displeased with the service he has received, he will tell many people. Since the ED often is the entry point for many inpatient admissions, it is crucial that EDs welcome patients and provide them with excellent service. The ED generates 12%–13% of inpatient admissions on average, and annually that translates into important revenue for hospitals (Nawar et al., 2007; Pitts et al., 2008).

Many hospitals are spending a great deal of capital to improve the design and decor of their EDs, to entice paying customers to use their emergency services. Patient and customer-centric ideas, such as

expanded treatment and waiting rooms equipped with flat-screen tele-
visions and laptops, and "comfort rounds" (Kershaw, 2008) distribute
up-to-date reading material, pillows, snacks, toys and games, and sometimes even art therapists for children appears to be a growing trend.

There are, however, pros and cons to touting customer service as a
core competency. The necessity to *keep it positive* is perhaps the major
reason that hospital and ED incidents of violence or disruptions are significantly underreported. Generally, when an incident is described on
the news or in print media, you can be sure that the content has been
carefully edited by public relations professionals to create the message
that the hospital is taking immediate, corrective action to rectify the situation. They want to be sure to communicate the perception that the
hospital and ED are safe environments for its customer, the patient. It is
a well-documented fact (Harmacinski, 2003) that many hospital administrators ignore or de-emphasize situations of unrest within the hospital
in order to convey the message of a safe place for patients to come for
care.

Violence changes the perception of the welcoming image that the
hospital wishes to project to gain the competitive edge and to perhaps
add that one additional paying patient to its bottom line "A lot of hospitals worry about their image, but with one bad incident all their good
PR is gone in a heartbeat" (as quoted by Fred Roll in Thrall, 2006). Physicians and hospitals alike are clued into the critical nature of patient
satisfaction, just as hotels focus on customer satisfaction. Physicians and
hospital administrators are graded and compensated on the scores that
their patients give them. And, to be sure, if you have a negative experience in a hotel, or encounter a situation that has not been resolved to
your satisfaction, will you choose to visit that hotel again? Probably not.
Hospitals also face much of the same scrutiny. Each is focused on creating a memorable and problem-free experience for its customers. Molly
Rowe tells us that Jonathon Tisch, CEO of Lowes Hotels, is convinced
that hotels and hospitals strive for the same outcome "taking care of individuals who are entrusting an experience to you." Rowe shares several
of Tisch's customer-focused tips including providing "basic comfort" in
an environment that may be unfamiliar and often frightening, such as a
busy Emergency Department. By offering small tokens of comfort and
concern, your customer—the patient—will feel taken care of and will return to your ED again if the need arises. Tisch, the author of *Chocolates
on the Pillow Aren't Enough: Reinventing the Customer Experience*, believes that a positive attitude along with the "willingness of the staff to

understand service and [to] be able to offer value" will ensure repeat business from your customer (Rowe, 2007).

An example of market-need customer service is exemplified by the Rochester (New York) Gun Violence Task Force. The task force is a crisis intervention team that is composed of 13 members, including members representing the Rochester Police Department, social workers, psychologists, and clergy. Members of the task force approach every young gunshot victim with an objective of not only helping the victim but also attempting to prevent intervention of gangs and their retaliation. The ultimate goal is to steer the victim away from the gang and to provide the youth's family with working strategies to shield their youth from the effects of the gang and their influence. Although this approach at first may not appear to fit the model of customer service, the Gun Violence Task Force is providing an extremely valuable service to the residents of the community, its customers (O'Brien, 2008).

It seems rational, although unacceptable, that episodes of violence in an Emergency Department are downplayed. "We appear to be waiting until someone is killed before we take the right security steps in emergency rooms. What is happening here is just insane," says Dr. David Golan an Emergency Department physician. "We give people who say they're going to kill people a chance to do it" (quoted in Harasim, 2005, pp. 1, 2).

CASE STUDY

THE REALITY: VIOLENCE CAN HAPPEN IN YOUR EMERGENCY DEPARTMENT

One spring evening in a typical suburban Emergency Department, a man walks into the ED with a concealed .44 magnum handgun. He has come to seek revenge on the physician who treated his girlfriend several days before. The ED has no walk-through metal detector or security guard posted at the entrance to the ED. The security guard position was eliminated during the previous quarter to cut costs in the hospital budget. Metal detectors have not even been considered. (This is a nice part of town, after all, and there have not been any incidents of violence, so why would we need

(Continued)

metal detectors?) Consequently, there is nothing to deter the man from walking directly into the main part of the ED with his hidden weapon, there is no mechanism to detect the weapon, and no reason for anyone to be suspicious of this man. The evening is a very busy one in the ED, so no one takes particular notice of this man.

Back-to-back critically ill or injured patients have been brought into the Emergency Department by the paramedics. Several staff have called in sick and there is no replacement staff. Twenty-two patients have waited for hours to be seen by the triage nurse and/ or medical staff. The nursing staff in triage is busy managing the constant arrival of new, walk-in patients, and there has been little opportunity to reassure or communicate with the patients who are waiting. As a result, patient and staff tension is high.

Several staff members notice the man, but they assume he is the family member of a patient and continue their activities. The man walks into the ED. He catches sight of the physician who is the target of his intended revenge. The man immediately pulls his gun and shoots the physician several times. Nurses, hearing the gunshots coming from the hall, and who step cautiously out of various patient rooms, are shot by the man who is now out of control and firing wildly. The physician and one nurse are dead; the second nurse is critically wounded with a gunshot wound to her head.

The man continues his unrestrained carnage, running from room to room, randomly shooting at patients and staff. The ED secretary and other staff cower beneath the reception desk. The ED has no panic alarm with which to send an SOS or to notify security or police of their frantic need for help. The video cameras, trained on the entrance of the ED, are unmanned.

No one, it seems, is aware of the chaos. A few moments later, a laboratory technician walks into the main ED. When he realizes that he has walked into the scene of a homicide in progress, he quickly retreats to summon help. Within minutes the police arrive and attempt to subdue the man.

The perpetrator has confined himself to a room and has taken three hostages with him. Four members of the ED staff are dead, including a physician and two nurses. A patient and his wife are critically wounded.

(Continued)

CASE STUDY DISCUSSION

Is this scenario a fantasy or a possibility?

Unfortunately it could become a reality for your Emergency Department. A majority of Emergency Departments are vulnerable to precisely this type of violence and tragedy.

Hospitals aren't in the business of preventing patients from coming to their hospital for care. Traditionally, hospitals are places that "help people get better and haven't given much thought to stopping others from coming in to do [them] harm" (Amy, 2005).

Although you may not read about an incident like this or hear it on the news, this is a scene that could be occurring in Emergency Departments all over the U.S.—and throughout the world—every day. U.S. Emergency Departments are in crisis, and hospital leadership needs to take action now.

PATIENT DUMPING: EMTALA, THE ANTIDUMPING LAW

EMTALA was intended to prevent hospitals and EDs from refusing patients for treatment, or to limit the transfer of patients to another facility, based strictly on the ability of the patient to pay for services. The concept of patient dumping is repellent to health care professionals. The fact is that some hospitals were found responsible for unceremoniously discharging patients who had no appropriate place to go. One hospital was charged with calling a cab for a patient and dropping her off in her stocking feet in a less-than-desirable area of town. It can be argued that the majority of health care professionals did not go into health care to injure or dispose of patients, especially those patients who need health care. It is irrational to consider patient dumping as a strategy for decompressing EDs.

The EMTALA may be somewhat accountable for the closure of more than 500 Emergency Departments since 1990 (Andrews, 2003), because patients who do not have the financial resources to pay for primary or emergency medical care are now authorized to use the ED for situations that are not emergencies. EMTALA may also be part of the reason that patients are overutilizing Emergency Departments. There is evidence that between 1996 and 2001 individuals with private health care insurance have generated a 24% increase in ED use, partly due to difficulty getting timely appointments with their own physicians. The ED is the logical place to go when an individual has a health care concern and PCP appointments are scarce. The EMTALA regulation opened the ED door for all to enter, not just to regulate and legislate against unethical EDs who try to unload financially burdensome patients. A discussion of EMTALA is summarized in Exhibit 3.1.

Exhibit 3.1

EMTALA DEFINITION AND INTERPRETIVE GUIDANCE AND PROPOSED CHANGES IN FISCAL YEAR 2009

- In 1986, Congress enacted the Emergency Medical Treatment and Labor Act (EMTALA) to ensure public access to emergency services regardless of ability to pay. Section 1867 of the Social Security Act imposes specific obligations on Medicare-participating hospitals that offer emergency services to provide a medical screening examination (MSE) when a request is made for examination or treatment for an emergency medical condition (EMC), including active labor, regardless of an individual's ability to pay. Hospitals are then required to provide stabilizing treatment for patients with EMCs. If a hospital is unable to stabilize a patient within its capability, or if the patient requests, an appropriate transfer should be implemented.

- There must be a list of physicians on-call for consultation who are available, by law, following the initial examination to provide further evaluation and/ or treatment necessary to stabilize an individual with an EMC; (Interpretive Guidelines: §489.20 (r)(2))

  Section 1866(a)(1) of the act states that, as a requirement for participation in the Medicare program, hospitals must maintain a list of physicians who are on-call for duty after the initial examination to provide treatment necessary to stabilize an individual with an EMC. The on-call list identifies and ensures that the Emergency Department is prospectively aware of which physicians, including specialists and subspecialists, are available to provide care.

  A hospital can meet its responsibility to provide adequate medical personnel to meet its anticipated emergency needs by using on-call physicians either to staff or to augment its Emergency Department, during which time the capability of its Emergency Department includes the services of its on-call physicians.

(Continued)

Exhibit 3.1

EMTALA DEFINITION AND INTERPRETIVE GUIDANCE
AND PROPOSED CHANGES IN FISCAL YEAR 2009 (*Continued*)

- The Centers for Medicare and Medicaid Services (CMS) does not have requirements regarding how frequently on-call physicians are expected to be available to provide on-call coverage. Nor is there a predetermined ratio CMS uses to identify how many days a hospital must provide medical staff on-call coverage based on the number of physicians on staff for that particular specialty. In particular, CMS has no rule stating that whenever there are at least three physicians in a specialty, the hospital must provide 24-hour/day 7-day/week coverage in that specialty. EMTALA requires Medicare-participating hospitals with Emergency Departments to screen and treat the EMCs of patients in a nondiscriminatory manner, regardless of the patient's ability to pay, insurance status, national origin, race, creed, or color.

- A technical advisory group was convened in 2005 by CMS to study EMTALA. The advisory group focused on incremental modifications to EMTALA but also envisioned a fundamental rethinking of EMTALA that would support development of regionalized emergency systems. A new EMTALA would continue to protect patients from discrimination in treatment while enabling and encouraging communities to test innovations in emergency care system design, for example, direct transport of patients to non–acute care facilities, such as dialysis centers and ambulatory care clinics, when appropriate.

The Institute of Medicine in 2006 recommended that the Department of Health and Human Services adopt regulatory changes to EMTALA and the Health Insurance Portability and Accountability Act (HIPAA) so that the original goals of the laws are preserved but integrated systems may further develop.

EMTALA CHANGES: HIGHLIGHTS

- Technical Advisory Group (TAG) recommendation #53: to create funding mechanism for EMTALA regulations and requirements

- The American College of Emergency Physicians (ACEP) proposes reconsideration of the imposition of EMTALA rules on a receiving facility when an admitted inpatient is transferred to a facility that has specialty service for that particular patient need

- Move the EMTALA on-call requirement from the EMTALA regulation to a more-appropriate "hospital provider agreement" regulation that essentially regionalizes specialty physician resources by rotating specialty physician coverage among regional hospitals

- Removal of legal and financial barriers to initiate community call plan to share specialty (physician) resources

- Revise (make technical correction to) the provision for EMTALA to be temporarily put on hold relative to the implementation of emergency preparedness plan or a declared public health emergency

- Shared approaches with National Quality Forum (NQF) to reduce avoidable hospital readmissions while recognizing that some patient readmissions will occur

EMTALA has produced unintended consequences. A second provision of EMTALA is that EDs are required to provide specialty care for patients who need it, by having physician specialists on-call for patient needs. EDs are having difficulty complying with the physician on-call portion of the EMTALA regulation. Patients who require specialty care, such as plastic surgery, gastroenterology, or pediatric surgery, must be evaluated for the purpose of stabilization of the current medical condition. The on-call specialist compliance with EMTALA is typically achieved through hospital contracts with specialty physicians who are affiliated with the hospital or with hospitals in the local area.

Obtaining on-call agreements with certain physician specialties, such as neurosurgery and ophthalmology, is difficult because there are a limited number of specialists in certain fields and in certain areas of the nation. Specialists, such as trauma surgeons, whose skill is required to treat injured patients, may be particularly difficult to contract for on-call services because of their high demand, especially if the hospital is a trauma facility (*EMTALA and On-call Responsibilities for Emergency Department Patients,* 2006). The percentage of ED patient visits for traumatic injury has been fairly constant: 24.3% of total patient visits in 2006 and 24.9% of patient visits in 2005 were classified as traumatic injury (Pitts et al., 2008). Most of these patient visits would require the services of physician specialties. Overall, the top five specialist groups that are in limited supply (per the American College of Emergency Physicians [ACEP]) include: orthopedics; plastic surgery; neurosurgery; ear, nose, and throat (ENT) specialists; and hand surgeons, a subspecialty of orthopedics.

CHALLENGES TO MAINTAINING EMPLOYMENT OF SPECIALIST PHYSICIANS

There are several issues that contribute to the difficulty in securing the services of specialist physician coverage in EDs. They include the following:

1. Availability. There is a widespread lack of specialists. The specialists who are on-call for a specific hospital often take calls at other hospitals and are permitted to perform surgery or other time-consuming procedures during the time they are on-call, per a recent EMTALA clarification of the rule. The result is that specialists often are not available as the need arises. ED

physicians can spend valuable time trying to locate a specialist for a highly acute patient who is at risk when the specialist is not readily available.

2. Liability. All physicians, including specialists, are incurring higher costs for liability insurance for their general practices and for their ED coverage. The cost of malpractice is increasingly high, especially for surgeons, the type of specialty that is in greatest demand for an emergency setting. The choice that a specialty physician makes to evaluate a patient who is not known to him, as in the case of an ED patient, elevates the physician's risk and may affect the cost of his malpractice insurance.

3. Compensation. On-call physicians have been enticed to accept on-call coverage at hospital EDs through the payment of stipends or other monetary packages. Fewer hospitals are able to budget or offer a stipend as an incentive since the specialty physicians are charging high, premium rates to hospitals and EDs to be on call. Additionally, on-call physicians are experiencing growing difficulty in receiving reimbursement for their services and may receive no compensation for so-called unassigned patients or charity care. Evidence suggests that more than 75% of all on-call physicians surveyed in 2006 did not receive timely reimbursement for services rendered in EDs (*EMTALA and On-call Responsibilities for Emergency Department Patients*, 2006). Providing on-call services is often not economically feasible nor reasonable for specialty physicians because the physician often is required to see an emergency patient during the time that either surgery or office hours are scheduled. A survey conducted in 2003 revealed that, on average, ED physicians provided $138,000 in EMTALA-related charity care annually. One-third of all ED physicians provided more than 30 hours/week, and specialists provided more than 6 hours/week in uncompensated EMTALA-related care. It was determined that in 2001 specialists serving in an on-call capacity in the ED incurred $25,000 in bad debt for EMTALA-related medical services (*The Impact of Unreimbursed Care on the Emergency Physician*, 2003).

4. Work–life balance. Physicians are beginning to recognize the value and benefits of balancing their work with their need to enjoy non-work-related activities and families. ACEP lists the life-balance factor as one that is increasingly important in the choice that physicians make to limit their on-call availability.

5. Inefficient facilitation. Emergency Departments often struggle with efficiency, due not to the inefficient practices of the department but to system (hospital) inefficiencies, including long turn-around times in laboratory or other ancillary service departments; lack of specific instruments or procedural expertise; unavailability of inpatient beds; and the physician's unfamiliarity with the specific hospital and equipment, processes, and staff.

Several years ago, physician organizations and advocacy groups initiated conversations with the Centers for Medicare and Medicaid (CMS), which regulates EMTALA, to ensure that all stakeholders were acutely aware of the problem of limited specialists available for on-call ED duty/responsibility. Additionally, the groups attempted to engage CMS in discussions to create solutions and perhaps alter the intent of the regulation while protecting the patient against discriminatory practices.

Becoming a physician has always been an honorable aspiration and a highly compensated choice of careers. Physicians-in-training paid more than their share of dues to achieve one of the most highly regarded careers in the U.S. and in the end, the financial and lifestyle benefits made the sacrifices worthwhile. In the 1980s, as the financial systems supporting health care in America, along with the intrusion of managed care organizations taking much of the patient-focused decision making away from the physician, coupled with the meteoric expense of malpractice, the choice of a career as a physician became less tantalizing. For these reasons, it is not surprising that physicians are in limited supply.

Currently, CMS has proposed a flexibility option to EDs to create a pooled resource that could be shared by regional facilities. CMS is considering allowing hospitals to engage in the regional coordination of physician resources to help alleviate problems of limited specialty resources. If the revision to EMTALA is approved, hospitals within a defined region would be able designate one of the hospitals as the on-call hospital for a certain time period, or for a specific service. Each hospital must have a back-up plan in the event that an on-call physician is not available. If EMTALA violations should occur, CMS retains the right to review the back-up plan (Centers for Medicare and Medicaid, 2008).

According to ACEP, EMTALA requires Medicare-participating hospitals with EDs to screen and treat the emergency medical conditions of patients in a nondiscriminatory manner to anyone, regardless of their ability to pay, insurance status, national origin, race, creed, or color. EMTALA was enacted as a method to outlaw and regulate against patient dumping. Hospitals and EDs are at a crisis point, complicated by solutions for disposition of patients, and plans to discharge patients to the next level of care or follow up are stymied by limited community resources and long waits for appointments. Further driving the problem of overcrowded EDs is the lack of good, viable, and accessible primary care alternatives and extremely limited treatment options for discharged, nonemergent, uninsured, and psychiatric patients.

The EMTALA regulation is not a direct cause of violence in the ED. However, the consequences that have been created by the enactment of EMTALA are likely indirectly responsible for the overutilization of the ED. Crowded waiting rooms, long patient waits, and boarded patients who cannot be moved to inpatient beds in a timely manner are documented causes of agitation, aggression, and violence in the ED.

CASE STUDY

The case study regarding the issue of patient dumping was written in 2007 by Richard Hinton of the *LA Times*.

Despite the public outrage over the dumping of homeless patients on Los Angeles's skid row, there is growing debate about whether criminalizing the practice would solve the problem. As the number of suspected dumping cases reached 55 last week, a state senator announced legislation that would make it a misdemeanor for hospitals to transport patients and leave them on the streets against their will.

But some legal experts question whether the law could be effective without a parallel effort to provide more shelter and services for chronically ill homeless patients who are well enough to leave the hospital but have no place for continuing medical services.

There are only about 40 "recuperative beds" available in L.A. for homeless people who need medical attention after being discharged from hospitals, officials said, and there is general agreement that's not enough. The proposed law, legal experts say, might be vulnerable, because it seems to make hospitals alone responsible for finding care for these patients.

"It is more complicated than it first appears," said Russ Korobkin, a UCLA law professor who teaches health law. "Requiring hospitals to be responsible for the patients and not leave them in the gutter is

(Continued)

a first step. But you've got to have a second step of providing some government-funded beds for recovery." Otherwise, he and others said, the law essentially creates an "unfunded mandate," which could be challenged in court, that hospitals must not only treat the sick but also find housing for them upon their release.

Another expert on health law, USC law professor Alex Capron, said the proposed legislation could leave a hospital on the hook for services that go well beyond how it provides treatment for homeless people. "If someone lives in a one-room flophouse alone, would that even be an appropriate discharge under this law and to what extent would a hospital be responsible?" he asked.

The proposed legislation, by state Sen. Gil Cedillo (D-Los Angeles), would make it a misdemeanor for a hospital facility or worker to transport patients anywhere other than their residences without their informed consent. Individual offenders could be punished by up to two years in county jail and a fine of up to $1,000. Healthcare facilities could be fined up to $10,000.

Cedillo and others said the law would give city prosecutors better tools to prosecute hospitals for dumping. City Atty. Rocky Delgadillo has filed criminal charges against just one hospital, Kaiser Permanente, saying the dumping of a homeless woman on skid row in 2006 amounted to false imprisonment. That legal strategy, however, hasn't been tested in court. "We had great faith in hospitals' commitment to their patients," Delgadillo said. "We have great faith in the Hippocratic oath. We had great faith in people's adherence to common decency. We hoped hospitals would adhere to those ideals. But it doesn't appear so.

"These dumping incidents aren't aberrations, and they certainly make it necessary for us to make a clear and powerful statement about what is appropriate behavior for the health community and anyone dealing with fellow members of society," he added. But some question whether it makes sense to focus only on hospitals when they are just one piece of the puzzle.

Homeless services officials said there is not enough money for long-term housing of homeless people, especially those with medical conditions or mental problems.

L.A. civil rights attorney Carol Sobel questions the validity of a law that would make hospitals liable for how they treat the homeless while not extending that liability to other groups.

"This is the last person in a chain that has failed these indigent patients," she said. "Where's the county social worker? Where are the

(Continued)

nursing homes? Where are the missions? Where's the rest of the system that is supposed to care for these people? Why don't the police criminally charge the mission that turns somebody away?"

Hospital officials argue that they are being singled out even though medical centers in Los Angeles County provide care for 18,000 homeless patients each year. They say it's difficult to find places to send those who are well enough to leave the hospital but have no place to go where they can receive care.

But Delgadillo and others say that although hospitals often face a dilemma, there is no excuse for leaving patients on skid row if they have nowhere else to go. Earlier this month, a 54-year-old man in a soiled hospital gown, his colostomy bag still attached, was found crawling in the gutter after being dropped off outside a skid row park, far from homeless services.

Police say that as onlookers demanded help for the man, the driver of the van for Hollywood Presbyterian Medical Center applied makeup and perfume before driving off. The hospital said it is investigating but acknowledged that it didn't follow its own release policies.

The Kaiser case involved a 63-year-old patient who was discharged early last year from Kaiser Permanente's Bellflower medical center. A short time later, video at a downtown mission captured her stepping out of a taxi in a gown and socks and then wandering aimlessly down San Pedro Street. Kaiser has denied any wrongdoing, saying the woman was discharged by mistake. The hospital said it has revamped its release policies.

Delgadillo said that about 10 of the 55 dumping cases have the potential to lead to further action. He said dumping isn't unique to skid row, adding, "We suspect it is happening in other parts of the city."

Andy Bales, executive director of Los Angeles's Union Rescue Mission, said hospitals make facilities for the homeless a social services safety net, dumping patients at the mission's doorstep or in the lobby without even calling first.

But the mission doesn't have the medical facilities for the people, leaving them nowhere to go. The proposed law, he said, "will not only overcome indifference, but evil." (Hinton, 2007)

IS THERE A SOLUTION TO OVERCROWDING IN THE EMERGENCY DEPARTMENT?

Many hospitals have attempted to expand the capacity of their EDs in an effort to decrease the wait time for patients who have come to the Emergency Department for care. But as the old adage goes, build it and they shall come, and this seems to play out in every ED that has expanded its capacity: more patients come!

In addition to a growing number of emergency visits, patients are sicker, requiring the time-intensive and cost-intensive use of high-tech equipment that is often in excessive demand, highly utilized, and a scarce resource (ACEP Foundation, 2004).

As described previously, when an ED is at capacity, a backlog is created in the waiting areas and in the ED that mushrooms to the inpatient units, in turn producing a very real and a very serious new problem of patient holds or patient boarding in EDs.

EMERGENCY DEPARTMENT SECURITY

As the demand for emergency services increases so does the risk of violence and the need for security personnel, policies, training, and equipment. Even the federal government, aware of the critical need for improved security in the Emergency Department, is considering the deployment of so-called red teams to visit hospitals to assess their security gaps. The federal government may not anticipate the serious problems that they will encounter. Jeff Aldridge, health care security consultant and expert, believes the government will find that hospitals are severely lacking in constructive security activities. Mr. Aldridge tells us that although "hospitals want to be a warm, open atmosphere . . . they can't do that anymore" (quoted in Harris, 2006).

CASE STUDY: ENVISIONING SOLUTIONS

SELF-REGISTRATION

The escalating problem of more patients visiting the ED for care is producing some creative tactics for desperate, action-oriented EDs. One such solution is the installation of a self-serve PC/Mac kiosk for the purpose of self-registration and check-in for patients arriving in the ED. If automation can reduce the time it takes for the patient

(Continued)

to be registered, the assumption is that the patient can complete the paperwork quickly, which will shorten the time it takes for the ED staff to identify those patients who need immediate attention.

However, this assumption is somewhat flawed and may not have the positive, time-saving outcome that is anticipated for the following reasons:

1. Many individuals, especially older patients, are unsure how to use a computer or may be intimidated to try.
2. Patients may not recognize that their symptoms demand immediate attention, and care could be delayed while they enter their name and symptoms into the computer.
3. Computer kiosks cost money in terms of capital expenditures and/or ED personnel and training time.
4. Triage RNs are required to conduct a face-to-face, 30-second evaluation of each arriving patient, as soon as the patient arrives. A visual assessment of each patient by a trained professional is essential, and this assessment expertise is the purpose for triage: to sort the non–critically ill patients from those who require immediate treatment. It is important, for the purpose of an educated patient assessment, that only RNs be assigned to a triage post, because patient assessments may only be performed by an RN.[4] A kiosk-as-triage-nurse will delay care and may cause unnecessary deaths in the waiting room.
5. Reducing registration time does not improve the time it takes for a patient to be seen by the physician. If a patient has a routine or nonurgent problem, the waiting time to be seen by a medical professional will be just as long as in pre-kiosk days (*Emergency Department Kiosks Offer Short Patient Check-Ins*, 2007). However, any innovative attempt to reduce the time that it takes to document and complete the required registration tasks is always a good thing.

Dr. Arthur Kellerman, chairman of Emergency Medicine at Emory University School of Medicine and a practicing emergency room physician at Grady Memorial Hospital, both in Atlanta, Georgia, was the key subject of one of a 2006 National Public Radio (NPR) three-report series, titled "The Future of Emergency Care," covering the impending breakdown of emergency services in the U.S. (Institute of Medicine, 2006). The NPR series, presented to highlight the findings in the report by the Institute of Medicine, explores many of the issues presented in this chapter, including the impact of uninsured patients, EMS service gaps, and ED challenges, as the series walks with Dr. Kellerman through a busy night in an Atlanta Emergency Department. "The Future of Emergency Care" is a scathing criticism of U.S. EDs' operational failures and the failure of the health care system to provide appropriate, timely, and necessary care to its citizens. Not even one ED in the U.S. received a passing grade in the report.

STRATEGIES TO REDUCE ED CROWDING

The American College of Emergency Physicians conducted a study in 2005 focused on the problem of ED crowding and provided an extensive list of suggestions for improving the flow of patients through the ED to help reduce crowding. Many of the suggestions require time, resources, and a risk and may end up not having the impact that was intended (*ACEP Task Force Report on Boarding. . .*, n.d.).

One approach that has the potential for decreasing boarding within EDs is the concept of transferring patients to overflow units, or the boarding of waiting patients in the hallways of the units to which they will be assigned as inpatients—once a bed becomes available.[5]

There are several advantages to a plan of this kind. First, the patient gets the same level of care as if he were already an inpatient because the sheer volume in the overflow unit is less; specific nursing caregivers are assigned to the unit, providing better care for the patient; and the burden of caring for the boarded patient is removed from the ED staff, allowing them to focus on treating emergency patients. Another important benefit is that the expense of boarding and caring for the patient shifts to another unit or department, preserving the tenuous ED budget.

OVERFLOW: OBSERVATION AND TRANSITIONAL UNITS

The concept of overflow units (observation unit, transition unit, decision unit) may be one key to preventing medical errors or the unintended death of boarded patients in the emergency room. As an added benefit, if the overflow unit is in the hallway of the planned inpatient unit, the patient may be admitted sooner because the presence of the patient and his needs may drive efficiency (Holmberg, 2007).[6]

Full capacity protocol has been in use at Stony Brook University Hospital in Stony Brook, New York, since 2001, with good results. The plan utilizes specific criteria for patients being transferred from the ED and requires the concurrent use of a written plan by the accepting unit. For a patient to be transferred from the ED, the accepting unit must be able to offer each patient safe care, privacy, access to a nurse, wireless telemetry, and a bathroom. To sweeten the deal, aligning with the hospitality model of retaining patients as customers, each patient receives flowers from the hospital within 12 hours. "It's all about making the patient feel better," says Dr. Peter Viccellio, ED physician and the creator of full capacity protocol (Viccellio, 2008).

A 6-month retrospective study (October 2005 to March 2006) revealed that 18% of patients who arrived in the ED and required admission were shunted to the boarding unit while awaiting an inpatient bed. ACEP attributes the serious and dangerous practice of boarding patients in the ED to unnecessary deaths; 13% of ED physicians admit knowing a patient who died in the ED due to ED boarding (Gelles, 2008). The larger issue of ED crowding, which is a true crisis, may be downplayed by administration or other leaders in the hospital. Aside from generating inpatients, who are a source of revenue for hospitals, EDs are not moneymakers.

ACEP has proposed three solutions to ED boarding:

1. Move ED boarded patients who are waiting for an inpatient bed to the inpatient unit, even if the bed is not available. This solution allows for patients who need emergency care to utilize an ED treatment bed and removes the responsibility for (adequately) caring for that patient from the ED physicians and staff. Another benefit is that this action shifts the impetus to find longer-term solutions from strictly an ED problem to a system (hospital) problem.

2. Level the operating room scheduling over the entire week instead of lumping all surgeries into Monday, Tuesday, and Wednesday; this action will smooth the demand for ICU beds and will open up more inpatient beds.

3. Discharge patients from inpatient units before noon so that the ED will have a projected number of available inpatient beds to use for waiting ED patients by noon every day. Several hospitals have created discharge units consisting of a pleasantly appointed room, staffed by RNs who educate discharged patients and family caregivers about medication and follow-up visits and can leisurely answer questions or clarify information. An additional benefit to discharge units is that patients can be escorted to patient accounting to settle up or make payment arrangements for the hospital bill before leaving (*ACEP Task Force Report*, n.d.).

Crowding is one documented reason for anger and frustration in the ED. Crowding and boarding are dangerous practices that have evolved from an essential need, but the emotions that crowding and boarding create also direct the potential for violence in the ED.

It is illogical that, in general, health care has not adopted the tools of business management, such as queuing theory to help decipher demand and fixed capacity, and other similar manufacturing predicaments.[7] While management tools may not seamlessly correlate to the circumstances of people and of life and death, there are many lessons that can be learned.

CASE STUDY

Encouragingly, a recent article in the Journal of Emergency Nursing *(Tanabe, 2008) highlighted a research project titled, "Should You Close Your Waiting Room?" that used queuing theory methodology, among others, to provide solutions for the project.*

The capacity monitor described in the article utilizes four simple questions that ED staff can ask themselves to discern, beyond gut feeling, if they can safely see additional patients, or if they need to divert the patient(s) to another facility. A "no" answer to any of the four questions definitively tells staff that they are at overcapacity in staff (too many patients and too few staff); treatment area; overflow/ observation/boarding unit or urgent care/fast-track area; or whether the higher acuity levels of current patients puts them at risk for a higher utilization of time and resources of medical personnel.

The outcomes of the study will be published in the future, but the method developed for ED staffs to use, to determine whether

(Continued)

the ED has the capacity to see one more patient, was derived from several scientific and management methods, including, notably, queuing theory. High-volume, non–fixed demand businesses, like fast-food restaurants, utilize queuing theory principles to determine how many cash registers to have open at lunchtime and how many employees need to be on hand to manage the unknown demand of the hungry public. Fast-food restaurant segments have much competition in the marketplace, and the focus on operational excellence and responsiveness to its customers is necessary for them to be successful (Litvak, 2007).

   A simple solution, or at least the start to a solution, is for hospital administration to accept the assumption that ED crowding is not isolated to the ED alone. Once the problem of ED overcrowding is acknowledged as a system problem and is understood and acknowledged by the entire hospital, opportunities for improvement will be enhanced. An idea as simple as enacting a standard and consistent checkout time for inpatients will help free up inpatient beds, making the transfer of boarded ED patients (those waiting for an inpatient bed) more efficient and timely. Accomplishing a standard checkout time will require the commitment of all physicians on staff at the hospital and of all nurse managers of the inpatient hospital units. This commitment may necessitate that the discharging physician complete the patient's exit paperwork and instructions the evening prior to the actual discharge of the patient. Identifying and thoroughly educating all hospital stakeholders in the rationale for a standard checkout time will help smooth and catapult the success of the new process. (See Exhibit 3.2 for guidance for managing capacity in the waiting room.)
   EDs need to invest in creative, proactive solutions now or the unintended consequences of diverting patients away from the ED completely is an all-too-real possibility. Wal-Mart has installed a pilot program of urgent care clinics (Solantic) inside three of their Jacksonville (Florida) area stores. Urgent care clinics are a viable and attractive option to the Emergency Departments in terms of time and cost savings for patients. Solantic's three-tier pricing maxes out at $189 and includes the cost of the visit, more than one procedure, treatment, injections, X-rays, IV fluids, and eye numb and wash. Urgent care clinics are typically staffed by physicians, as opposed to the drug-store based clinics that are staffed by

Exhibit 3.2

ED CAPACITY CHECKLIST TOOL

CAN WE SAFELY ACCEPT ONE MORE PATIENT?

1. Does either team (MD or RN) have an available staff member to initiate care for a new patient?
2. Is there adequate treatment area/room space to accept a new patient directly from triage (immediate bedding)?
3. Is the acuity of the patients in ED treatment rooms reasonable enough to accept immediate bedding patients?
4. Is there additional capacity in urgent care/fast track/observation units?

A "no" response to any of the questions guides the staff—beyond gut instinct— to determine if the ED is at overcapacity in staff, space, patient acuity, or observation units.

Adapted from "Questions to Guide the Use of the Waiting Room," by P. Tanabe et al. Copyright © by Elsevier. Adapted with permission.

nurse practitioners and provide targeted primary care services. Clearly, patients now have three distinct options for nonprimary or urgent/emergent care: EDs, urgent care clinics, and retail health clinics (so named because they typically reside within retail pharmacy/grocery establishments and were initiated to support the pharmacy trade).

Dr. Linda Lawrence, immediate past president of the American College of Emergency Physicians (ACEP), encourages patients to be cautious when making a choice between time and cost savings or the opportunity to have a condition evaluated. The majority of problems belong in the Emergency Department. "One of our concerns is that people can't recognize when they have an emergency or don't," says Dr. Lawrence. "A patient who says they are having indigestion and goes to an urgent-care clinic may really be having a heart attack," she warns (Landro, 2008, p. 2).

According to the CDC, of the 115.3 million emergency room visits in 2005, only 5.5% were medical emergencies that needed to be seen and evaluated immediately (Landro, 2008, p. 2). (See Table 3.2 for a comparison of emergency department utilization 2005, 2006; see Figure 3.1 for a comparison of ED patient visits by Triage Level, 2005, 2006.)

Table 3.2

EMERGENCY DEPARTMENT UTILIZATION 2005, 2006

	2005	2006
# Emergency Departments in the U.S.	3,795 (down from 4,176)	3,833 (down from 4,019)
# ED visits	115.3 million	119.2 million
# ED visits per each U.S. ED	30,000	31,098
# patient visits per minute— all U.S. EDs	219	227
ED utilization rate	Up 7% (increase of 20% in 10 years)	Up 18%
Highest ED utilization rate	Infants <12 months (91.3 visits/100 infants), 3.8 million	Infants <12 months (84.5 visits/100 infants), 3.5 million
# patients arriving via EMS	18 million (15.5%)	18.4 million (15.4%)
# minutes wait to see provider (mean)	56.3	55.8
Total ED length of stay (not including wait time)	2.4 hours	2.6 hours
% of ED visits resulting in admission	12	12.8
Hospital LOS in days of inpatients admitted through ED	5.2	5.3
% of Emergency Departments utilized that were located in an urban area	85.9	85.5
% of admission to designated trauma hospital	36.9	35
% of ED visits due to injuries	41.9	35.6
Payment sources		
% private insurance	39.9	39.7
% Medicare	16.6	17.3
% Medicaid/SCHIP (State Children's Hospital Insurance)	24.9	25.5
% uninsured	16.7	17.4

(Continued)

Table 3.2

EMERGENCY DEPARTMENT UTILIZATION 2005, 2006 (*Continued*)

	2005	2006
LPT (Left Prior to Triage)— % patients who left ED without seeing provider	2	2
% of patients who were seen again in the ED within 72 hours of initial ED visit	1.9	3.6
% ED visits admitted to ICU	1	1.9
Triage		
% triage level I (highest acuity)	5.5	5.1
% triage level II (emergent acuity)	9.8	10.8
% triage level III (urgent acuity)	33.3	36.6
% triage level IV (semi-urgent acuity)	20.7	22
% triage level V (nonurgent acuity)	13.9	12.1
% unknown triage level or no triage done	16.7	13.4

There is some evidence that the growth of retail health clinics is slowing. Some of the retail health care providers that had clinics inside Wal-Mart have closed, along with three other brands that have discontinued operations in selected outlets. According to industry executives and developers, the supply was simply greater than the demand. "Too many clinics opened too quickly" (Yee, 2008, p. 1) citing a growth of from 200 to 800 retail clinics of all brands opening in 2008 (Yee, 2008, p. 2). "Retail clinics," says NOW Medical CEO Patrick Dunleavy, "can't grow faster than the country can understand what they're for" (Yee, 2008, p. 3). Some of the problems the retail clinic industry has experienced has been the longer-than-expected profitability timeline, the glut of competitors and the "winning over" of new customers (Yee, 2008, p. 2). A distinction must be made between retail/walk-in clinics that are typically staffed by

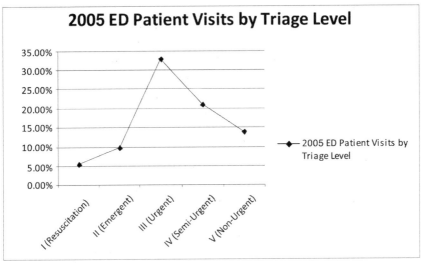

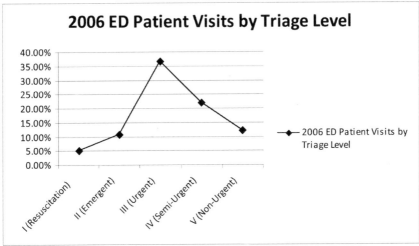

Figure 3.1 2005, 2006 ED patient visits by triage level.

nurse practitioners and urgent care clinics that are traditionally manned by physicians. Both types of clinics can evaluate a condition and refer to the emergency department when required. Both the retail clinic and the urgent care clinic offer quick care at a lower price than emergency departments and provide low-acuity care, the type of care that should be directed away from emergency departments. (See Table 3.3 for emergent/ urgent care options to avoid the Emergency Department.)

Table 3.3

PATIENT OPTIONS FOR EMERGENT/URGENT CARE

COMPARISON: OPTIONS FOR EMERGENT/URGENT CARE				
	URGENT CARE SERVICES AVAILABLE	QUICK THROUGHPUT	PATIENT CENTRIC	INSURANCE ACCEPTED	HIGH VIOLENCE POTENTIAL
Emergency Department	Yes	No	No	Yes	Yes
Urgent Care Clinic	Yes	Yes	Yes	Yes	No
Retail Health Clinic	Yes, but focused on low-acuity primary care	Yes	Yes	Yes	No
Which would YOU choose?					

CASE STUDY

REDUCING PATIENT FRUSTRATION—AND THE POTENTIAL FOR VIOLENCE—BY DIVERTING PATIENT INFLUX INTO THE EMERGENCY DEPARTMENT

A large hospital system has decided to take on the issue of patient crowding in the ED. Crowding in the ED creates long wait times for patients because patients who do not have emergency conditions are also coming to the ED for care. And one of the most documented reasons for violence in the ED is patient frustration caused by the long waits that can escalate from frustration into anger and violence.

Americans who have no health insurance and are suddenly confronted with a medical problem that frightens them, but may

(Continued)

not be a true emergency, often come to the ED for care. And EDs are pulling out all of the stops to become more efficient, saving time and frustration for the patients. Often, the internal processes are so muddled that it is difficult to carve away even small amounts of time.

The plan that one large hospital system has implemented is to assess and then re-assess patients visiting the ED. The triage nurse first assesses the patient to evaluate whether the patient has an emergent condition that must be seen and treated as an emergency. Next, the ED physician evaluates the patient, rendering the EMTALA-required or medical screening examination (MSE). If the patient does not have an emergent condition, the patient is referred to a clinic or another health care resource outside the ED for further evaluation and treatment. The patients apparently appreciate the advice, especially if they are able to save money by not having their condition treated in the ED. And, often, patients are relieved to know that their condition is not life-threatening and can wait to be treated. If the patient prefers to stay at the ED and receive treatment for the condition, the hospital requests payment up front to offset the time and the expense incurred.

CASE STUDY DISCUSSION

For this hospital system, crowding is a very big problem. In creating a plan to limit crowding and still provide excellent care to all patients, the hospital had to carefully work within the EMTALA guidelines to avoid giving the impression that the hospital and the ED were dumping the patient. They were not. However, if any hospital fails to meet the EMTALA guidelines, CMS could impose huge fines against the hospital.

Patient crowding is an enormous patient safety and patient care issue. Patient crowding can cause patients to respond violently because of the pain and stress they are experiencing. Only time will tell if this hospital's plan will decrease patient boarding in the ED. If even marginally successful, other hospitals may benefit by choosing to adopt this creative plan (Moewe, 2008).

CASE STUDY

A COUNTER TO REDIRECTING NONEMERGENCY PATIENTS IN THE EMERGENCY DEPARTMENT

Senator Charles Grassley (R-Iowa) apparently does not understand the rationale for diverting nonemergency patients away from the Emergency Department. A comment attributed to Grassley was quoted in the Washington Post *on September 2, 2008. The article stated that Grassley believes that the University of Chicago Medical Center, by redirecting nonemergency patients to more appropriate clinics in the community, was attempting to "cull the least profitable patients away from its emergency room" (Stephens, 2008).*

One hundred nineteen million patients visited U.S. EDs in 2006, an increase of 3.9 million patients from the previous year. EDs were created to care for patients with emergency, life-threatening conditions and not for patients who are assessed, by ED physicians, to be nonemergencies. Often patients who come to the ED use the ED for primary care needs because they cannot get a timely appointment with their own physician or, a more common reason, do not have health care insurance to cover a primary care visit. Thirty-four point one percent of all patient visits to the ED in 2006 were classified as semi-urgent or nonurgent.

Emergency Departments are closing at remarkable rates, as is the situation in New Jersey, because they can no longer support the numbers of patients who are requiring charity care. One hundred eighty-six Emergency Departments closed in the U.S. in 2006, potentially eliminating capacity and access for nearly 6 million patients.

EMTALA requires that all patients entering the ED must receive an MSE and be stabilized. Nonemergency patients who are directed away from the ED to community clinics have been evaluated by a physician and the patient has been determined to not have a medical or surgical emergency. This is appropriate care. The proactive approach of the University of Chicago Medical Center and several other hospitals in Florida may be the one action that will prevent the complete meltdown of Emergency Department services in the U.S.

The clear point is that our government appears to have no understanding of the problem that EDs face in today's environment. Along with former President Bush's inaccurate belief that all U.S. citizens have access to care by using Emergency Departments (Rollins, 2007a), Senator Grassley's comment is troublesome in that he would make an assumption that not-for-profit hospital EDs have not provided enough required charity care. Senator Grassley ought to request a meeting with the ACEP to gain a true understanding of the rationale behind the redirection of nonemergency patients to more appropriate care (Stephens, 2008).

EMS, DIVERSIONS, AND OTHER PATIENT-MANAGEMENT STRATEGIES AND OUTCOMES

Ambulance diversion was initiated as a method to reduce the progression of overcrowded Emergency Departments. By diverting trauma or emergency patients to another Emergency Department that has fewer patients in treatment areas or in the waiting room, the assumption is that the patient will receive better care, more rapidly.

Currently in the U.S., EMS/ambulance systems have four provider sources, city or county, fire departments, private providers, and not-for-profit providers. Six thousand 911-centers manage calls to 15,000 EMS system providers (rigs or units) and 800,000 EMS responders. The system is dangerously under capacity to manage 18.4 million transports annually (in 2006), averaging 6.2 transports per 100 persons. EMS utilization has increased by 17%, or by 5.4 per 100 persons since 1997 (Pitts et al., 2008).

EMS/ambulance providers are plagued by system fragmentation partially due to the organization of the EMS services that are currently managed and regulated by three departments: public health, public safety, and emergency services. Ideally, one municipal authority should manage the EMS services. None of the providers use the same equipment or communication devices, which exacerbates the fragmented delivery of emergency services. The disparity in communication device function and operation seriously affected response coordination and capabilities in New York during the 9/11 disaster because fire department providers could not speak with the EMS/ambulance providers or with hospitals. The attempt at coordinating a group effort and response was severely limited.

Adding to the frustration, EMS services do not coordinate among providers, services do not work together, EMS has no educational or operational standards, there is a lack of communication or joint learning among the providers, EMS services vary widely in performance, EMS care delivery is not evidence-based, EMS services are unprepared for large disasters or large-scale emergencies, and emergency providers may not be adequately trained in basic or in advanced emergency care.

One serious problem facing the EMS/ambulance services is the dramatic federal funding cut that has occurred progressively over the past 30-plus years. Funding in the 1970s created the 911 system, but by 1980, budget reductions led to disorganization of emergency equipment and response capability and the imprecise way that EMS systems have developed over time (Jagim, Ojanen, & Neis, 2006).

The U.S. is at tremendous risk for pervasive violence in the form of a national emergency if another terrorist attack occurs. Entities who wish to harm or control the U.S. may be developing biological weapons, devising sophisticated nuclear arsenals, and are, perhaps, scouting our water system and our food supply for a defect that could give them a quick entry into a vulnerable system. EMS/ambulance systems need funding and organization to develop capacity, interoperability, and coordination to enhance the U.S.'s ability to be fully ready to react to a surge capacity that may occur in the U.S. or in Emergency Departments during a national emergency.

Currently, ambulances are diverted away from crowded Emergency Departments at alarming and dangerous rates. An ambulance/EMS diversion strategy was a good resolution to the problem of overcrowded EDs, at least for awhile, but a 2004 editorial from the *Annals of Emergency Medicine* has wisely said that "diversion is a solution with its own problems" (Zigmond, 2006). Now, with the closure of many emergency rooms and the growth of nonurgent patients visiting Emergency Departments, emergency rooms with few patients may not exist. Diversion may result in an emergency patient being redirected to an Emergency Department that is distant from the patient's home and family and may no longer be a viable resolution to the problem of overcrowded EDs. In the U.S. today, ambulances are turned away from Emergency Departments at the average rate of once every minute (*EMS Fact Sheet*, n.d.).

Eighteen million, or 15.5%, of all ED patients arrived by ambulance to Emergency Departments in 2005, according to statistics that have been compiled by the CDC (Nawar et al., 2007). Patients covered by Medicaid use the Emergency Department at a rate of 82 per 100 persons versus the rate of 21 per 100 persons for those with private health care insurance (*More Than 1 Billion Healthcare Visits*, 2008). Public education regarding the appropriate use of EMS/ambulance services and promoting the use of alternate community services may be necessary to help the public understand the crisis that is occurring in the EMS service and Emergency Departments in the U.S.

Diversion, in and of itself, is not a direct cause of increased violence in the ED. Indirectly, diversion policies can create circumstances that put EDs at risk, by transporting large numbers of patients to an already-overcrowded Emergency Department, thus increasing the chance that aggression or violence will occur in the ED. Some policy and practice considerations for hospitals and Emergency Departments are:

1. No diversion. When the Emergency Department becomes saturated with patients and the hospital or ED has no diversion plan for managing the patients who continue to arrive, the ED waiting room and treatment areas have no option but to have patients wait longer in the waiting room and/or to place patients on stretchers located in the hallways of the treatment areas. When EMS arrives with another patient, EMS offloading may be significantly delayed while the ED staff attempts to manage space to make room for one more patient. A patient who is currently occupying a room or a space in the treatment area of the ED may need to be moved out of the room to accommodate another patient requiring more acute resources.

2. Diversion is not a four-letter word. Diversion is occasionally a necessary evil. The ED must guard against accumulating massive numbers of people in the waiting room and treatment areas that may create aggressive and violent situations. It is a vital responsibility of Emergency Departments to manage patients in the waiting room and ED treatment areas and to protect patients from harm. Frequently, number-driven CEOs or hospital administrators must be educated to understand that EDs will be confronted with a decision to go on diversion to ensure the safety of the patients and staff. The Emergency Department needs to retain the authority to make the decision to divert if it becomes essential to do so.

3. The enforcement of short off-load times for EMS. The goal of both EMS and the Emergency Departments is to accept— offload—all EMS patients within a strict, short period of time. Typically, EMS and Emergency Departments have good, co-operative working relationships and both work to solve the ED

problems of capacity. Emergency Departments and EMS can sometimes become stymied with a sudden surge of patients, especially as Emergency Departments are implementing the no waiting or no waiting room concepts.

4. Creating win-win policies and pre-arrival protocols can help. Teamwork among EMS, Emergency Department management, and hospital management can effect creative solutions that benefit both services and patients. Several hospitals in Miami have worked with EMS to enact a short door-to-doc protocol for patients who have the symptoms of impending strokes or heart attacks. This arrangement provides the best and quickest treatment for patients and ensures that the hospitals have the benefit of the patient admission. Additional efficiency-driven protocols can include coordinated information technology (IT) systems among all ambulance providers and Emergency Departments within a defined area of a city or county. The Emergency Departments communicate information about diversion or available ED capacity into a Web-based tool so that the ED capacity of each local hospital Emergency Department is available to the EMS. With the advance of IT and Web-based applications, systems and procedures will improve. One benefit of tools of this type is time-saving, and very likely patient-saving as well, eliminating the need for EMS to make frequent telephone calls to the EDs to evaluate capacity. EMS providers can direct and coordinate the efficient utilization of ED capacity for all of the hospitals in the region at any given point in time.

5. Hospital home. A recent trend among medical providers and several health plan providers is to facilitate a medical home for all patients. The medical home concept is an old concept initiated by the American Association of Pediatrics in 1967 as a method to coordinate care for patients (Rosenthal, 2008). The medical home model provides continuity of care for patients and smoothes the process for all stakeholders to have coordinated services and in most cases, updated and available medical records and other information. The medical home model saves providers time while enhancing the quality of care for the patient. An additional benefit is that the patient and the health plan incur a lower cost of delivery. Hospital home works much the same way, taking patients who need emergency care to their predesignated hospital home. This idea is particularly beneficial because integrated electronic

medical records are currently in the early stages of development. Even if the hospital is on diversion, patients who have a designated hospital home are taken to the Emergency Department of the hospital home where the patient is "known to caregivers" and where the patient's medical records are conveniently available. The hospital home concept often can help "prevent a transfer" to another facility (Erich, 2008, p. 4).

6. Community public service announcements (PSAs). A large number of waiting patients or a surge in patients can create an overflow situation in the waiting room or ED treatment areas to the point that the volume of patients can be a threat to patient safety. PSAs can be made via local television and radio and perhaps even by way of the Internet. As an example, Grady Hospital in Atlanta, the safety-net hospital for mental health admissions in the city, recently issued PSA-like announcements to the Atlanta medical community to warn that they were experiencing a dangerous overcapacity situation in their Emergency Department and in the inpatient psychiatric unit and warned that they could not accept additional patients with mental illness. Typically, Grady has accepted and assessed all patients with mental health crises for emergency medical conditions before transferring the patient to a state mental health facility. Because the state mental health facilities are "dealing with their own capacity issues," the transfer rate to these facilities, from Grady, has slowed, often requiring seriously ill mental health patients to board in the acute-care Emergency Department for as many as 40 hours, according to a recent article in the *Atlanta Journal Constitution*. The crisis situation put patients needing both mental and physical emergency treatment in peril (White, 2006, p. 1).

7. Advice nurses. A strategy that EMS and Emergency Departments are employing is to add advice nurses as an adjunct to 911 services with the objective of having nonemergency needs redirected away from ambulance transport to an Emergency Department, and instead to community services. The concept of advice nurses is not new, but utilizing advice nurses in conjunction with the 911 service is a new application. Advice nurses, similar to telephone, hotline, insurance or physician office ask-a-nurse services, or pediatric triage nurse services provide a prescribed set of advice to patients in an attempt to direct the patient to the appropriate health care provider and/or location, including urgent

care, the patient's own physician/PCP, Emergency Department, outpatient mental health facility, and so forth. The advice nurse initiative is also an attempt to control utilization of the Emergency Department by offering an alternative to care. According to the article *Diversionary Tactics*, Montreal (Canada) and some U.S. cities have implemented the advice nurse service (Erich, 2008).

In 2007, ACEP sponsored a bill in Congress numbered and named S. 1003: Access to Emergency Medical Services Act of 2007. The bill was introduced in 2007 with a three-pronged objective:

1. To improve access to emergency medical services and the quality and efficiency of care furnished in Emergency Departments.
2. To provide for additional payments for certain physician services furnished in such Emergency Departments.
3. To establish a CMS Working Group.

The bill is designed to improve access to EMS services and to improve the quality of care in Emergency Departments. The bill will allow the examination of facts that affect the effective delivery of EMS and emergency services. Currently the bill is in the first step of the legislative process (S. 1003: Access to Emergency Medical Services Act of 2007, 2007).

CASE STUDY

Finding and initiating creative solutions to prevent a backlog of patients in waiting rooms is a constructive and proactive step in preventing patient and visitor agitation that could escalate into violent situations.

A process improvement team at Oakwood, a large Emergency Department in Michigan, joins many other hospitals that, in past years, have vigilantly tried to develop a solution to keep patients flowing quickly through the emergency room, a process

(Continued)

that promises to prevent patients from having to wait in the waiting room to see a medical provider. For the past 6 years, the ED has made good on a 30-minute guarantee for its ED patients; the hospital now promises its public "zero wait times."

The idea for the no-wait plan was generated by patients who have completed many surveys and participated in marketing telephone calls over the past years in an effort to give the community the best service—the type of service they are wanting—and to keep them coming to Oakwood ED for care.

To accomplish the no-wait policy and service, planners at Oakwood ED put their heads together, bringing in "800 people" including lab, radiology, and other ancillary departments whose own "test turnaround time" was a critical piece to achieving success for the ED no-wait time and throughput. The cadre of people on the process improvement team were able to add more monitored beds and a "transitional unit" (often two reasons that ED patients cannot get moved out of the ED), implement a 10-minute turnaround for X-rays (a process that typically can require up to 1 hour), improve guideline development and orientation metrics, and ratchet up the triage procedure.

The new process has been a smash success, resulting in increased ED volume and inpatient admissions. The best indicator of accomplishment has been the dramatic rise in patient satisfaction scores. According to the nurse manager of the ED, any ED of any size can make similar improvements. Inpatient bed management along with the unfailing support of administration are the keys to making it happen.

A process and system improvement with patient care in mind is a win-win solution. The importance of responding to patient needs while they are in the ED, waiting to see a medical provider, is essential in preventing frustration and anger that can lead to violent outbursts. The additional step taken by Oakwood to strengthen and reinforce triage services—thereby focusing their ability to observe patients entering the ED and controlling the activities of the patients, families, and visitors in the ED waiting room—can further diminish opportunities for violence ("System Says ED Patients Will Have Zero Wait Time," 2007).

NOTES

1. The Emergency Medical Treatment and Active Labor Act (EMTLA), finalized in 2003, is a Center for Medicare and Medicaid Services (CMS) requirement that obligates all Emergency Departments to accept, screen, stabilize, and treat or transfer all persons presenting for care in the Emergency Department. For more information, please see http://www.medi-smart.com.

2. *Length of stay* refers to the segment of time from patient arrival in the ED until that patient is discharged from the ED.

3. Acuity describes the level of illness of an individual. A high acuity indicates a very sick patient with perhaps many comorbidities and complex health conditions. Comorbidities refers to one or more additional diseases or disorders that are present in addition to the primary disease. An example would be cardiovascular or heart disease and diabetes mellitus.

4. The Nurse Practice Act is written and legislated in each state. However, RNs only are permitted to perform actual patient *assessments*. Licensed practical nurses (LPN or LVN), as valuable members of the health care team, can work in tandem with the RN or may independently collect pertinent data and review findings with the RN who is responsible for authorizing the findings.

5. The ACEP defines this process as *full capacity protocol*.

6. Hospital Corporation of American (HCA) was an early adopter of the concept of off-ED boarding. Often because of the limited real estate of HCA's EDs, the hallway (either ED or inpatient unit hallway) became the location of necessity for boarded patients waiting for an inpatient room.

7. Queuing theory is a theoretical study of waiting lines, expressed in mathematical terms.

REFERENCES

ACEP Foundation. (2004, March 15–25). *Cover the uninsured week.* Retrieved November 16, 2007, from www.covertheuninsured.org/media/research/ERsurvey.pdf

ACEP task force report on boarding and Emergency Department crowding; ACEP's suggested boarding solutions generate national support. (n.d.). Retrieved August 13, 2008, from http://acep.org/advocacy.aspx?id=33074

Amy, J. (2005). *Security and crime news from the Mobile (Alabama) Register.* Retrieved June 1, 2007, from www.jrrobertsecurity.com/security-news/security-crimenews0025.htm

Andrews, M. (2003, September 21). *Uncertainty inside emergency rooms.* Retrieved September 22, 2008, from http://proquest.umi.com/pqdweb?index=2&did=867061 02&SrchMode=1&sid=2&Fmt=10&VIns=PROD&VType=PQD&RQT=309&VName=HNP&TS=1240691953&clientId=2335

Appleby, J. (2008, June 16). *Mentally ill face extra-long ER waits.* Retrieved August 22, 2008, from http://www.usatoday.com/news/health/2008-06-16-ERwaits_N.htm

Cracks in the foundation: Averting a crisis in America's hospitals. (2002, August). Retrieved August 22, 2008, from http://www.aha.org/aha/content/2002/pdf/cracksreprint08-02.pdf

Centers for Medicare & Medicaid. (2008). Retrieved August 24, 2008, from http://www.
 cms.hhs.gov
Docs note rise in emergency department crowding. (2007, October 9). Retrieved April 17,
 2009, from http://www.modernhealthcare.com/apps/pbcs.dll/article?AID=/20071009/
 REG/310090013
ED workforce appears stretched to its limits. (2006). *ED Management, 18*(7), 80–81.
Emergency department kiosks offer short patient check-ins. (2007, September 19). Re-
 trieved October 4, 2007, from wwwmedicalnewstoday.com/articles/02769.php
Emergency Department violence. (n.d.). Retrieved November 6, 2007, from http://www.
 acep.org/advocacy.aspx?id=21830
EMS fact sheet. (n.d.). Retrieved September 1, 2008, from http://www3.acep.org/
 Access_to_EMS_Fact_Sheet[1].pdf
EMTALA and on-call responsibilities for Emergency Department patients. (2006). Re-
 trieved November 6, 2007, from http://www.acep.org/practres.aspx?id=29434
Erich, J. (2008, April 1). *Diversionary tactics.* Retrieved September 12, 2008, from
 http://www.emsresponder.com/print/EMS-Magazine/Diversionary-Tactics/1$7430
Gelles, K. (2008, May 30). Our view on medical treatment: Ailing ER's threaten patients,
 leave communities vulnerable. *USA Today.*
Harasim, P. (2005, March 21). *Concern from healthcare workers over hospital violence.*
 Retrieved June 1, 2007, from http://www.securityinfowatch.com/article/printer.
 jsp?id=3381
Harmacinski, J. (2003). *Emergency room violence growing concern for Nurses.* Salem,
 MA: The Salem News.
Harris, M. (2006, July 17). Hospitals face intrusion of violent world into facilities; both
 urban, suburban cope with security risks. *The Baltimore Sun.*
Holleran, R. S. (2006). Preventing staff injuries from violence (R. B. Tomi St. Mars, Ed.)
 Journal of Emergency Nursing, 32(6), 523–524.
Holmberg, D. (2007, June 10). The patients in the hallways. *The New York Times,*
 p. 14NJ.3.
Hospital closures. (2007). Retrieved November 15, 2007, from http://www.treatmentad
 vocacycenter.org
Institute of Medicine (2006). *The future of emergency care.* Washington, DC: Author.
Jackson, F. J., & Flinn, R. J. (1994). The emergency room view on violence. *Security
 Management,* 25–26.
Jagim, M., Ojanen, D., & Neis, F. (2006). *IOM Report: Future of emergency care in the
 US health system.* Des Plaines, IL: Emergency Nurses Association.
Judd, A. M. (2008, August 21). *Mental health system may cut back, privatize.* Retrieved
 August 21, 2008, from www.ajc.com/metro/content/stories/2008/08/21/mental_
 health_privatize.html
Kershaw, S. (2008, February 12). *City hospitals reinvent role of emergency.* Retrieved
 March 22, 2008, from http://www.nytimes.com/2008/02/12/nyregion/12er.html?_r=1
 &scp=12&sq=health+care&st=nyt&oref=slogin
Kowalenko, T. W. (2005). Workplace violence: A survey of emergency physicians in the
 state of Michigan. *Annals of Emergency Medicine, 46*(2), 142–147.
Landro, L. (2008, August 8). Options expand for avoiding crowded ERs. *The Wall Street
 Journal,* p. D1.

Litvak, E. (2007). *Applying queuing theory to healthcare: Managing random capacity in a fixed demand environment.* Retrieved October 18, 2007, from http://www.ihi.org/IHI/Programs/ConferencesAndSeminars/ApplyingQueuingTheorytoHealthCareSept2007.htm

Lothian, D. (2007). *Nurses confront violence on the job.* Retrieved November 12, 2007, http://www.cnn.com/2007/HEALTH/07/11/nurse.violence/index.html

Lubell, J. (2007). *MHA press room: Emergency Department visits hit record high.* Retrieved May 27, 2008, from http://mhanewsnow.typepad.com/pressroom/2007/07/emergency-depar.html

Moewe, M. (2008, August 11). Memorial turns non-emergency patients away from ER. *Jacksonville Business Journal.*

More than 1 billion healthcare visits. (2008). Retrieved August 6, 2008, from UPI: http://www.upi.com/Health_News/2008/08/06/More_than_1_billion_healthcare_visits/UPI-66361218050055/

Nawar, E.W., Niska, R.W. , & Xu, J. (2007). *National Hospital Ambulatory Medical Care Survey: 2006 Emergency Department.* Hyattsville, MD: Centers for Disease Control, U.S. Department of Health and Human Services, National Center for Health Statistics.

NJ hospitals going under as state bailout cash ends. (2008, February 13). Retrieved August 1, 2008, from www.fiercehealthcarefinance.com/story/nj-hospitals-going-under-as state-bailout-cash-ends

Nursing shortage growing worldwide. (2007). Retrieved November 14, 2007, from http://www.about.com/Nursing

O'Brien, T. (2008, May 14). *Crisis team plan counters gun violence.* Retrieved August 11, 2008, from http://timesunion.com/ASPStories/storyprint.asp?StoryID=688379

Pitts, S. R., Niska, R. W., Xu, J., & Burt, C. (2008). *National Hospital Ambulatory Medical Care Survey: 2006 Emergency Department Survey.* Hyattsville, MD: Centers for Disease Control.

Psych ED helps speed throughput time by 9%. (2006). *ED Management*, p. 52. Atlanta, GA: AHC Media.

Reavy, P. (2007, October 1). *ER nurses fall victim to increasing violence.* Retrieved September 30, 2008, http://www.deseretnews.comarticle/1.5143.695214458.00.html

Rollins, J. (2007a). A statement from Donna L. Mason, MS, RN, CEN President of the Emergency Nurses Association. *Pediatric Nursing, 33*(4), 373.

Rollins, J. (2007b, March 1). Tension in the waiting room: 86% of ED nurses report recent violence. *ED Nursing.*

Rosenthal, T.C.M. (2008, December 22). *The medical home: Growing evidence to support a new approach to primary care.* Retrieved December 31, 2008, from http://www.medscape.com/viewarticle/585208_1

Rowe, M. (2007, September). *Personalities: It's all about the service.* Retrieved January 22, 2008, from http://www.healthleadersmedia.com/content/92130/topic/WS_HLM2_MAG/Personalities-Its-All-About-the-Service.html

S. 1003: Access to Emergency Medical Services Act of 2007. (2007). Retrieved August 12, 2008, from http://www.govtrack.us/congress/bill.xpd?bill=s110–1003

Silberner, J. (2006). *Emergency Departments at the breaking point; your health; morning edition.* Retrieved November 16, 2007, from http://www.npr.org/templates/story/story.php?storyId=5486114

Sills, M. (2008, August 10). *Mental health emergency room extension creates model.* Retrieved August 21, 2008, from www.theadvertiser.com/apps/pbcs.dll/article?AID= 2008808100309&template=printeart

Statement of proposal. ABX3 5 (chapter 3, statutes of 2008) third extraordinary session; California Medi-Cal. (2008). Retrieved February 20, 2008, from Medi-cal.ca.gov/ pubsdoco/newsroom/newsroom_9299.asp: http://files.medi-cal

Stephens, J. (2008, September 3). Grassley seeks information about hospital with ties to Obamas. *The Washington Post*, p. A13.

Study: Uninsured population grows with immigration. (2008, August 5). Retrieved August 5, 2008, from www.kansascity.com/382/story/734235.html

System says ED patients will have zero wait time. (2007). *ED Management, 19*(1), 4-6.

Tanabe, G. M. (2008). Should you close your waiting room? Addressing ED overcrowding through education and staff-based participatory research. *Journal of Emergency Nursing, 34*(4), 285–289.

The Impact of Unreimbursed Care on the Emergency Physician. (2003). Retrieved November 6, 2007, from www.acep.org

Thrall, T. H. (2006, September). *Stopping ED violence before it happens.* Retrieved November 14, 2007, from http://www.hhnmag.com/hhnmag_app/jsp/articledisplay. jsp?dcrpath=HHNMAG/PubsNewsArticle/data/2006September/0609HHN_FEA_ Safety&domain=HHNMAG

Torrey, E. E. (2008). *The Shortage of Public Health Hospital Beds for Mentally Ill Persons.* Arlington, VA: Treatment Advocacy Center.

Viccellio, P. (2008, June 4). *Reducing emergency department crowding through the full capacity protocol.* Retrieved August 12, 2008, from http://www.rwjf.org/quality equality/product.jsp?id=28816

Weber, E. S. (2008, August). Are the uninsured responsible for the increase in emergency department visits in the United States? *Annals of Emergency Medicine, 52*(2), 108–115.

White, G. M. (2006). *No room for new mental patients.* Retrieved August 12, 2008, from www.ajc.com/metro/content/metro/atlanta/stories/2008/08/06/grady_mental_health_ patients.htm

Winton, R. (2007, February 25). *Patient dumping may seem criminal, but. . .* Retrieved September 12, 2008, from http://articles.latimes.com/2007/feb/25/local/me- dumping25?pg=1

Yee, C. (2008, August 11). *Some walk-in clinics closing after boom.* Retrieved September 12, 2008, from http://www.startribune.com/business/26850829.html

Zieger, A. (2008). *NJ hospitals in dire straits after charity budget cuts.* Retrieved August 1, 2008, from http://www.fiercehealthcare.com/story/nj-hospitals-in-dire-straits- after-charity-budget-cuts

Zigmond, J. (2006, February 13). No more room: Overcrowding blamed for ambulance diversions. *Modern Healthcare, 36*(7), 28.

4   The Cost of ED Violence

REAL LIABILITIES

Preventing the death, maiming, or loss of career of even one physician, nurse, or Emergency Department staff member justifies the cost related to the prevention of Emergency Department violence. Data suggest that staff members who spend the most time with patients are at the greatest risk of experiencing an assault (Erdos, 2001). Nurses rocket to the top of this list. But there is little data to support the extent of fatal assaults on Emergency Department staff.

The greatest expense of all is borne by those Emergency Departments whose philosophy is "it can't happen here."

The true cost of violence migrates into the lives of victims and their families who have also become casualties of Emergency Department violence. In 2001, 40 nurses who had incurred harm from random patient assaults responded to a survey to inform the researchers that 21% had multiple or life-threatening injuries, including fractures, lacerations, bruises, and loss of consciousness. Forty-five percent of the respondents required time away from work, and 73%, or 29 of the victims, reported work absenteeism ranging from 1 week to 1 year. Thirty percent of the nurse victims reported symptoms suggestive of posttraumatic stress disorder, which implies a long-term cost impact (Erdos, 2001).

More recently, the Paramus Medical Center in New Jersey reported that 72 staff members who were injured in patient assaults in 2006 required at least 1 day off work. The 72 injuries represented 29 additional injuries from the previous year. The injuries included bites, scratches, and kicks in the stomach, yet this amazingly large number does not reflect the true cost of violence in the ED.

Workplace violence can take an organizational toll, such as low worker productivity and increased stress, leading to high employee turnover, and it can affect the trust that employees have with management (Ray, 2007).

The cost impact for medical services in the ED and hospitals is high. The cost for treating nonfatal assault injuries that resulted in hospitalization was an average of $24,353 per person in medical costs and $57,209 per person in lost short-term productivity for each U.S. hospital treating nonfatal assault injuries. Recent 2007 statistics from the Centers for Disease Control (CDC) reveal that all U.S. hospital Emergency Departments treat an average of 55 people for injuries every minute (Nawar, Niska, & Xu, 2007). The results are summarized in Exhibit 4.1.

Violence in the United States generates a massive cost to society. While the CDC report did not define interpersonal violence, it is assumed to mean any act of violence against another person, including intimate partner violence (IPV), dating violence, lateral violence, elder abuse/violence, and child abuse. This total cost accounts for $37 billion annually for medical expense and lost productivity (CDC, 2007). These direct costs can be interpreted to mean the dollar amounts for the general treatment of violence for emergency evaluation, ongoing medical care, and for the lost productivity of the victim.

Indirect costs include the costs for the long-term loss of productivity and psychological trauma experienced by the victim and the cost for treating this trauma via medications, hospitalizations, and/or psychotherapy. Additional costs of violence are identified as:

- Loss of morale
- Anger
- Loss of confidence
- Increase in sick days and leave
- Change in job status
- Burnout (Kuhn, 1999)

The average cost for a female victim of IPV, according to a 2005 CDC report, is $948 per incident. Costs for a male victim of IPV are

Exhibit 4.1

ANNUAL COST OF VIOLENCE IN AMERICA

50,000 deaths

   $1.3 billion in lost productivity

   $4,906 per person in medical costs

2.5 million injuries

   $57,209 in lost productivity

   Average hospitalization cost: $24,353 per person intimate partner violence (IPV)

   16,800 homicides

   2.2 million injuries

   $37 billion cost

      $33 billion in lost productivity

      $4 billion in medical costs

EDs in U.S. treat 55 injuries every minute

   Self-inflicted injury

      $32 billion in lost productivity

      $1 billion in medical costs

   Suicide

      $1 million in lost productivity

      $2,596 average medical cost

   Nonfatal self-inflicted injury

      $9,726 in lost productivity per person

      $7,234 average medical cost per person

not well-documented, but in general, the direct medical cost of IPV per episode averages $387 (Schneider, 2005).

In 2007 a study was conducted to determine the costs and utilization rates for children whose mothers were either current victims of IPV or had a history of IPV that ended before the child was born. Children whose mothers had a history of IPV that occurred prior to the child's birth demonstrated high dollar and utilization rates for mental health services, primary care visits and costs, and laboratory expenses. Those children who were born during the time that the mother continued to experience IPV had high utilization for Emergency Department visits and primary care, and the children were three times more likely to incur costs for mental health services, even after the abuse had ended. The study concluded that IPV screening should become routine in the Emergency Department in an attempt to identify abuse and to provide initial and ongoing intervention (Rivera, 2007).

The Texas Health Resources has created a Domestic Violence Cost Calculator and has made the calculator available on their Web site, http://www.texashealthresouces.com (Texas Health Resources, 2008). Data and assumptions, attributed to the research team of Murray Straus and Richard Gelles, applies a female victimization rate of 116 employees per 1,000 and is able to project the number of women expected to be assaulted and the number of times annually that this number of women can anticipate being assaulted every year. In addition, the calculator computes health benefit costs, lost productivity (absentee) costs, and total costs associated with female IPV.

The statistics produced by the IPV calculator are comparatively cut and dry and depict astronomical costs for the treatment of violence against women in the U.S. The IPV calculator may provide a method that Emergency Departments can use to project staffing and budgetary needs for at least one segment of violence appearing at the ED door. Since the costs of male IPV cannot be accurately determined, only female statistics and projections can be determined.

PHYSICIAN SHORTAGES

The Association of American Medical Colleges (AAMC) Web page heralds the plea: "Help Wanted: More U.S. Doctors" (www.aamc.org). Their message is clear: the concern is that the demand for physicians in the very near term will be greater (by 30%) than the supply. The organization is calling for a 30% increase in physician education. In October 2008, the AAMC Center for Workforce Studies released a report regarding physician shortages in the U.S. (*Recent Studies and Reports on Physician Shortages in the United States*, 2007). The study predicts the current and future needs for physicians in certain specialties, varying in the degree of need by state. The AAMC report concludes that many areas of the U.S. have the potential for serious or critical shortages. The populations that are most likely to be affected are the underserved and the elderly. Nationally, there are shortages in the following specialties: allergy and immunology, cardiology, child psychiatry, dermatology, endocrinology, neurosurgery, primary care, and psychiatry.

State-by-State Reports of Physician Shortages (American Association of Medical Colleges)

Arizona: Arizona has a limited number of medical school training options and has determined a reduction in the numbers of physicians in the following specialties available in the state: allergists, cardiovascular surgeons, endocrinologists, gastroenterologists, hematologists, and infectious disease physicians.

California: The growth in demand for physicians is likely to outpace the physician supply by percentages between 4.7% and 15.9%. The population of California continues to grow rapidly, and serious physician shortages are predicted by 2015. Currently, 60% of all practicing physicians work in only five counties of the state. In 2000, 25% of all physicians were greater than 55 years of age.

Florida: All agree that demand outstrips production of physicians in Florida. Ten percent of all physicians are less than 35 years of age. Twenty-five percent of all physicians are greater than 65 years of age. Florida predicts a population increase of 60% by 2020, and the aged population is projected to grow by 124% during the same timeframe. In 2006 the Florida Board of Governors approved the establishment of two new medical schools.

Georgia: In 2006, only 77% of new physicians had received an offer for employment and had accepted the offer, and only 50% of new physicians were choosing to stay in Georgia to practice.

Iowa: In 2007, the state developed a plan with the University of Iowa to improve the supply of physicians in the state, including a decision to slightly increase educational and training opportunities and to improve recruiting and retention strategies. The five specialties that are in low supply in the state of Iowa are psychiatry, neurosurgery, general internal medicine, orthopedic surgery, and cardiology.

Kentucky: In 2005, the state reported that physician shortages would continue to pose a major challenge. Currently 66% of the counties are designated as health professional shortage areas (HPSAs) for primary care. Four hundred physicians who are practicing family physicians are aged 60 years or older and are projected to retire in the near future.

Massachusetts: Annually since 1992, the Massachusetts Medical Society has conducted a study about the physician workforce in the state and each year the data supports "strained" health care market conditions. The 2007 report concluded that Massachusetts was experiencing critical or severe shortages in neurosurgery, anesthesiology, cardiology, gastroenterology, family practice, internal medicine, psychiatry, vascular surgery, and urology. Massachusetts is concerned that they will have difficulty meeting physician demand for the above-mentioned physician services.

Michigan: Michigan reports that there will be a significant gap between supply and demand within 12 years. The aging population will continue to require more physicians than will be available, particularly in those specialties serving the elderly. The specialties that are at risk for shortages are general surgery, radiology, urology, otolaryngology, and ophthalmology.

Mississippi: In 2003, Mississippi reported that 66% of its counties were officially designated as HPSAs. Mississippi has high levels of chronic illness and poverty.

Nevada: In 2006, Nevada reported a very low physician-to-population ratio. A consulting firm has recommended that Nevada increase its medical school and graduate medical training opportunities.

North Carolina: In 2007 the state reported shortages of physicians, nurse practitioners, physician assistants, and certified midwives. The state reports that without strategic changes, the shortages of health professionals are likely to become very severe. The projected gap in providers is due to a growth in the population, aging of both the population and the providers, and the increasing prevalence of chronic illness.

Texas: In 2002 the state reported that the physician-to-population ratio was extremely unfavorable. In 2007, the Texas Tech University Health Sciences Center of the El Paso School of Medicine was approved for development. Over a 20-year span of time, the number of graduates from medical schools has remained flat, and the population has increased by 50%. The state is seriously underrepresented by Hispanic and African American physicians, and the communities of these ethnic groups are seriously underserved.

Oregon: The state has determined that they have a "looming shortage of physicians." In 2004, the state said that the current population growth exceeds growth in the number of physicians. The current physician shortages, particularly in rural areas are in the specialties of rheumatology, nephrology, gastroenterology, allergy immunology, and pediatrics. Nearly one-half of the state's practicing physicians are greater than 50 years of age and approaching retirement.

Utah: In 2003, the state revealed current shortages in pediatric neurology, child psychiatry, adult psychiatry, obstetrics and gynecology, general surgery, dermatology, urology, and cardiology. Utah has a plan in place to recruit 270 physicians annually, but with the nationwide shortage of physicians the state is concerned that it will not be able to maintain or meet its current recruiting level.

Wisconsin: In 2004 the state reported shortages in primary care, general surgery, and radiology in rural areas. The demand for primary care is projected to increase by 13.5%, and the demand for all other physicians will be greater than 20% (www.aamc.org).

Report of Physician Shortages by Specialty

The demand for specialty physicians is already a recognized need in Emergency Departments. Because of critical shortages of specialty physicians, the Centers for Medicare and Medicaid (CMS) is considering allowing Emergency Departments to comply with the CMS requirement of having a full-complement of on-call specialists to provide consultation services to Emergency Department patients having a need for a specific specialty physician via a regional plan that would allow hospitals to share on-call physicians. CMS is evaluating the efficacy of Emergency Departments using a regional plan because of the difficulty that hospital Emergency Departments are encountering recruiting on-call specialty physicians.

AAMC has determined that there is a national shortage for primary care physicians in the U.S. Physicians providing care specifically to the geriatric population will continue to be affected as demand grows. The geriatric population is projected to continue to grow as the geriatric-specialist physician supply is decreasing.

The specialty physician shortages, as determined by AAMC, are listed here.

Allergy and Immunology: In 2000, the shortfall in this specialty was anticipated within 10 years, as determined by the American Academy of Allergy, Asthma and Immunology at the State University of New York (SUNY) Albany Center for Health Workforce Studies. Many physicians are retiring and the replacement of the retiring workforce with new specialty physicians will not be equal and will fall short of the demand for allergy and immunology specialties.

Anesthesia: In 2003, the AAMP study revealed a shortage of anesthesiologists. There was not enough data to determine how the need for this specialty would progress in the coming years, but the conclusion was made that if demand increased "above one point five percent (1.5%)," that there would be a shortage of anesthesiologists through 2015.

Cardiology: In 2004, the American College of Cardiology Task Force on Workforce determined that there is a serious shortage of cardiology specialists in the U.S. More than one source has predicted a shortfall in cardiologists of up to 20% by the year 2020 due primarily to the aging population and the propensity of obesity in the U.S.

Child Psychiatry: There is an "evident shortage" in this specialty. The demand for child psychiatry has steadily grown but the supply of specialists in adolescent and child psychiatry has grown slowly. This shortfall has been recognized since 1990, when a report from the U.S. Department of Health and Human Services (DHHS) determined that (in 1990) there was a need for 30,000 practicing psychiatrists but that only 7,000 psychiatrists were currently in active practice in the U.S.

Critical Care: A 2003 report by the U.S. Health Resources Services Administration (HRSA) determined that the demand for critical care intensivist physicians would be greater than the current and projected supply and that a shortfall would continue through the year 2020 if the "current supply and demand trend continues."

Dermatology: In 2004, it was determined that there were inadequate numbers of dermatologists to meet the current demand. The American Academy of Dermatology included the utilization of "physician extenders (Nurse Practitioners and Physician Assistants)," and would continue the search for employees who had the "experience of recent graduates entering the workforce."

Emergency Medicine: The Institute of Medicine (IOM) has determined that there is a critical shortage of emergency medicine physicians. Three reports in 2006 outlined "overburdened; underfunded and highly-fragmented" Emergency Departments and ambulatory services and the surge in ED utilization by the uninsured population and those in rural areas who have few options for care. The on-call specialists needed by patients in the Emergency Department are not available because of physician shortages, adding to long patient waits in the Emergency Department waiting rooms.

Endocrinology: In 2003, a joint study among the journals *Endocrine Practice, Diabetes Care*, and the *Journal of Clinical Endocrinology and Metabolism* revealed that newly trained endocrinologists are insufficient and will not meet the demand for diabetes care in the coming years. The current workforce will be retiring. In 2003, the demand was determined to exceed supply by 15%. The primary causes for the shortfall is physician retirement and limited new supply of trained specialists in endocrinology. They predict that "demand will exceed supply from now until [the year] 2020."

Geriatric Medicine: From the study results that have been presented in this report, it is apparent that primary care demand is rising and that the supply of physicians is currently limited enough to not meet the needs of the aging population. In 2004, it was determined that the lack of geriatric specialists was "severe and worsening"; there were only 7,000 practicing geriatric specialists meeting only 35% of the current demand. Fourteen thousand geriatric specialists are "needed to adequately care for the existing (2004) elderly population." Twenty-six percent of the currently available positions in this specialty are un-filled, and 54% of the positions now available in geriatric psychiatry are unfilled. The greatest barrier to enticing physicians into this specialty and retaining geriatric specialists is the low Medicare reimbursement rates.

Medical Genetics: In 2004, the current workforce study by AAMC revealed that the "situation is critical" stating that 58% of available po-sitions are unfilled. The scope of the practice of medical genetics is expanding and has relevance to health concerns today, such as some (American College of Physicians, 2006) types of cancer, neurology, and cardiology disorders.

Neurosurgery: In 2005, the *Journal of Neurosurgery* reported that there is a "severe decline in the number of active neurosurgeons and a static supply of neurosurgical residents." The typical law of supply and demand is keeping the need for this specialty high. The available positions for specialists in neurosurgery have effectively doubled since 1994.

Oncology: The U.S. will face a shortage of oncologists if "current can-cer rates and practice patterns continue." By the year 2020, demand will increase by 48%. No solution has been devised to reverse the trend.

Pediatric Subspecialties: The Federal Expert Panel was created by the DHHS in 2003 to address the concerns of pediatric subspecialty de-mand nationally. The greatest concern is the access to care for pediatric needs in certain pediatric specialties. Because of the limited number of pediatric specialties, children with specific needs are seeking the care of adult providers in these specialties.

Primary Care: "Primary Care is on the verge of collapse" said the American College of Physicians (ACP) in 2006 in its report, "The Im-pending Collapse of Primary Care Medicine and Its Implications for the State of the Nation's Health Care" (American College of Physicians, 2006, p. 10). Chronic illness, aging population, fewer medical school entrants, and fewer resident/intern physicians in training are some of the reasons highlighted for the potential collapse. The ACP has several critical recommendations for "averting a crisis" (p. 10), including the implementation of the advanced medical home model of care coordina-tion, an urgent plan to reform reimbursement policies, and the creation of financial incentives to improve quality and efficiency to maximize payouts via the pay for performance incentives currently in place.

Psychiatry: In 2003 the Academy of Academic Psychiatry, in their journal, stated that the "rate of growth of psychiatrists will not be able to keep up with the rate of growth of demand" (American College of Physicians, 2006, p. 10). In 2003 the average age of psychiatrists in active practice was 55.7, and the percentage of young psychiatrists aged 40 or less was only 8%.

Rheumatology: There is a predicted high demand and low supply of rheumatology specialists projected between the years of 2005 and 2025. Several reasons given for the projection include the aging of the population and an increase in the incidence of musculoskeletal diseases. Currently, shortages result in patients having to wait an average of 38 days to obtain an appointment with a rheumatologist (American Association of Medical Colleges, n.d.).

A report from the HRSA predicts that the shortfall of all physicians will be 55,000 by the year 2020. The specific calculations they have made compare the FTE (full-time equivalent) physician supply as 866,400 to the demand of 921,500, disclosing a significant gap of over 55,000 physicians in 10 short years. The data are replicated in Exhibit 4.2.

The U.S. Council on Graduate Medical Education in 2005 has recommended that the U.S. increase medical school graduates by 3,000 by or before the year 2015 based on predictions of current (Moore, 2004)

Exhibit 4.2

PHYSICIAN SHORTFALLS BY 2020

In 2004, Merritt, Hawkins, and Associates published their work, *Will the Last Physician in America Please Turn Off the Lights? A Look at America's Looming Doctor Shortage,* predicting a shortfall of 90,000 to 200,000 physicians in the U.S. Reasons cited for the tremendous gap in medical health care providers are:

- The demise of managed care
- The aging of the U.S. population
- The changing practice patterns of physicians
- Increasing numbers (and complexity) of regulations
- Massive amounts of paperwork

and projected physician supply and demand in both general medicine and surgery and in specialties.

A staggering forecast from Merritt, Hawkins and Associates, a leading physician recruitment and consultation firm, was made in 2004 and projects a shortfall of 85,000 physicians by the year 2020 due to the "demise of managed care; the aging population; a change in [physician] practice patterns; an increase in regulations; and the ongoing increase in paperwork" (*Summary Report: 2006 Review of Physician Recruitment Incentives*, 2006, p. 9). These are the deficiencies in our system that government health care planning groups need to take note of in order to begin to provide leadership and solutions (*Summary Report: 2006 Review of Physician Recruitment Incentives*, 2006).

The results of these reports are alarming and dismal; the data support and explain the current situations in which Emergency Departments find themselves, with excessive numbers of low-acuity and primary care patients, very high numbers of potentially dangerous psychiatric patients subjecting patients and staff to violence, and a low and dwindling supply of specialists to evaluate Emergency Department patients. The result is that Emergency Departments have encountered the crowding and boarding effect that is responsible for the substantial risk to which patients and staff are exposed. Emergency Department nurses, physicians, and staff are in jeopardy of violence from the amplified emotions and tension that are prevalent in congested, inefficient environments. Crowded conditions and few workable solutions are a tangible and grave problem for Emergency Departments.

The Inconsistent Workforce: The Lack of Continuity of Care Due to Nurse Shortages and the Effect of Agencies

In this era of nursing shortages, the nurse staffing agency—a company providing per diem or temporary staffing to health care facilities—has become the norm. Currently in the U.S., the registered nurse (RN) vacancy rate for U.S. hospitals is estimated at 8.1%, or the lack of 116,000 RNs (*Nursing Shortage Growing Worldwide*, 2007).

A 2008 article in the *Charlotte Business Journal* (Charlotte Business Journal Staff, 2008) featured William Cody, PhD, the dean of the Presbyterian School of Nursing at Queens University in Charlotte, North Carolina. In the article, Dr. Cody shares his interpretation of the current state and predictions relative to the shortage of nurses in the U.S. and confirms that the nursing shortage is not going away anytime soon.

According to Dr. Peter Buerhaus of Vanderbilt University, Nashville, Tennessee, 1 million new and replacement RNs will be needed by the year 2016. In fact, when asked, 81% of all MDs and 82% of all RNs perceive that there are current nursing shortages where they work (Charlotte Business Journal Staff, 2008).

The Joint Commission, an independent, not-for-profit organization that "accredits and certifies more than 15,000 health care organizations and programs in the United States," revealed in a 2008 statistic that a decreased nurse staffing level was the reason implicated in 24% of all hospital deaths. Ninety-three percent of hospital nurses reported major problems relative to having enough time to maintain patient safety. This fact adds credence to the fact that nurses perceive having difficulty providing all of the care that their patients need (Nowakoski et al., 2008, p. 8).

Nurse staffing agencies are a necessary evil. Nurse staffing agencies are not evil in their intent, of course, but evil in that they have to exist at all. But the nurse staffing agency is necessary; it is an essential gap filler for hospitals, nursing homes, home health agencies, and all places that provide patient care and cannot fill their many open nursing positions. Nurses, especially those with young children at home or the nurses who wish to keep their hand in their craft but, on their own terms, can work as many or as few shifts or assignments as they like. The salary, too, for nurses employed through nurse staffing agencies is higher because the agency typically does not provide traditional insurance or other benefits to their nurses. Hospitals are willing to pay premium dollars to fill their empty nurse slots in order to provide a basic level of patient care.

As a result, hospitals and other facilities and health care services that temporarily employ the nurse staffing agency nurse expend a large amount of their personnel dollars on the agency nurse so as to provide a safe level of nurse staffing. Staffing ratios must meet certain guidelines for facilities to provide adequate care for the patients for whom the facility is responsible. Basic economics tells us that when there is a lack of supply (nurses) and an increase in demand (many patients) the cost to provide the limited resource (nurses) is high.

Temporary agency nurses cannot supply the same consistency of care for a patient as can the regular nurse, who often cares for the same group of patients every day that he or she is working. There is a great deal of benefit to consistency that is called continuity of care. As an example, there is great benefit to both the nurse and the patient when the nurse knows the patient and knows his routine and the medication that he is receiving. Recognizing that a certain patient behavior is typical behavior for that individual patient, and that the physician has been enlightened, is an enormous benefit to the patient.

A second primary risk to the patient with temporary or agency nurses is that medication errors are more likely to occur when the nurse is not familiar with the patient. The nurse has to rely on one or two other people, often a clerk or secretary, to interpret a written physician order and to write it correctly onto the medication administration record. If this process is not done impeccably, erroneous medication order information can likely be communicated. If the nurse is not familiar with the patient or his usual dosage of a medication, errors can occur.

Fortunately, a lot of the risk of misinterpretation or misreading the physician order has been eliminated through electronic ordering, but often only large hospitals or health care systems have fully ascribed to and implemented electronic methods and support because of the high entry cost of electronic systems.

Inconsistency of the nursing staff may not be directly responsible for an increase in violence in today's hospitals and Emergency Departments. However, the overall nursing shortage is a key in the potential occurrence of violence in Emergency Departments. When there is a shortage of nurses or physicians to care for the patients, the pace is slowed and the time that a patient must wait to see a provider is extended. Any increase in the amount of time a patient is expected to wait increases the opportunity for patient or visitor frustration to mount and for a potential violent outburst to occur.

DECREASING THE COST OF VIOLENCE

Many experts suggest that improving the rapidity and continuity of emergency or trauma care and shoring up recognition and treatment of violence-related injuries in the Emergency Department will improve patient outcomes, both in patient well-being and in reduction of health care expense. Providing early and consistent education about the prevention of interpersonal injury is a strategic step in rewriting the culture of domestic violence or abuse that, over a generation, could reduce the incidence of abuse and resultant trauma. "A large-scale assessment of community risk for violence and the implementation of violence-prevention strategies has been shown [to be] successful in reducing injury" (CDC, 2007).

Individuals who experience interpersonal violence are likely to acquire secondary accompanying medical conditions, or comorbidities, along with the mental health issues of depression and posttraumatic stress diagnoses. Psychological stress can increase the physiologic impact of chronic diseases such as hypertension, diabetes mellitus, and cardiovascular disorders. Comorbidities exacerbate chronic illnesses and drive up the time and cost of caring for these individuals.

A 2007 report by the CDC reveals the impact of child abuse on health care costs of female adults, conducted over a 7-year period, definitively supports that violence is a key driver in health care utilization and costs.

The study, from a large sample group, revealed that women who experienced physical abuse during childhood used primary health care services 16% more than did women who did not experience physical abuse as children. Physical abuse is defined as physical (battering), sexual, or psychological abuse. Adult women who experienced physical abuse during childhood utilized health care services 22% more often than did adult women without a history of physical abuse in childhood. The impact of both physical and sexual abuse in childhood had the greatest utilization rate and accompanying costs, as did this cohort of women who used mental health services. The women in this study group also utilized Emergency Department services, outpatient and specialty care services, and pharmaceuticals at a 36% higher rate than did women who reported no history of either physical or sexual abuse in childhood (see Figure 4.1).

Healthcare Utilization & Costs for Adult Women Who Experienced Abuse in Childhood

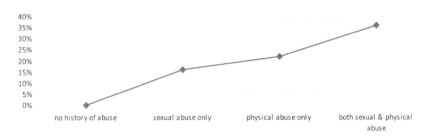

Figure 4.1 Health care utilization and costs for adult women who experienced abuse in childhood.

CASE STUDY

HOW SAFE ARE OUR HOSPITALS?

"Safety is at the heart of the health care agenda with hospitals needing to make substantial service improvements to avoid the adverse events currently affecting one in ten people admitted [to health care services]," says the British Geriatric Society article in Age and Ageing.

It doesn't sound as though our close relatives and neighbors from across the pond are experiencing any better outcomes in the geriatric population, even in their environment of national health care. The journal is concerned regarding the reporting of adverse events ranging from "hospital-acquired infections" to "pressure sores and falls" in this population. The risk of adverse events occurring in the elderly who are admitted for inpatient treatment increases 3% every year. As they age, the elderly have a 3% increased risk for adverse events each year.

According to the article, 11% of all adverse effects were determined to be "preventable," and a similar study from Australian hospitals revealed a preventable adverse effect rate in the elderly of 51%. The U.S., according to this source, had a greater number of adverse effects in the elderly, and a "greater proportion" of these events led to disability or death, especially those events occurring in the elderly who had "complex medical procedures and falls."

Quality and safety appear to be the causative agent of adverse effects of inpatients in UK hospitals. The source reveals that attitudes and assumptions create barriers to improvement or change and are the result more of "system failures" of hospitals than of individuals. The article states that these barriers to improvement are enormous challenges for UK hospitals.

The experience of the aviation industry may yield some solutions for health care. Airlines emphasize "workflow management; the prevention of stress and fatigue; teamwork; and an individual responsibility to safety," and may suggest improvement strategies for the health care industry. Total quality management principles and incident reporting have been cited as a strategy to improve outcomes (Ramanath, n.d.).

(Continued)

The cost of violence in the U.S. is high in terms of hard costs relative to liabilities and lost productivity, but violence has an enormous economic cost to health care: loss of customer trust, direct costs of enhanced security requirements, unintended costs of regulatory oversight, and societal costs that are borne by the community and the hospitals that must provide extensive support, follow-up services, and education. The unfortunate prediction is that the cost of violence will continue to escalate, exacerbating the necessity for health care systems to build in violence protection for their consumers. Costs incurred by the closure of general medical-surgical and psychiatric facilities to care for the impaired and the loss of trained physicians and the lessening workforce will affect the U.S. for generations to come. Costs to enlighten elected officials and enhance national and state budgetary line items for violence ensures direct cost increases for citizens and residents.

Global violence, too, most particularly in health care systems around the world, is expanding and pulsing ahead of the U.S. in numbers of reported health care violence incidents. The addition of new jails and the erasure of inpatient health care facilities is not a situation known only in the U.S., but is a situation that exists throughout the world.

Theorists have written for decades about the growing trend of societal violence with implications of costs associated with violence. If the assumption is that history repeats itself and that the future is predicted by past occurrences, it isn't difficult to interpret a meaningful message that violence is here to stay. Furthermore, with inflationary change and additional costs relegated to the control, correction, and treatment of violence, the cost of violence will continue to scale upward, generating an uncontrollable and grave influence on U.S. economic stability.

REFERENCES

American Association of Medical Colleges. (n.d.). Retrieved April 9, 2009, from http://www.aamc.org/workforce/recentworkforcestudies2008.pdf

American College of Physicians. (2006, January 30). *The impending collapse of primary care medicine and its implications for the state of the nation's health care: A report from the American College of Physicians.* Retrieved April 9, 2009, from http://www.acponline.org/advocacy/events/state_of_healthcare/statehc06_1.pdf

Centers for Disease Control. (2007). *The cost of violence in the United States.* Retrieved May 18, 2008, from http://www.cdc.gov/print.do?url-http%3A//www.cdc.gov/ncipc/factsheets/CostOfViolence

Charlotte Business Journal Staff. (2008, August 8). *Nursing shortage growing critical as population ages.* Retrieved September 12, 2008, from http://www.queens.edu/news_detail.asp?press_id=2601&section=nursing

Erdos, B. H. (2001, September). *Emergency psychiatry: A review of assaults by patients against staff at psychiatric emergency centers.* Retrieved October 20, 2007, from http://psychservices.psychiatryonline.org

Kuhn, W. M. (1999). Violence in the Emergency Department 1999. *Postgraduate Medicine, 105*(1).

Moore, R. (2004, March 5). *Dkr shortage looms large on the stage for health care.* Retrieved April 9, 2009, from http://www.bizjournals.com/nashville/stories/2004/03/08/focus2.html

Nawar, E. W., Niska, R. W., & Xu, J. (2007). *National Hospital Ambulatory Medical Care Survey: 2006 emergency departments.* Hyattsville, MD: Centers for Disease Control, U.S. Department of Health and Human Services, National Center for Health Statistics.

Nowakoski, N., O'Leary, D., Reno, K., Safian, K., Sample, S., Sengin, K., et al. (2008, July 12). *Health care at the crossroads: Strategies for addressing the evolving nursing crisis.* Retrieved April 12, 2009, from http://www.jointcommission.org/NR/rdonlyres/5C138711-ED76-4D6F-909F-B06E0309F36D/0/health_care_at_the_crossroads.pdf

Nursing shortage growing worldwide. (2007). Retrieved November 14, 2007, from www.about.com/nursing

Ray, M. M. (2007). The dark side of the job: Violence in the Emergency Department. *Journal of Emergency Nursing, 33*(3), 257–261.

Recent studies and reports on physician shortages in the United States. (2007). Retrieved July 2008, from http://www.aamc.org/workforce/recentworkforcestudies2007.pdf

Ramanath, R. H. (2008). How safe are our hospitals? *Age and Ageing, 10*(1093), 243–245.

Rivera, M. A. (2007). Intimate partner violence and health care costs and utilization for children living in the home. *Pediatrics, 120*(6), 1270–1277.

Schneider, M. E. (2005, December 1). Costs of intimate partner violence. *OB GYN News,* p. 31.

Summary Report: 2006 Review of Physician Recruitment Incentives. (2006). Retrieved April 9, 2009, from http://www.merritthawkins.com/pdf/2006_incentive_survey.pdf#search="will%20the%20last%20physician%20in%20america%20please%20turn%20out%20the%20lights&quot

Texas Health Resources. (2008). Texas Health.org. Retrieved May 19, 2008, from http://www.texashealth.org/main.asp-enorgid-684BA615301F4118AB23B2A946F7293D

5 Creating the ED as a Safe Haven

While it is very important to know, analyze, and understand the reasons behind the statistics related to Emergency Department (ED) violence, a superior strategy is to focus on the positive changes that can be made to create an atmosphere of sincere caring and concern for the patients who choose to come to your hospital for care during what may be the most stressful time of their lives—being in pain and fearful of what may be the cause.

Creating change is expensive. Making significant changes to your ED can often be outside the reality and possibility of budget constraints and perhaps out of your control. The executive team of your hospital may have decided that construction to add the 20 ED beds that are desperately needed to accommodate the growth that has occurred in the neighborhood cannot possibly be done for 2 more years.

Start small. Get all of the ED stakeholders including ED management, the physicians, the ED staff, and your patients involved in a plan consisting of 10 or so small, inexpensive changes that can be done quickly and with very little investment but that can make a huge difference. Involving your customers in making change is very powerful.

When patients arrive for care and must wait until they can be seen by a provider, the situation is probably something that you cannot change entirely with creativity. It may take more monetary investment such as additional staff, new equipment (telemetry monitors, for example), and both ED and inpatient staff, equipment, and capacity for the inpatient side to successfully collaborate to solve ED throughput issues. Putting yourself in your patient's shoes can help you understand how the patient feels and may provide you with a working strategy to improve the ED and waiting room environment for the patient.

Communicating often with waiting patients and families is essential to moderating their anxiety. Let the patients know that you haven't forgotten them and keep them apprised of where they fall on the *waiting list*. Offer refreshments if it is medically appropriate. Create multiple small seating sections. Provide fun and glossy updated reading material or movies on DVD. Purchase extra blankets, pillows, and refreshments and have them readily available. Simple additions can ensure success in turning your waiting room into a *welcoming* room and may convert a grumpy patient or family member into one who is—if not *content*—at least more tolerant of the wait to see the provider. Keeping your customer in the communication loop and updated will satisfy even the most demanding customer.

Concentrate on making changes that create security and safety for the patients and families. If your Emergency Department has experienced an episode of serious aggression or violence or a near-miss episode of violence, chances are that hospital administration has added one or two layers of security to the Emergency Department. If not, work closely with hospital administration to demonstrate the need for security and safety for the patients and for the staff. The perception—and the reality—of having a safe haven in your ED will ensure that your Emergency Department continues to attract patients/customers, especially if an episode of violence has occurred.

HOSPITAL VIOLENCE AGAINST PATIENTS

Recently, two tragic episodes of patient deaths in hospital Emergency Departments have been told in graphic detail in the news media. The circumstances of the deaths illustrate the crisis that U.S. EDs are facing. For psychiatric patients, EDs have very limited options for patient transfer or referral to either inpatient psychiatric treatment facilities or to outpatient mental health community services. The severe lack of services is forcing Emergency Departments to board patients in the ED often for up to 4 days. One Emergency Department nurse reports that the many ED boarded psychiatric patients in her ED were crying and bellowing for nearly 20 hours a day. Imagine if you can what the stress must be like for staff and for patients in a similar circumstance. The mentally ill who are not treated with the appropriate medications often end up in Emergency Departments and very often incite violence. Inpatient psychiatric services have closed because of lack of government funding and low reimbursement rates driven by patient inability to pay. Patients who are experiencing serious psychiatric and/or mental health issues are predictably unable to hold a steady job, so they have no opportunity to participate in an employer-funded health plan and have limited ability to purchase health insurance. Large numbers of mentally ill patients may have no place to live because of their inability to work, causing a surge in homeless, mentally unstable individuals out on the streets of many cities. The shortage of inpatient psychiatric beds in the United States has ensured that the streets will continue to be the repositories for the mentally ill and that Emergency Departments will be their "defacto" asylums and "mental health centers" (White, 2006, p. 2). The mentally ill who have no place to go usually end up in Emergency Departments. This patient population is typically responsible for a large share of the violent episodes against nurses. The many shuttered hospitals and diminishing numbers of psychiatric facilities, services, and psychiatrists is a serious crisis for U.S. health care and for U.S. citizens and residents who find themselves in need of such services.

CASE STUDY

USA Today *published the unforgettable story of a 49-year-old female patient who died on the floor of the psychiatric Emergency Department waiting room in Kings County Hospital, New York ("Family to Sue Psych Ward," 2008). The daughter of the deceased woman is seeking damages of $25 million and criminal prosecution against the psychiatric/health care workers who "did nothing to help her." The daughter believes that "whoever committed [this] criminal act should be held responsible" ("Family to Sue Psych Ward," 2008).*
A video recording showed that the woman collapsed face-down on the floor many hours after she had arrived. She allegedly had

(Continued)

been waiting for medical assistance in the waiting room for over 24 hours. For over 1 hour after her collapse, no one came to her assistance, although the videotape evidence revealed that several security guards and at least one hospital staff came to view the woman's "prone body" ("Family to Sue Psych Ward," 2008). It is unknown why no one in the Emergency Department would help the woman. Eventually, someone who was identified as a "member of the medical staff" approached the woman and realized that the woman was deceased ("Family to Sue Psych Ward," 2008).

The president of the corporation that oversees Kings County Hospital issued a statement about the incident, saying that "new staff, procedures and training" had been implemented since the death and that these measures would likely be "supplemented by further reforms" ("Family to Sue Psych Ward," 2008).The corporation referred the case to law enforcement and regulatory authorities. The hospital assured cooperation and support of any and all investigations.

The woman, originally from Jamaica, had moved to the U.S. in 2000 to find employment. None of her children or family lived in the U.S. One of the daughters described herself as being "heartsick" at the thought of her mother dying in such a way, alone and thousands of miles from her home and family.

Part of the bigger problem in a situation similar to that described in the preceding paragraphs is that the evidence in the medical record may have been altered. This hospital has been accused of covering up the neglect that is so apparent on the videotape recording of the real-time events. The video record is evidence of the lifeless form of the woman on the floor of the ED, yet the medical record reflects that the patient was "awake and up and about" at the same time ("Family to Sue Psych Ward," 2008). Six hospital personnel have been fired. The hospital is already mired in complaints and lawsuits from other investigations of patient mistreatment and will most likely incur irreversible financial duress and may be forced to close ("Family to Sue Psych Ward," 2008). The concern, aside from the sad commentary on the dismal treatment of human beings in need of help, is the public health and safety emergency created by the severe shortage of therapeutic psychiatric services for the mentally ill.

Thirty-Six Compelling Reasons for ED Personnel and Administrators to Know and Understand Violence in the ED

1. Twenty-six physicians, 18 registered nurses, 27 pharmacists, 17 certified nursing assistants (CNAs), and 18 other health care workers were killed on the job between 1980 and 1990, according to the Department of Labor (*Emergency Department Violence,* 1995).
2. Two hundred twenty-one hospitals in the U.S. and Canada reported 42 homicides, 1,463 physical assaults, 67 sexual assaults, 165 robberies, and 47 armed robberies against health care workers, according to the International Association for Healthcare Safety and Security in 1995 (*Emergency Department Violence,* 1995).
3. Verbal threats, physical assault, and even stalking are common occurrences in EDs. Of 171 ED physicians surveyed, 76% report experiencing at least one violent act over the previous 12 months and nearly one-third were victims of physical assaults ("Assaults Against ED Nurses Are Largely Unreported," 2005).
4. Ninety percent of Emergency Department managers at VHA member hospitals cited patient violence as the greatest threat to ED personnel ("Poll: ER Violence," 2003). (VHA is a 24,000-member national health care alliance providing supply-chain management and support by assisting its members in performance improvement relative to operations and clinical issues.)
5. The average annual rate for nonfatal violent crime against physicians is 16.2%, and the average annual rate for nonfatal violent crime against nurses is 21.9% according to a 2007 report by the Emergency Nurses Association and taken from the 2004 Bureau of Labor statistics ("ENA Members to Participate in Survey," 2007). Health care and social services workers have the highest rate of nonfatal assault injuries (Cooper, 2005). The average annual rate for nonfatal violent crime against mental health professionals is 68.2% ("ENA Members to Participate in Survey," 2007).
6. Thirty-five percent to 80% of all hospital staff have been physically assaulted at least once (Clements, 2005).
7. Eighteen percent of all Emergency Department physicians obtained a gun for protection, and 31% of those surveyed have their own form of "personal protection" (*Emergency Department*

Violence, 2005). Of 475 respondents, 99% of male and female surgical residents surveyed in 1997 reported carrying a gun or knowing someone in a hospital environment who does (Barlow, 1997).

8. Less than 3% of all hospital facilities surveyed had 24-hour security, and 11% had no security in the Emergency Department ("Dealing With Violence in the Emergency Department," 1998).

9. Screeners found 1,400 knives in the course of 1 year, screening only at night in the Emergency Department. This data is from a small-town hospital in Minnesota (Amy, 2005).

10. Greater than one-quarter—26.7%—of major trauma victims presenting to level-one trauma hospital Emergency Departments were carrying lethal weapons (14-year period, reported in 1999) (Kuhn, 1999).

11. Eighty-nine percent of physical assaults toward physicians were initiated by a patient (*Emergency Department Violence*, 2005).

12. Alcohol, drugs, and prescription pain medication abuse, along with psychiatric disorders, are several factors that contribute to violence in the Emergency Department (Kuhn, 1999).

13. Emergency Departments are vulnerable to violence because of the 24-hour accessibility of drugs and potential hostages (Kuhn, 1999).

14. Nurses "are probably even more on the front line than physicians when it comes to confronting potentially violent patients and may be at even higher risk" ("Assaults Against ED Nurses Are Largely Unreported," 2005).

15. Long wait times and delays in care can increase hostility (Kuhn, 1999). "Long waits at hospital (Emergency Departments) are a major factor in provoking hostile behavior among people who are already under stress" (Harasim, 2005; McPhaul, 2008).

16. In 1995, the greatest number of physical assaults and the second largest number of homicides occurring in a hospital occurred in the Emergency Department (*Emergency Department Violence*, 1995).

17. Nine hospitals reported violence that resulted in death in a survey of 170 U.S. teaching hospitals, each with 40,000 patient visits annually (Kuhn, 1999).

18. Physical violence can be preceded by a period of increasing tension characterized by a tense, threatening posture or loud,

profane speech accompanied by increased motor activity or restlessness (Kuhn, 1999). Violence may be a sudden and unpredictable event, especially in patients with medical conditions that cause delirium or confusion (*Emergency Department Violence*, 2005; Kuhn, 1999).

19. Emergency physicians report that 45% of physical assaults stemmed from patients who were believed to be intoxicated. The true incidence of significant episodes of violence is unknown, since violence in the Emergency Department is underreported (*Emergency Department Violence*, 2005).

20. Occupations with the highest proportion of respondents experiencing physical assault were nurses and protective services (security) personnel (*Emergency Department Violence*, 2005).

21. During a 6-month period, the National Institute for Occupational Safety and Health (NIOSH), a government organization, reports that stationary and hand-held metal detectors used to screen entrants to a Detroit, Michigan, hospital found 33 handguns, 1,234 knives, and 97 Mace containers. *The study did not report whether the hospital was a trauma center* (Harasim, 2005).

22. A study of violence in hospitals (not specifically of Emergency Departments) reported 8.3 nonfatal assaults per 10,000 hospital staff, compared with the rate of nonfatal assaults for all private-sector companies that report 2 nonfatal assaults per 10,000 workers (Harasim, 2005).

23. In 2001 the Joint Commission on Accreditation of Healthcare Organizations (JCAHO), which sets standard operating requirements for hospitals, ruled that any type of restraint, to control violent behavior, should seldom be used (Harasim, 2005; *JCAHO and CMS—Patients' Rights and Use of Restraints*, 2008).

24. The average time that a patient must wait in the emergency room to be seen by a medical professional ranges from 6 hours to as much as 24 hours (Rollins, 2007). In 2006, the Centers for Disease Control (CDC) reported an average wait time of 56 minutes, on average, for a patient to wait prior to seeing a medical professional in the ED (Stobbe, 2008).

25. "De-institutionalization" of mentally ill patients relies on a 24-hour open access to emergency care. The personnel in Emergency Departments must now manage patients who have psychiatric illnesses and were cared for, in the past, in psychiatric hospitals and facilities (Kuhn, 1999).

26. Eighty-six percent of all ED nurses describe some form of violence committed against them while on duty over the past 3 years (Reavy, 2007).

27. Violence may be a sudden and unpredictable event, especially in patients with medical conditions that cause delirium or confusion (Kuhn, 1999).

28. In 2005, the Massachusetts Bureau of Labor Statistics reported more than 4,000 hospital employees had been assaulted while working in the ED. A 2005 survey of ED doctors in Michigan revealed that 28% had been physically assaulted, while 75% had been verbally abused (Reavy, 2007)

29. A survey of Emergency Department physicians revealed that 82% said their EDs are operating at or over capacity on weekdays and 9 in 10, or 91%, said their EDs were at or over capacity on weekends (American College of Emergency Physicians, 2004).

30. Emergency Department visits have grown by 20% since 1992, amassing 102 million ED visits in 2001 and escalating to 115.3 million ED visits by 2005. Patient visits to U.S. Emergency Departments in 2006 were 119 million (Pitts, Niska, Xu, & Burt, 2006).

31. The total number of EDs in the U.S. has declined by 14% since 1993 (*Emergency Department Violence,* 1995). Between 1993 and 2003, ED visits grew by 26%, the number of EDs declined by 425, and the number of hospital beds dropped by 198,000 (Silberner, 2006).

32. In 2005, 242 employees at five hospitals in Cincinnati were surveyed regarding their experience with violence or abuse from a specific cohort of patients. Most of the 242 employees reported verbal abuse at least once from patients or visitors; there were 319 patient assaults and 10 visitor assaults. Sixty-five percent of the employees did not report the violence/abuse to the hospital authorities. Sixty-four percent of the employees had not received violence prevention training in the prior 12 months. The employees reported concerns about the violent experiences, their feelings of safety, and job satisfaction following the assaults (Gates, 2006).

33. More than 40% of nurses indicated that their workplace was somewhat safe or not safe at all (Rollins, 2007).

34. Violence in the U.S. has reached epidemic proportions (*CSPV Overview,* 2008).

35. Violence is the second leading cause of death in the workplace (Keely, 2002).

36. A GE Security/AHSS Healthcare Benchmarking study of EDs found that 45% do not issue visitor passes; 28% do not have video surveillance in the ED; 47% cannot electronically lock down the facility; 57% state that the ED accounts for one of the top 3 locations requiring the majority of security officer time (Howard, 2008).

There are many stakeholders who benefit from Emergency Department working strategies and policies against violence including the patients/customers and their families, the community, vendors and visitors, the hospital owners/stockholders, the board of directors, the business owners who have the long-term goal of revenue growth, and, of course, the Emergency Department staff. Strategies must be dynamic and adaptable to meet the needs of current and future circumstances. The overarching goal of a violence prevention strategy is to create barriers to violence and add layers of security that will safeguard all stakeholders against violence or from the fallout from violence.

CASE STUDY

LETTER TO THE EDITOR: GUNS DON'T BELONG IN THE EMERGENCY ROOM!

Do You Agree?

August 16, 1994

A letter to the editor of the New York Times *in the mid-1990s was written by a pair of Emergency Department RNs. The women were concerned that the presence of weapons in the ED could lead to a dangerous trend and a potentially tragic outcome for patients, visitors, or staff at Bellevue Hospital. The nurses purport that "this proximity of a large number of loaded weapons and violent people is asking for trouble," especially because the hospital is the evaluation point for many types of patients including "prisoners, psychiatric patients, substance abusers and the general public."*

(Continued)

The nurses agree with me when they tell the editor of the Times *that "violence in the emergency department setting has been escalating in recent years (Kohler, 1994)." Recently, a Bellevue Hospital staffer was wounded by a bullet when he was shot in the hand by a police officer. The officer was attempting to wrest the gun away from a prisoner at the time that the gun went off. The nurses believe that episodes such as the one described above are "predictable" because of the volume of dangerous weapons and the numbers of people who are carrying armed and lethal weapons.*

The nurses are concerned for the safety of the general public who visit the Emergency Department at Bellevue Hospital where "dangerous criminals and psychotic patients are within reach of loaded weapons."

Emergency departments today are strained to overcapacity and are in the presence of patients who are emotionally unstable, are acting out, who are under the influence of illicit drugs, or are members of violent street gangs (Kohler, 1994).

REFERENCES

American College of Emergency Physicians. (2004). *As uninsured patients turn to Emergency Departments for care of untreated illness, emergency physicians call for coverage for all Americans.* Alexandria, VA: Public Opinions Strategies.

Amy, J. (2005). *Security and crime news—from the Mobile (Alabama) Register.* Retrieved June 1, 2007, from http://jrrobertssecurity.com/security-news/security-crime news0025.htm

Assaults against ED nurses are largely unreported: Act now to prevent violence. (2005, June 1) *ED Nursing*.

Barlow, C. R. (1997, August). Violence against surgical residents. *Western Journal of Medicine, 167*(2), 74–78.

Clements, P. D. (2005, June). Incidence of violence in the workplace. *Nursing Economics, 23*(3), 119–124.

Cooper, J. R. (2005). *Letters to the editor.* Retrieved May 19, 2008, from http://www.nursingworld.org/MainMenuCategories/ANAMarketplace/ANAPeriodicals

CSPV overview. (2008). Retrieved July 21, 2008, from http://www.colorado.edu/cspv

Dealing with violence in the Emergency Department. (1998, September). Retrieved May 14, 2009, from http://findarticles.com/p/articles/mi_qa3689/is_199809/ai_n8811262/

Emergency Department violence. (1995). Retrieved November 6, 2007, from http://www3.acep.org/Content.aspx?id=21830

Emergency Department violence. (2005). Retrieved November 6, 2007, from http://www3.acep.org/Content.aspx?id=21830

Emergency Department violence. (n.d.). Retrieved October 12, 2006, from http://www. acep.org/advocacy.aspx?id=21830

ENA members to participate in survey on violence in the Emergency Department. (2007, April). *ENA Connection*, p. 12.

Family to sue psych ward for $25M in watched-death case. (2008, August 14). Retrieved August 14, 2008, from www.usatoday.com/news/health/2008-07-08-hospital-death_N.htm

Gates, D. R. (2006). Violence against emergency department workers. *Emergency Medicine, 31*(3), 331–337.

Harasim, P. (2005). *Concern from healthcare workers over hospital violence.* Retrieved June 1, 2007, from http://www.securityinfowatch.com/article/printer.jsp?id=3381

Howard, E. (2008). *Security for the Emergency Department.* Retrieved October 28, 2008, from http://www.facilitycare.com/SecurityfortheEmergencyDepartment

JCAHO and CMS—patients' rights and use of restraints. (2008). Retrieved May 22, 2008, from http://www.premierinc.com/safety/topics/patient_safety/index_3.jsp# JCAHO%20and %20CMS

Keely, B. (2002). Recognition and prevention of hospital violence. *Dimensions of Critical Care Nursing, 21*(6), 236–241.

Kohler, T. M. (1994, August 16). *Guns don't belong in the emergency room.* Retrieved August 8, 2008, from http://www.nytimes.com/1994/08/16/opinion/l-guns-don-t-belong-in-the-emergency-room-973998.html?scp=1&sq=%22Guns%20don't%20 belong%20in%20the%20Emergency%20Room%22,%20August%2016%20 1994%20&st=cse

Kowalenko, T. W. (2005). Workplace violence: A survey of emergency physicians in the state of Michigan. *Annals of Emergency Medicine, 46*(2), 142–147.

Kuhn, W. (1999). Violence in the Emergency Department. *Postgraduate Medicine, 105*(1).

McPhaul, K. L. (2008, May 26). *Environmental evaluation for workplace violence in healthcare and social services.* Retrieved August 28, 2008, from http://www.cdc.gov/ niosh/topics/PtD/pdfs/McPhaul.pdf

Pitts, S., Niska, R., Xu, J., & Burt, C. (2006). *National Hospital Ambulatory Medical Care Survey: 2006 Emergency Department Survey.* Centers for Disease Control, Health Statistics.

Poll: ER violence tops concern of terrorism. (2003, January). *Healthcare Purchasing News*, p. 20.

Reavy, P. (2007, October 1). *ER nurses fall victim to increasing violence.* Retrieved September 30, 2008, from http://www.deseretnews.comarticle/1.5143.695214458.00. html

Rollins, J. (2007, March 1). Tension in the waiting room: 86% of ED nurses report recent violence. *ED Nursing.*

Silberner, J. (2006). *Uninsured patients, few beds keep ERs maxed out.* Retrieved May 28, 2008, from http://www.npr.org/templates/story/story.php?storyId=5486114

Stobbe, M. (2008). *Average ER waiting time nears 1 hour, CDC says.* Retrieved August 12, 2008, from http://ap.google.com/article/ALeqM5ilSq6tBqDRxCxXyajBdg-ZG0ekbAD92CVG3G1

White, G. M. (2006). No room for new mental patients. *Atlanta Journal Constitution*, p. 2.

Assessing Violence in the ED: The Victims and the Perpetrators

## PART II

Violence is a tool of the ignorant.

—*Flip Wilson*

## 6

Assessment of Your ED: Identifying Your ED Risk for Violence

IDENTIFYING PRE-AGGRESSIVE BEHAVIOR AND CLUES TO POTENTIAL VIOLENCE

The lack of economic opportunity may be one contributing factor responsible for the growth of violence in the United States. Unfortunately, individuals who have limited educational prospects or who lack parental guidance may inadvertently become high-risk individuals, inclined to commit violence. Individuals with violent tendencies or those who have learned the traits of violence on the street from peers or from life experiences turn up on the doorstep of every Emergency Department (ED) in the U.S. every day. It is of critical importance that health care professionals, who welcome and care for these individuals in the ED, are alerted to any potential for violence.

What does an individual who possesses the key components of violent tendencies and who may be wired to commit a violent act look like? Current literature quantifies the typical violent aggressor prototype into four broad categories:

1. An individual's history of violent behavior or being the prior or current victim of violence is the one element acknowledged as a reason for an individual to exhibit violence or to have violent

tendencies (*Emergency Department Violence*, n.d.; Rollins, 2007a).

2. A young, urban male from a lower socioeconomic group who has a poor school and/or job record carries the risk factor for the potential of violence. Violent behavior is most often triggered by males who are 30 years of age or less, who have access to weapons, and who are plagued with alcohol or substance abuse problems. The violent individual often has a limited family support system and generally has experienced run-ins with the law including multiple arrests for violent crime (Kuhn, 1999). It is well known that the two major demographic predictors of violent behavior are male sex and younger age (Grunberg, 2007).

3. A clinical diagnosis of substance abuse, acute manic/depressive states, acute schizophrenia, acute organic brain syndrome, personality disorders, temporal lobe epilepsy, or other seizure disorders should cue the health care professional to take fundamental precautions when interacting with this individual.

4. Specific behavioral activity can present as clues for violent acts, including tense posture and clenched fists and loud, threatening, and insistent speech. A restless demeanor or pacing can indicate an increasing potential for an individual to instigate violence (Kuhn, 1999).

Currently, there is no tracking mechanism, reporting network, authority, or collection point in which to receive or enter data of patients who exhibit violent tendencies or to identify those individuals who seek emergency services as a result of an aggressive or violent crime. Emergency Department personnel have limited local or regional resources in which to verify a previous history of violence, which leaves ED personnel oblivious and vulnerable to the violent actions of individual patients.

Emergency staff needs to be aware that incidents of violence occur mainly at night and most frequently between the hours of 11:00 P.M. and 7:00 A.M. Ironically, and fortunately, it is during this time that fewer numbers of patients are coming to Emergency Departments across the U.S. See Exhibit 6.1 for general guidelines when assessing potentially violent patients.

Michael O'Malley, a former police officer and owner and president of Management of Aggressive Behavior Training International (MOAB), recommends intervention at stage 1 because "the early management of behavior" is critical, says O'Malley (Thrall, 2006). In stage 1, if an indi-

Exhibit 6.1

GENERAL GUIDELINES FOR COMMUNICATION AND PERSONAL SAFETY WHEN ASSESSING OR TREATING POTENTIALLY VIOLENT PATIENTS

ED STAFF AND PHYSICIANS ARE TO ENTER ONLY WHEN ACCOMPANIED BY ANOTHER PERSON

- ○ Limit eye contact
- ○ Approach the patient only from the front
- ○ Maintain a safety zone of four times greater than normal (approximately 4 feet)
- ○ Ask the patient where he would like you to stand, especially if the patient retreats from you
- ○ Stand at an oblique angle to the patient
- ○ Stand with your back to the door for easy escape if this becomes necessary
- ○ Post security staff who have been trained in de-escalation techniques outside the door at all times

vidual is, or becomes, increasingly anxious he may need simple reassurance. Be proactive and don't ignore the signs.

When an individual reaches stage 2, or verbal aggression, he may yell and use profanity. O'Malley cautions against using wit or joking with the upset individual because the individual may construe your response as a reactionary tactic. Instead, validate the person's feelings and use an assertive, calm, but authoritative approach. "Maintain eye contact and have hands in an open position," he urges (Thrall, 2006). O'Malley suggests saying, "I realize that you are upset, but I can't help you when you are yelling and upset. Let's work on this together." O'Malley recognizes this is a difficult task and that to become proficient you may require training to recognize the right time to intervene and how to say things correctly. Your goal is to avoid the escalation of a potentially aggressive situation.

O'Malley stresses that most physical aggression can be prevented if the signals given by the individual are understood and responded to. It is important to know what to say and when to say it (Thrall, 2006; see Exhibit 6.2).

Researchers in Australia spent three hundred hours in an ED in Western Sydney to assess the ED staff as they attempted to diminish the

Exhibit 6.2

ASSESSING LEVEL OF RISK TOOL

THREE PROGRESSIVE STAGES OF VIOLENT BEHAVIOR

Stage 1: Anxiety

Stage 2: Verbal aggression

Stage 3: Physical aggression

impact of violent episodes created by patients. Multiple interviews with the staff and the results of their research resulted in the development of the STAMP Tool. STAMP is the acronym for Staring and eye contact, Tone and volume of voice, Anxiety, Mumbling, and Pacing (Luck, 2007).

One of the signs noted by the researchers was *staring*, which was a very important and precise symptom of impending violence. The researchers noted this symptom in 56% of the potentially violent patients. Interestingly, many of the nurses, during the interview, remarked that their interpretation of patient staring was thought to be a method patients used to "intimidate [the nurses] into some form of action" (Luck, 2007). Generally, the nurses responded to staring and inadvertently circumvented a violent act.

Tone and volume of voice were significant factors in assessing the level of anxiety demonstrated by patients. Most everyone can recognize that an elevation in tone and loudness of the voice, similar to what occurs during yelling, indicates distress. Tenor and volume of voice were present in 81% of the potentially violent patients (Luck, 2007).

In 69% of the violent patients, they were observed to "mumble; use slurred or incoherent speech; repeatedly ask the same questions or make the same statements" (Luck, 2007). The presence of these symptoms were determined to be a precursor to violence, as the manifestations indicated "mounting frustration" (Luck, 2007). Similarly, pacing suggests escalating anxiety, frustration, or agitation and was noted to be present in 56% of the patients in the study (Luck, 2007).

The STAMP assessment tool can be used as an effective checklist to guide nursing personnel in assessing patients whose agitation or frustration may result in a violent act (Luck, 2007). A summary of key elements of the STAMP tool are found in Exhibit 6.3.

Exhibit 6.3

ASSESSING SIGNS OF POTENTIAL VIOLENCE IN PATIENTS WITH THE STAMP TOOL

- **S = Staring and eye contact**
- **T = Tone and volume of voice**
- **A = Anxiety or agitation level**
- **M = Mumbling**
- **P = Pacing**

The presence of even one of the indicators can signify an escalation in apprehension that may lead to violent activity.

From Judith Tindale, 2007; STAMP Violence Assessment Tool (Luck, 2007).

STREET GANGS AND THE ED

Street gangs are spreading and their resulting violence is proliferating. Cities, towns, and workplaces have become common arenas for the macho street mentality of the gang member. No longer can a blind or naïve eye be turned toward street gangs and their violent tendencies. Understanding and awareness can help thwart and avoid violent situations while saving the lives of staff, patients and visitors alike. (Redfern, 2006)

From 1993–2003, according to the National Crime Victimization Survey, gang members committed 373,000 of the total 6.6 million violent victimizations disclosed by the most current data available (U.S. Department of Justice, 2003).

The propagation of street gangs is possibly the greatest challenge faced by U.S. Emergency Departments today. There exists no primer on street gangs or gang activity, so we must all rely on as much expert experience, published knowledge, and statistics as are available to help design a plan to prevent the migration of street gangs and violence into our Emergency Departments and hospitals.

Gangs are regarded as a product of the 1930s or 1940s, but the first evidence of gangs in the U.S. appears in the history books in 1783 just after the Revolutionary War. Confirmation of the presence of violent and criminal street gangs was in the 1800s in New York City, whose members were comprised mainly of immigrants. Following the U.S. Civil War, many ethnic and religious gangs originated composed of Jews, Italians, African Americans, and Irish. "Asian gangs formed in California in the mid-1800s" and were joined by "Hispanic gangs in the 1920s and 1930s" (Moffatt, 2002). In the early part of the 20th century and today, gangs originate among socioeconomically disadvantaged youth who form gangs in response to exclusion from—and the understanding that they may never achieve—middle-class status. These youths were typically from large, culturally diverse neighborhoods and among immigrant populations. The neighborhoods were characterized by deteriorating housing, poor employment opportunities, and limited social control (Moffatt, 2002).

Today, all U.S. cities with populations of 250,000 or more, and 86% of all cities with at least 100,000 residents, are known to have active street gangs. In total, there are 731,500 street gang members and 21,500 specific street gangs in operation in the U.S. (Grossman, 2003). According to the Department of Justice, the count is much higher, with as many as 24,500 known gangs in the U.S., with 770,000 members (Bureau of Justice Assistance, 2005).

A *gang* is defined as a group or association of three or more individuals who may have common identifying signs, symbols, or names and who collectively or individually engage in, or have engaged in, criminal activity that creates an atmosphere of fear and intimidation (Bureau of Justice Assistance, 2005).

The type of individual who is at risk for gang participation may be the youth who is misunderstood or does not fit in with his peers. He or she is seeking an identity and a status to meet some unfulfilled need. Most gang members experience poverty, unemployment, and dysfunctional families. He or she may feel singled out or discriminated against because of his or her ethnicity. Educational opportunities for this individual are probably limited. Gang membership may substitute for the middle-class status that most aspire to but realize may be unattainable (Redfern, 2006).

Risk factors for gang membership include:

1. Male gender
2. African American and/or Hispanic youth
3. Low socioeconomic status/poverty

4. Unemployment
5. Need for status and identity
6. Alcohol and/or drug use
7. Weapon ownership
8. Exposure to violence
9. Hopelessness or fatalism
10. Victimization

Gang membership fills an important gap for the disenfranchised individual, providing a sense of fitting in or belonging. The gang becomes a platform for improved self-esteem for individuals who are seeking attention from society. Violence is the way of life for a gang member. When confronted with circumstances in which he or she has no control, such as being injured and taken to the Emergency Department, the gang member is pushed to react with violence, which may be the only response or reaction that the gang member knows. Rationally, if street gangs are present, especially in an Emergency Department waiting room, the opportunity for violence increases radically.

Emergency Departments located in cities are at the highest risk for violence from street gangs. Staff can often become unknowing victims of drug or gang-related feuds (Kuhn, 1999). Injured gang members feel threatened when they are suddenly thrust into an environment that is controlled by their perceived enemies such as law enforcement or medical personnel, and they will not hesitate to impose their dominance with violence.

According to Louis Savelli, a former sergeant for the New York Police Department and commander, Gang Unit, NYPD, hospitals are *not* neutral territory for street gangs. Hospitals are at enormous risk of finding themselves in the middle of gang warfare or a gang dispute (L. Savelli, personal communication, August 20, 2008). But potential attacks are not relegated to gang threats alone. Drug dealers, substance abusers, and routine criminals will attack for even simple reasons if those reasons are perceived as circumstances beyond their control. Health care workers have been attacked for making an individual wait for an extended period of time in the waiting room (Harris, 2006).

Hospitals must train Emergency Department staff to recognize potential gang activity. Street gangs can generally be recognized by unique *gang identifiers* such as the consistent use of the same color or symbol worn by a group of individuals or clothing designed by a specific designer or clothing representing a specific sports team. The presence of particular tattoos can define membership in a gang, and the appearance of a symbol that is displayed in a tattoo may identify an individual as the member of a gang. In addition, gang identifiers can be exhibited on clothing, in jewelry or on items that the gang member has in his possession such as telephone books, bandanas, or other items (Lewis, 2008). Other identifiers among gang members may be unusual body piercings, hand signals, language, hairstyles, specific brands of tennis shoes, and the types and colors of shoelaces. Encourage staff to pay particular attention to tattoos because certain tattoos are a clear and distinctive gang trait and can pinpoint the gang in which your patient may be a member. Remember the details of tattoos, including colors, symbols, and placement so that you can report information to the police department. Tattoos are catalogued so that the police and other law organizations can identify gangs and can anticipate or recognize gang activity and crime in certain areas (Lewis, 2008).

Gang members typically use special hand signals to communicate with each other. ED staff must also be educated about impending signs of potential violence from street gangs or from any individual. Caution and awareness are essential watchwords for the safety of the Emergency Department staff. Agitation is a hallmark of impending danger. Agitation as a symptom may be easy for ED professionals to identify in a patient because a physiologic state of agitation may be due to pain, anoxia, or fear in an individual who has come to the emergency room for care.[1] It is critical that the alert triage and ED staff also consider agitation as a potential warning sign of impelding gang violence that may be about to erupt. Agitation can expose a gang member who has been in a recent fight or who is looking to start a fight (L. Savelli, personal communication, August 20, 2008).

Gang members are notorious for so-called mad dogging, or staring down one another as a display of dominance. If rival gang members mad dog, the situation will usually result in violence, according to Savelli, who is President of the Homefront Protective Group, a gang information and consultation group. If mad dogging by members of a gang is directed toward emergency or hospital staff, it is an unambiguous indicator of imminent violence. Assume, unless there is a valid reason otherwise, that anyone who is mad dogging, using hand signals, or arrives on the scene after a violent fatal or nonfatal shooting victim and/or is thought to be the member of a gang will have a weapon and/or drugs in his or her possession. Be warned that the gang member will not hesitate to use a weapon on anyone for any reason, whether this is a logical conclusion or not.

It is essential that judicious vigilance be used when interacting with an individual who may be a gang member. Gang members may be reluctant to remove clothing or surrender possessions. Savelli warns that the removal of the gang colors is considered disrespectful and may result in an attack by the gang member. Anyone who challenges the gang member's beliefs or need for respect is at imminent risk for injury or death.

The one unfailing tenet that the gang member possesses is the demand for respect. If a gang member perceives disrespect from anyone, including Emergency Department staff, the outcome can be deadly. Gang members have an overarching requirement for respect and for saving face in all encounters and from every individual with whom they come in contact. The gang member will not hesitate to injure or kill someone if he believes that someone has shown disrespect to himself or his gang.

All gangs have three characteristics and three purposes. The characteristics are as follows:

1. Gangs have specific initiation rituals or activities that a potential gang member must submit to, or do, to be accepted by the gang. Initiation could include beatings by other gang members or the performance of a criminal activity. Pay close attention to patients who come into the Emergency Department who are victims of a beating because a patient who has received a beating may point to important clues about potential gang activity.

2. All gangs have a required dress code that may be represented by certain colors or sports team clothing (jackets, hats, shoes) or may be only displayed in unique tattoos or body piercings.

3. The purpose of a specific gang involves the activities that gangs do when they are together, such as activities designed to take the control of one geographical area or the painting of gang-identifying graffiti in certain areas to mark a gang's territory and to warn rival gangs of the danger they will encounter if they trespass or attempt competitive activities in this area (Moffatt, 2002). An example of gang-related graffiti can be seen in Figure 6.1.

The three purposes for gang (and for group) membership are identification, affiliation, and cohesion.

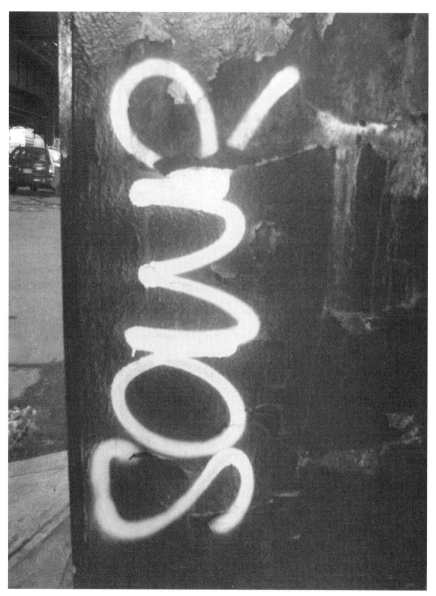

Figure 6.1

1. The identification of a gang member with a specific gang is important for the gang member to outwardly demonstrate that he belongs to a group and that his participation is valued. As discussed earlier, identification may be the driving force for membership in groups, to feel as though one belongs and is involved and committed to the activities of a group, whether as a member of a gang or as a charity volunteer. It is important for the member to have others recognize that his activities benefit the group and to have like-minded affiliation with others who think and act as he does. Teenagers seek to identify with certain things such as designer clothing, popular types of music, and the music groups or movie actors they admire and seek to emulate. Identifiers among teenagers are called peer trademarks, which are typical and normal for teenagers—even for adults—and are to be expected. Peer trademarks do not indicate participation in a violent street gang (Moffatt, 2002).
2. The second purpose of gang membership is affiliation or the need for socialization in a group of people who think and act as the gang member does. Individuals join gangs to meet needs that have not been met by society or families. Gang membership is an aberrant form of socialization and belonging.
3. Cohesion can be best described by the connection that individuals in groups or gangs have for one another. "Cohesion develops through [a] uniformity of purpose and [the recognition of] similar likes and dislikes" within the affiliations that are established. Violent gangs connect through cohesion and affiliation that tend to "provide security in a violent or dangerous environment" (Moffatt, 2002, p. 68).

The human resources departments in hospitals need to be educated about gangs, most specifically the gangs in the city and in the geographic location of your hospital. Establish a pre-employment policy stating that all potential employees must have a rigorous background check. Background checks are nearly always required by employers or companies prior to employment, but obtaining a pre-employment background check is a critical procedure for hospitals. A gang member may seek hospital jobs in the areas of pharmacy or in security as a means to gain access to drugs or guns. Make human resources aware of the possibility of gang infiltration for applicants of these two positions in particular, and educate the human resources staff about being alert to gang member identifiers such as unique tattoos or specific clothing (Mc-Adams, 2004).

When dealing with a patient who is suspected to be a gang member, remember the three Rs that will help staff understand the mentality of gangs:

1. Reputation. Reputation for a gang member is the number one requirement. The reputation of the gang is of utmost importance to each gang member; the reputation is the status marker of the gang and is to be defended at all costs. Each member of the gang expands his own personal reputation and the collective reputation of the gang through action and accomplishments.
2. Respect. Respect from all—individuals outside the gang, such as health care workers, and from other gang members—is demanded. Violence will ensue if the gang member interprets disrespect. Gangs will show disrespect to other gangs through hand signals, defacing gang graffiti, or by mad dogging.
3. Retaliation. Retaliation is the consequence for disrespect. Gangs will ultimately *always* retaliate for perceived damage to the gang reputation or for disrespect shown the gang. Retaliation is the gang tactic used to repair and restore the gang image and reputation (Grossman, 2003).

STRATEGY: TRUST YOUR GUT INSTINCTS

When Something Doesn't Feel or Look Quite Right, It Probably Isn't

Types of Street Gangs

1. Social Gangs—nonviolent gangs. The gangs may have benevolent values and purposes. Organizations such as Girl Scouts or Boy Scouts are considered gangs because these groups have the unique characteristics of gangs such as initiations, similar and identifiable clothing/uniforms, and the group provides "meaning and purpose to each other" through their association (Moffatt, 2002, p. 66). Boy and Girl Scout groups function as *social* gangs because they have beneficial service goals and support nonviolent activities.

2. Delinquent Gangs—also called tagger gangs. Typically, tagger gangs are nonviolent gangs of adolescents. This type of gang breaks the law by marring or disfiguring public property such as bridge overpasses and so forth with graffiti, which is their main activity. Tagger gangs wear baggy clothes worn as a uniform to hide spray paint and painting supplies.

3. Violent Street Gangs—violent gangs tend to glamorize violence by using violence in gang initiation, for purposes of gaining higher rankings in the gang, and for retention of gang members. Violence is not only "desirable, but necessary" (Moffatt, 2002, p. 64) for this type of gang. Another facet of gangs is that they provide the social membership and respect that the members may not ever attain in other ways, such as the esteem and acceptance from society, school peers, or parents or siblings in the home. The member of this type of gang can gain the admiration of his gang members through violence, by "enduring beatings . . . and risk[ing] prison or death" (Moffatt, 2002, p. 64).

- Racial gangs are generally violent gangs. The purpose of racial gangs is to promote the identity of the race—Black, Asian, or Hispanic—and to provide a method and direction for the anger that may be created from racism against the race or the members of the gang. Moffat explains that very youthful members are enticed to join racial gangs and often stay active for many years. Specifically in Hispanic gangs, fathers may encourage their sons' participation and propagate the family involvement in the gang. Neo-Nazi or skinhead gangs are White supremacist gangs and are extremely violent and angry because of their strong, radical beliefs that the White race is the dominant, perfect race. Skinheads have shaven heads to demonstrate their association with the gang, which explains the gang name *skinheads.* Typically skinheads use Ku Klux Klan symbols, swastikas, and other Nazi symbols in their tattoos and other items. Hate groups often wear colored shoelaces to identify their association with the gang and to indicate their views: white shoelaces demonstrate so-called White power, red shoelaces warn that the gang member is "prepared to harm or kill" (Moffatt, 2002, p. 65), and green shoelaces demonstrate that the gang member is a gay basher.

- The Ku Klux Klan is another White supremacist gang in which members clothe themselves in white hoods and robes that are well-known symbols recognized primarily for terror and violence directed toward African American populations, especially in the U.S. South from the 1950s through the 1970s. The violence of the Ku Klux Klan consisted of cross burnings, intimidation, lynchings, and bombings and burning of African American places of worship, businesses, and homes. The Ku Klux Klan, or the KKK, has been in operation since 1865 with its origin in Pulaski, Tennessee. The KKK is classified as a hate group although it was not initially formed for the purposes of conducting hate crimes. The anti-KKK Act was passed by Congress in 1971. Today the KKK has 5,000 to 8,000 members ("A Brief History of the Original KKK," 2009).
- Motorcycle gangs can be violent gangs, such as the gang of Hell's Angels, but can also simply be the affiliation of like-minded individuals who enjoy camaraderie with other motorcycle owners. Often these gangs wear specific uniforms and promote similar causes.
- Ethnically diverse gangs such as Folk Nation or People Nation are violent gangs. Gangs that have different ethnic members are unusual because part of the function of gangs is to strengthen the ethnicity within the gang for a strong united front.
- Female gangs are sometimes referred to as gangsta-lettes, and membership in female gangs is growing rapidly. In the past, the female role in a gang was that of the girlfriend of the gang member. The female supported the male gang member by carrying his weapons, driving a getaway car, or committing burglary. Between 1981 and 1997, female arrests for various illegal gang activity increased 103%, and aggravated assault by females increased by 57% between 1990 and 1999 (Moffatt, 2002, p. 66). Until very recently, females used knives or their fists to commit violence and assault, but the incidence of violent criminal acts and homicide is rising among the female gang population. There were 8,000 female gang members in California in 2000 with the majority of them (75%) located in Los Angeles (Moffatt, 2002, p. 66).

GANG VIOLENCE = COLLECTIVE VIOLENCE

Gangs are considered by sociologists to be a collective of perpetrators of violent behavior. The development of gangs and specific gang culture is dependent on the section of a city in which the gang was formed. For example, gangs that form within a ghetto or inner city are primarily comprised of members who are of lower socioeconomic status. The members of this gang appear to function as if they live in a society that they have created, acting with indifference to the police and leaders of the U.S. society and government. The gangs do have active and frequently violent transgressions with police authority, but the members of the inner-city gangs seem to act and believe that they are "independent of society and its laws" (Moffatt, 2002, p. 72).The middle-class gangs, on the other hand, tend to be left of center and aggressive toward the upper social class and age structure (Moffatt, 2002).

Lou Savelli has worked with gangs since he was young and a member of a local gang himself. Back then, Savelli recounts, all young kids were involved in some type of hoodlum youth gang (tagger gangs), but the gangs in the 1970s were very different from the gangs today. The gangs today are much more violent and have specific agendas of violence and control (L. Savelli, personal communication, August 20, 2008). Gangs have "increasingly violent behavior and use sophisticated weapons" according to Greg Moffatt (2002, p. 72), who adds that part of the activities of violent street gangs in U.S. cities today are turf wars, illegal drug trafficking and trade, and robbery (p. 69).

Savelli credits his parents with their unconditional involvement in his life, insisting and pushing him to choose the good path and not the path that would have resulted, perhaps, in his participation in violent street gangs or in the mafia in his primarily Italian neighborhood in Brooklyn (L. Savelli, personal communication, August 20, 2008).

All of us who are of a certain age group probably remember our first exposure to street gangs from the movie *West Side Story*. The blockbuster musical portrayed the Puerto Rican and White gangs in New York City in the 1960s. The gang members, amidst their lively group dancing and singing, blatantly boasted and portrayed their power, giving the audience a view of the potential danger of gangs by wielding big switchblades and instigating aggressive activities. The typical citizen's awareness of gang activity that is present in U.S. cities today may be relegated to the uniform of baggy, low-slung jeans that may represent the youth's interest or membership in a gang. Or citizens may be aware of graffiti that has popped up even in more-affluent neighborhoods. The perception that gang activity in a given city is low or nonexistent is a very dangerous perception. Likewise, Emergency Departments who believe that gang activity and violence *can't happen here* leave themselves open and vulnerable to the unplanned and unexpected incursion of gangs. It can happen, and it will, especially for those EDs that are not prepared. Having a plan to recognize and manage gangs, even if potential gang incidents are—or are perceived to be—rare is the very best defense strategy.

Recently in Nashville, Tennessee, Savelli was the featured speaker at a convention of 1,500 law enforcement officers, security officers, and other individuals who attended the seminar to learn more about gangs in the Southeast. Savelli confirmed that gang involvement and the potential for gang violence in the city are generally downplayed by law enforcement professionals in Nashville.

STRATEGIES FOR DEALING WITH LOCAL GANGS

The best strategy for learning about the infiltration of local gangs in your hospital's geographic area is to have ongoing communication with the local police department. There may be several officers who are the gang specialists or experts in your city or geographic region or who have a particular interest in gangs and gang culture. The local police officers who deal with gangs on an everyday basis can be dynamic resources. Ask the gang specialist at the local police department to speak to your Emergency Department staff for a hospital or Emergency Department in-service. Videotape the presentation so that the information can be dispersed and communicated easily and frequently throughout the hospital. Your most important strategy is to know that gangs exist and be prepared—in advance—to deal with all and any gang infiltration into your hospital. Pay attention to all clues, such as types of injuries being treated in your ED, graffiti on the hospital campus, incidents occurring at other hospitals, and briefings from the local police department that may present strong evidence of gang activity or the increase in gang activity.

Your hospital's security staff/department is a critical partner with the Emergency Department staff for protection against gang infiltration. Security rounds in and around the Emergency Department must include being on the lookout for graffiti markings. Graffiti is the gang's method for marking a territory or for warning away other gangs. If graffiti is found, it is important to photograph the graffiti and communicate the presence of graffiti to the security staff and the Emergency Department. It is highly recommended that the graffiti is not crossed out because this action is seen as disrespectful to the gang and may result in retaliation by the gang. Have the graffiti professionally covered or removed or replace the item that has been permanently defaced if necessary (McAdams, 2004).

Ask security to e-mail the photograph to the local police department and request help, if necessary, to identify specific information about the gang and the interpretation of the graffiti symbols. Ask the security staff to catalog the graffiti by date and location and keep a record of all photographed graffiti in the security office. It is essential that the Emergency Department and the security staff have an established and consistent method for communicating information about gangs or other violent activity between departments (McAdams, 2004).

Communicate the presence of graffiti to all stakeholders within the hospital and share any information that has been received from the local police department. Also communicate to staff when the graffiti has been removed so that all staff can be alerted to new graffiti markings on property around the hospital campus, specifically in the area of the Emergency Department (McAdams, 2004).

CHECKLIST OF BEHAVIORS TO ANTICIPATE FROM A PATIENT WHO MAY BE A GANG MEMBER

Remain constantly aware of potential threats in the form of:

- Hostile cues, especially the apparent use of hand signals
- Body language that may indicate aggression (see Exhibit 6.2)
- Restlessness, agitation, or pacing
- Loud speech, especially the progression of loud speech to shouting or yelling
- Profanity
- Staring or mad dogging (L. Savelli, personal communication, August 20, 2008).

CHECKLIST OF HOW TO COMMUNICATE WITH A PATIENT WHO MAY BE A GANG MEMBER

- Be very patient
- Be very professional
- Do not show fear
- Minimize eye contact
- Avoid the use of hand gestures
- Give the gang member patient a sense of control
- Allow the gang member patient to make as many decisions as possible (e.g., choosing to have an IV in the left arm or right hand)
- Don't preach or parent
- Be nonjudgmental and open-minded
- Be a good listener
- Treat the gang member patient's belongings with respect
- Be cautious and vigilant
- Clear the room of any items that could potentially be used as a weapon
- Post security guard or police immediately outside the door
- Ask the local police gang experts for advice on how to remind the gang member that EDs are not to be used for gang warfare and that hand signals are not permitted in the ED (Grossman, 2003).

Savelli suggests that the Emergency Department staff pay close attention when a patient who may be a member of a gang arrives in the Emergency Department. Notice any clues that the belongings may provide, such as a clue about what may happen next, and be alert to the possibility that other gang members or a rival gang may show up in the ED. Does the patient have a weapon? Is it possible that he has committed a crime? What type of injuries does he have?

Savelli says that rap music and videos have a significant influence on youth and entice youth to get involved in gangs. Popular professional football, basketball, and other sports figures often flaunt their own gang membership. Displaying their multiple and specific tattoos and heavy chains and earrings, these aberrant role models underscore the notion that gangs are cool. Often schools can help propagate the correct messages that gangs are dangerous and crime-ridden and have an agenda that may lead to incarceration or death. Adolescents and teens, especially young boys, can mistakenly interpret that the fame, wealth, and success achieved by sports heroes/gang members as stemming from the active participation in a gang, which of course is not accurate. As with the other crime-based organizations, the allure of the unknown and the glamorous-appearing life of a gang member can be exciting and may appear to offer an opportunity to achieve the things in life that are otherwise unattainable.

Savelli encourages frequent and open communication with the police department, as they can share information about the gangs in the local area. The police departments generally have a gang task force or specialists who will be willing to provide education about gangs. Savelli's one final piece of information is to be certain that the Emergency Department is committed to making changes to protect the staff from the danger of gangs and to establish processes and enhance education and training so that circumstances that warrant communication with the police department are consistently reported to the authorities.

One important piece of advice from author Kelly McAdams is that when researching information about gangs on the Internet one should search only the sites that are sponsored by law enforcement, educational sites (National Education Association [NEA] for example), and gang-prevention groups (McAdams, 2004).

Lou Savelli and Kelly McAdams agree on one very important point: it does not matter where your hospital is located. Hospitals in cities, suburbs, small towns, and rural communities are not immune to gang violence. Savelli encourages all Emergency Departments, when it comes to the safety of the ED staff, to "err on the side of safety" (Savelli, 2008).

CASE STUDY

Kelly McAdams, RN, CCRN, MSN, CNS, at Palmetto Health/Richland, in Columbia, South Carolina, shares a gang experience in her 2004 article, Gangstas—Not in My Hospital! *(McAdams, 2004). EMS transported a young man to the Emergency Department for treatment of gunshot wounds to the chest. Soon after his arrival, the waiting room was filled with many individuals, all wearing similar red clothing and accessories. When a nurse went to the waiting room to update the family about the patient's condition, the crowd became rowdy and several began screaming and swearing. One of the people in the crowd, dressed in red, violently pushed a nurse.*

(Continued)

The scenario that Ms. McAdams depicts is precisely the type of situation that must be prevented and avoided in Emergency Departments. Circumstances similar to the one that Ms. McAdams describes can rapidly escalate to a violent free-for-all with ED nurses, physicians, and staff—and even patients—who may be caught in the middle of potential gunfire and unpredictable violence.

CASE STUDY

PRO-GUN LEGISLATION

"On July 1st," 2008, three days before the U.S. celebrated the 232nd anniversary of national Independence, *"Florida became the fourth state to allow people to bring guns to work"* (*"Gun Control,"* 2008). There is a requirement for a concealed weapons permit, and the gun must be locked in the owner's car. Nonetheless, guns have suddenly become a more prevalent issue in Florida. For the gun owner who is employed at a hospital, a school, a prison, or a power plant, guns are not permitted on the premises. Employers must adhere to a don't ask, don't tell restriction and refrain from asking their employees if they have a gun in the glove compartment of the car. The Economist *reports that Florida has issued one-half of a million concealed weapon permits in recent months and is now the U.S. state with the greatest number of gun-carrying citizens (*"Gun Control,"* 2008).*

Texas is buoyed by the recent news that the Supreme Court has acted to overturn the Washington, DC, gun ban. Texas has gone one step further, pushing for a measure that would permit the open carrying of handguns that is reminiscent of the Old West. An online petition supporting the change in law has garnered much interest. Eighteen thousand people, to date, have signed the petition encouraging legislators to pass the law. Texas citizens are interested in urging the passage of a law allowing individuals to be able to take their guns to work, as Floridians do.

(Continued)

Guns frequently fall into the hands of individuals who have evil or illicit intentions, those who wish to take matters into their own hands, or angry employees who do not consider the consequences of showing up at a former boss's office and doing him in. The other serious concern is the action of an unstable individual with a gun who may wish to influence those in unprotected Emergency Departments or the youth who is angered by a schoolmate or an unfair teacher and cannot or does not fully think through the consequences of such action. And what of Emergency Departments, not fortified by barriers of security staff or metal detectors, who admit a patient with a concealed weapon who has a plan to use it? Those are the circumstances that result in Emergency Department melees, leaving Emergency Department nurses and physicians at risk for injury and career-ending assaults—or worse.

VIOLENCE IN THE WORKPLACE: LATERAL VIOLENCE, HORIZONTAL HOSTILITY, OR WORKPLACE VIOLENCE

Violence is the second leading cause of death in the workplace (Cooper, 2005). Violence in the Emergency Department is most often caused by patients who are psychotic, feel vulnerable, or out of control (Butler, 2002) or who are frustrated by the lengthy wait to obtain medical care. Other direct causes of violence in the Emergency Department are those patients who are hemodynamically unstable or may be in pain. Violence can be caused by the families of patients or former patients, by an assailant without an identifiable reason, or by gang members.

Lateral violence is a type of interpersonal violence among workers and is a very serious sociological phenomenon deserving of attention and solutions, but lateral violence is not to be confused with violence in the ED. Lateral violence is only one aspect of violence that can occur in the Emergency Department. Emergency Department violence is a much broader issue.

Lateral violence, a relatively new term, refers to the incidence of violence in the workplace or the violence or abuse caused by a coworker. Lateral violence, sometimes called horizontal hostility, can occur in all workplaces and not only in hospitals or Emergency Departments. The

Occupational Safety and Health Administration (OSHA), involved in the promotion of violence-free workplaces, has defined a safe workplace as a work environment that is free of violent threats, actions, and hazards and a workplace devoid of events that are likely to cause death or serious emotional or physical harm (*Guidelines for Preventing Workplace Violence,* n.d.). In the past decade, we have become all too familiar with incidents of lateral violence occurring in post offices and in high schools and universities across the U.S., perpetrated by a fellow student or a former employee who apparently has gone berserk. Lateral violence can range from demeaning or belittling remarks to violent attacks and homicide.

According to Dr. Rosemary Erickson, a forensic sociologist, the majority of workplace violence is not the highly reported media event depicting shootings of innocent victims in public workplaces or on campuses (Kohl, 2006). Instead, 75% of lateral violence is related to robbery, while 25% of lateral violence constitutes those violent workplace incidents that we hear about all too frequently. Lateral violence can often result from a broadening of intimate partner violence (IPV) or the exacerbation of a psychotic episode. Coworker-against-coworker violence accounts for only 10% of the total occurrence of lateral violence in the U.S., but lateral violence is, nonetheless, a serious and growing concern for companies (Kohl, 2006). The 10% of coworker aggression/lateral violence is the type of violence that may affect Emergency Department personnel. These personnel need to be acutely aware of this danger, no matter how statistically extraordinary the occurrences can be.

Dr. Erickson noted in an article on the Web site SecurityInfoWatch. com that there has been a recent increase in this type of violence (Kohl, 2006). The difficulty lies in the fact that lateral violence does not correspond to typical criminal behavior and is not committed by individuals who represent commonplace criminals. Lateral violence is committed by ordinary individuals—your coworker or the guy sitting next to you in class.

The danger of lateral or workplace violence needs to be communicated more aggressively to individuals to arm them with tools to help staff, students, and workers recognize the type of individual in one's office, Emergency Department, or classroom who may be prone to acts of violence. Additionally, workplaces need to define clear expectations for workers to report suspicious individuals or behavior to help prevent potential episodes of lateral violence.

PROACTIVE SECURITY

Most workplaces, especially hospitals and Emergency Departments, have a plan for reacting when and if a violent episode erupts, but every workplace in the U.S. should throw out the book on crisis management and instead commit resources to the development of a proactive security plan that is designed to *prevent* the occurrence of violence in the workplace. The security goal of every company should be the proactive—not reactive—use of security. "We can get caught up . . . and too focused on the hardware and the gates and the cameras and need to consider the human element," says Dr. Erickson (quoted in Kohl, 2006).

A well-designed proactive security plan should contain:

1. Awareness plan, communicated to every employee
2. A focus on the human element, profiling the characteristics of a potential aggressor
3. Violence prevention training, including de-escalation tactics that include:
   a. Eye contact dos and don'ts
   b. Active listening
   c. Permission to vent, in appropriate settings, to dissipate anger and frustration
   d. Recognition of body language that may reveal frustration or aggression
   e. Self-awareness of our gestures, posture, and facial expressions
   f. Granting of personal space
4. Mitigation of the potential for violence in certain circumstances (e.g., during a firing or layoff)
5. Definitions of the different types of workplace violence
6. Reporting policies including an environment that encourages the reporting of violent incidents, episodes of aggressive, or violent lateral behavior and suspicious behavior or individuals

Profiling or identifying individuals who may exhibit the potential for workplace violence could be the key to preventing the horrific outcomes as experienced by Columbine High School, Virginia Tech University, the post office, and of many other less-publicized workplace injuries and homicides. Individuals who have the propensity for violence can display the following five characteristics:

1. May be angry
2. May be loners (have not made workplace relationships)
3. May have made threats against the company
4. May have an obsession with weapons
5. May be male (90% of all workplace aggression is committed by males) (Kohl, 2006)

An overall security plan should help every employee or student identify coworkers or classmates who may erupt in violence without active or intentional provocation.

LATERAL VIOLENCE IN THE ED

Lateral violence in the ED, as in other companies, can create emotional trauma and loss of employee morale and can result in the development of a hostile environment. Veteran nurses' reproachful or condescending comments to less experienced nurses, due perhaps to a lack of knowledge, or the harsh, derogatory comments to ED personnel from a frustrated physician, are only a few examples of lateral violence in the ED.

Donna Mason, immediate past president of the Emergency Nurses Association and former director of the adult ED at Vanderbilt University Medical Center, insists that her staff report any incidents of demeaning or belittling comments from anyone. "This kind of behavior [lateral violence] is . . . unacceptable" she has said ("Survey: Most ED Staff Victimized by Violence Never Report Incident," 2007). Creating an environment that encourages the reporting of any type of lateral violence is a critical and key step toward ensuring the safety and confidence of the personnel in the Emergency Department, in hospitals, and in all workplaces, according to Dr. Rosemary Erickson (Kohl, 2006). It is crucial that all employees are educated and made aware of the characteristics of the workplace aggressor who may have the potential for violence and to understand the definitions of lateral violence so that episodes of lateral violence can be recognized as such. It is essential for each employee to take responsibility for reporting any act of violence and to be trained in the reporting of any incident of lateral violence ("Survey: Most ED Staff Victimized by Violence Never Report Incident," 2007). Lateral violence is never OK.

The characteristics of lateral violence are replicated in Exhibit 6.4.

Exhibit 6.4

CHARACTERISTICS OF LATERAL VIOLENCE CHECKLIST TOOL

ARE YOU A VICTIM—OR A PERPETRATOR?

Aggressive or mocking body language such as raising eyebrows or rolling eyes

Making faces

Verbal retorts, abrupt responses, vulgar language

Undermining behavior such as ignoring questions, constantly criticizing, or excluding individuals from discussion

Withholding necessary information or advice

Sabotage, such as setting up a new hire for failure

Infighting and bickering

Scapegoating

Blaming and gossiping behind a colleague's back

Failure to respect privacy or breaking a confidence

Shouting, yelling, or other intimidating behavior

Judging others regarding age, gender, sexual orientation, ethnicity, or body size

Physical violence

CASE STUDY

As I learn more about lateral violence, I am surprised and very disappointed that the nursing profession seems to be at the forefront of this abusive and violent tactic. No matter what you prefer to call it, it is all the same. I could not imagine that the angels of mercy, the pet name that nurses have been called for many years, could purposely hurt each other. The top 10 types of lateral violence are nonverbal innuendo, verbal affront, undermining activities, withholding of information, sabotage, infighting, scapegoating, backstabbing, failure to respect privacy, and broken confidences.

I was stunned when I realized that I—and my other coworkers—had been victims of blatant lateral abuse from one of our supervisors. We knew that bullying was wrong; we just didn't know that bullying was lateral violence.

(Continued)

I encourage each of you to learn as much as possible about lateral violence and to spearhead education and initiate policies and workplace change to combat it. I further encourage you to view the YouTube video depicting nurse against nurse abuse or violence. Unfortunately, I think each of you may recognize what you see . . . http://www.youtube.com/watch?v=mBCRBaLHR1k and the following YouTube video from HCPro. http://www.youtube.com/watch?v=4MT8Wnb9ZY8&feature=related

We have all heard it for years, and I am beginning to believe it is true: nurses eat their young . . .

The case study of lateral violence among nurses is my own personal experience, illustrated here.

Each of us has been in the position of being the new employee. Being new is a very uncomfortable place to be, but I was excited about a new position with the opportunity to learn an entirely new set of skills and gain confidence and expertise. This is the job that I had been wanting—the one that I went to graduate school to find.

One of the directors of the department was in charge of a specific project that we would all be working on. I had no background in the essentials that I would need to know to function expertly, so I was excited to learn all that I could. When I approached the director to ask how I could begin to learn the procedures, I was surprised—and disillusioned—when she told me, in a mocking tone, to read the manual and to then ask for clarification for anything I did not understand. Because I had not known before this time that a manual existed, I did as she asked but refrained from asking additional questions, so as not to put myself in a position of feeling inept. Over the course of the next year, there were many bullying incidents from this same department director, against everyone with whom she interacted. I was resolute in knowing that I was not the only victim of her lateral violence.

I never was able to become comfortable or confident in the skills that I was expected to learn. Within 1 year, I resigned because I had found a position that I hoped would be supportive and empowering. If I had known then what I have since learned about lateral violence, I would have reported the incidents to my supervisor and

(Continued)

to the appropriate corporate human resources department at the company. Lateral abuse is as offensive as patient abuse and violence. Lateral violence is violence against you, and any transgression needs to be reported immediately!

COMBATING LATERAL VIOLENCE: NURSE AGAINST NURSE

Dr. Barry Stein, a psychologist in British Columbia, is a specialist in workplace aggression, harassment, and violence. Dr. Stein sums up the problem of nursing lateral violence:

"One of the real challenges is that most nurses are being worked off their feet.[2] Lateral violence may be due to nurses displacing stress and aggression on one another." Dr. Stein knows that nursing "workloads are reported to be at unsustainable levels, particularly in light of the fact that the average age of nurses is increasing at the same time that the industry is anticipating a significant staffing shortage." The nursing profession is depicted as the "pink ghetto." Dr. Stein explains that the [nursing] industry has had very little success recruiting men into the field because the image of nursing is that nursing is still a very female profession. (Pugh, 2005–2006)

Judith Tompkins, chief of Nursing Practice and Professional Services and executive vice president of the Programs at the Centre for Addiction and Mental Health (CAMH), in Toronto, reveals that a 2003 study conducted and reported in the *Journal of Advanced Nursing* discovered that "Fifty percent (50%) of newly qualified nurses report first-hand experience with lateral violence" says Linda Rabyj, a registered psychiatric RN in Canada (Pugh, 2005–2006). Part of the problem lies with the experienced nurses who have unrealistic expectations of new graduates, assuming and expecting that these new graduate nurses can "hit the ground running" says Judith Tompkins (Pugh, 2005–2006). We all know that this is not the case nor should any experienced nurse expect this of a new graduate RN. Unrealistic expectations can lead to a "lack of collegiality and mentoring from peers," according to Tompkins (Pugh, 2005–2006), leaving the younger or inexperienced nurse to feel thrown to the wolves.

Dr. Martha Griffin, a lateral violence specialist in Boston and at Brigham and Women's Hospital, believes that the high incidence of lateral violence in nursing is derived from the limited control that nurses have over their hospital work environment. She explains the problem as nurses having significant responsibility and "accountability" coupled with an insignificant amount of autonomy says (Pugh, 2005–2006). Dr. Griffin further explains that high accountability and low autonomy describes the behavior of "oppressed groups" whose conflicts, much like nurses and hospital nursing, develop because of limited involvement in the "power structure" (Pugh, 2005–2006). In other words, nurses are expected to control the good outcomes of their patients but have little input into the methods used such as diagnostics, treatments, hours of work, and expectations of work to improve the outcome of the patient. This is, after all, the nature of nursing. Physicians expect orders to be completed as they have designated, and the nurse manager of the Unit and the Chief Nursing Officer (CNO) rarely ask the nurse for her input relative to unit organization or hospital-wide problems and solutions (Pugh, 2005–2006). (The Chief Nursing Officer is the executive administrative leader of nursing for a hospital. Previously, when hospitals were organized differently, the Director of Nursing was the "nurse in charge" of nursing for a hospital. The Chief Nursing Officer has an expanded role from that of the Director of Nursing.)

Before lateral violence was identified as a problem at Brigham and Women's Hospital, Dr. Griffin reports that *60% of nurses left within a 6-month period of hire, specifically because of lateral violence.* Griffin implemented a "cognitive-behavioral-based awareness program" to address and combat the issue of lateral violence and achieved an improvement in retention rate from 60% to a remarkable 94% (Pugh, 2005–2006). The program begins by "naming the problem" (Pugh, 2005–2006). Much as with eating disorders, if people do not call workplace disorders, including lateral violence, what they are, there is no way to fix the problem because no one knows with what they are dealing. The other successful program attributes are a "zero tolerance for lateral violence" policy and the promotion of a healthy workplace as mandated by OSHA (Pugh, 2005–2006). Additionally, the empowerment of nurses to advocate for themselves and the introduction and application of tools or simple methods to combat lateral violence have been shown to have a positive influence on reducing episodes of nurse resignation. "Lateral violence cannot thrive when employers become ethically and legally responsible" (Linda Rabyj, quoted in Pugh, 2005–2006). One important aspect of a zero tolerance policy against lateral violence is to mandate that nurses report any incident of lateral violence to which they are subjected. Hospital (and other) administration officials have an obligation to ensure simple and quick reporting methods and guaranteed follow-up with the nurse reporting the abuse. The guarantee must include a statement that the nurse will have no consequence for reporting the abuse.

Unrestrained or ignored episodes of lateral violence in the workplace can result in behavioral side effects including the excessive use of alcohol, smoking (new habit), abuse of prescription medication, decreased productivity and/or creativity, an increase in orientation time, the use of excessive sick leave and benefits, and low staff retention (Pugh, 2005–2006).

TRUE ACCOUNTS OF VIOLENCE IN THE EMERGENCY DEPARTMENT

The account of the gunman presented in Chapter 3 who surreptitiously entered the Emergency Department and committed homicide was fabricated. The possibility of analogous accounts of violence is sadly not far from reality as revealed in the following real-life violence scenarios.

Patient Violence Against a Nurse

A gang member, for no apparent reason other than a long wait in the emergency room, smacked a nurse in the face. On another occasion, a prostitute threatened the lives of everyone in a doctor's waiting room just because she felt threatened by the way the other waiting patients were looking at her.

Gang Violence

Several years ago, at a local hospital in Brooklyn's Sunset Park neighborhood, an ED patient involved in a car accident would not relinquish his clothing to a nurse. He was later observed passing a bag to a friend (a fellow gang member). When officers responded, it was discovered that the bag contained two pounds of marijuana ready for sale and that the person who took possession of the bag was armed with a gun. Had a nurse or security officer intervened further, the drug dealers were prepared to kill.

Domestic Violence and Assault of Emergency Room Staff

Arriving home intoxicated, a 22-year-old man became angry when his wife questioned him about where he had been. He punched his hand through the glass-topped coffee table in his living room and proceeded to follow his wife to the bedroom where he rubbed the blood from his lacerated hand onto her face. When he finally agreed to be treated at the Emergency Department, he assaulted an emergency room staffer by throwing blood on her.

Threatened Assault of Emergency Room Staff

The waiting area of the hospital was evacuated when a woman told hospital security personnel that she had a bomb in her bag. A search revealed that there was no bomb.

Substance Abuse Violence

An Emergency Department RN in Las Vegas, Nevada, reports being thrown against the wall by someone on drugs according to the victim, a 50-year veteran RN. ED nurses are frightened and encourage action to control the events occurring in the Emergency Department. In a New Jersey general hospital that maintains a small five-bed behavioral health unit, nurses have endured direct punches and having youthful patients leap at them over a barrier and threaten to kill the nurse when the patient is released.

Substance/Alcohol-Related Abuse or Abuse by Mentally Ill Patient Toward an Emergency Room Physician

Dr. David Golan, Emergency Department physician in Las Vegas, Nevada, is a 6-foot-tall, 180-pound "fitness enthusiast." He reports having his face pummeled by a patient who shouted, "I'm going to kill you." The situation required Dr. Golan to subdue the patient in a headlock while security held the man and an RN injected a sedative to control the patient's outburst (Harasim, 2005).

Psychiatric Violence

Three emergency department physicians in Southern California were shot by a deranged patient. Two of the MDs can no longer practice medicine. Following the incident, the hospital installed metal detectors at the ED entrance.

Patient Violence Against a Nurse

A 28-year-old patient demanded attention from an emergency department RN in Memphis, Tennessee. The nurse responded that she would attend to him after she finished caring for another patient. The patient picked up a metal chair and beat the nurse with the chair. The nurse sustained a contusion to her arm and a dislocated thumb. When interviewed, the hospital stated that the episode was one that occurred rarely. The hospital further commented that its new security measures have helped prevent further injury.

A triage RN in New Jersey was taking a patient's history when the family of another patient approached, complaining and angry that his relative had not received care quickly enough. He pulled a gun on the nurse and demanded immediate care. The nurse complied; no shooting occurred. Security subdued the individual. The nurse was so traumatized that she could never work in an ED again.

Potential Violence Against a Physician

The adept assessment by a receptionist in the physician's office near Duke University may have thwarted a violent outburst by a patient when she recognized the patient's agitation in response to typical registration questions asked of a patient. The physician talked to the patient but was unable to get the man to answer any questions. A second appointment was made for the man, and the physician admits being very apprehensive at the thought of the patient's appointment. The patient would not allow blood to be drawn, and he later called the receptionist and complained that he was unfairly treated, adding that no one had treated him with such disrespect since Vietnam. An appointment made with the physician's partner was not kept. The physician hesitated to discharge the patient from his practice for fear the patient would become unruly and even dangerous. The physician recommends being realistic about potential danger from patients or families and urges advance preparation to elicit assistance if it becomes necessary.

Potential Visitor/Gang Member Violence Against a Nurse

Patricia, the ED RN, 8 hours into her 12-hour shift, attended to an Emergency Department patient who was a gunshot victim and had been transported to the ED by EMT/paramedics. Patricia was searching for the victim's family when she was approached by three individuals who informed her they were cousins of the victim. Fortunately, the nurse was suspicious enough to suspect the group was not related to the victim but surmised that they could be gang members. Patricia proactively contacted security for advice and protection. Both a gun and a knife were found on the unrelated visitors (Ray, 2007, p. 257).

Other Chronicles

- A 6-foot-4-inch-tall, 280-pound intoxicated man strikes and kicks his experienced Emergency Department nurse.
- A disgruntled family member kills a San Diego Emergency Department nurse and a paramedic student.
- A nurse is shot by her estranged husband while working in a clinic. A second nurse is killed as she tries to help her fatally wounded coworker.
- A nurse is thrown to the floor by her patient. A patient threatens his nurse with rape and murder. A nurses' aide is knocked unconscious by a patient (Cooper, 2005).
- A teenaged boy, a patient in the behavioral unit of an acute-care hospital, became enraged when a nurse requested to search his pockets. He vaulted over the wall of the nurses' station and lunged at her. "He went to punch me," she recalls. "He grabbed me by my glasses, which broke. A therapist tackled him and held him back until help could come. He threatened to kill me and my family when he got out" (Carmiel, 2007).

INTERNATIONAL PERSPECTIVE OF VIOLENCE IN ACCIDENT AND EMERGENCY DEPARTMENTS AND HOSPITALS

The U.S. does not hold the record for having the most encounters with violent crime committed in Emergency Departments and hospitals.

Canada, Australia, and Europe experience many violent episodes daily and, in fact, appear to have a greater number than the U.S. Is the reason that other countries seem to be subjected to more violence in the ED because there is more occurrence of violent crime in other countries or simply because they report more of the incidents that occur?

There is only a small amount of journalistic evidence of violence in U.S. Emergency Departments when compared with news from other countries. According to an article in the *Iraqi Journal of Nursing Scholarship*, "workplace violence has become an alarming phenomenon worldwide" (AbuAlRub, 2007, p. 281) and the article confirms that workplace violence occurs daily in the health sector in Iraq. Iraqi ambulance personnel incur the greatest exposure to violence, and hospital nurses are the second-most exposed individuals. Living in the midst of a war naturally creates stress among the population and may be responsible for the increase in abnormal psychological patient conditions that may show up in the local emergency rooms. Limited support from lawmakers is a significant risk factor for Iraqi nurses. Many nurses have requested training programs to assist them in learning ways to avoid violence and added that the enforcement of policies and legislation are two important steps that the government could take to help nurses control Iraqi hospital violence (AbuAlRub, 2007).

An interesting summary of an article from the Scottish journal *Applied Economics* has shown that an increase in the number of violence-related injuries treated in emergency rooms in Scotland equates to the price of beer. The research is from Cardiff University's Violence and Society Research Group and the study's conclusion is that a "1% rise in the real price of alcohol equates to an economy wide reduction in ED assault cases of 5000 per year" (Cardiff University Violence and Society Research Group, 2007, p. 670). The study, conducted in 2007, also determined that rising rates of poverty, unemployment, and the diversity of ethnic populations influenced the increase in violence-related injuries, which tended to also escalate in the summer months and during the occurrence of a major sporting event

A Tasmanian (Australia) newspaper, the *Mercury*, published an article in May of 2007 reporting that 350 "Code Black" alarms had been sounded in the past 12 months in response to threats of aggression or actual violence toward hospital staff or patients (Worley, 2007). Code Black alarms are similar to the U.S. 911 system, but Code Blacks are specifically activated for hospital violence or potential violence. Three hundred and fifty Code Black alarms average to nearly 90 per hospital for each of Tasmania's four hospitals, or one alarm per day for one entire week every month! When questioned, the health minister seemed as unaware of the violent occurrences in emergency departments and hospitals as is our own former president.[3] The health minister remarked that she did not want to "inflate this because it is not a huge issue." Clearly our public servants, globally, need to be educated about the reality of violence in emergency rooms and hospitals. The acting secretary of the Australian Nursing Federation retorted that nurses were "moving away from the profession because of aggression and violence in [their] workplace" (Worley, 2007).

In April, 2007, Israeli surgeons and entire hospital staffs throughout Israel went on strike for 2 hours in protest of increasing hospital violence, spurred by a recent episode of violence. A urological surgeon was stabbed by a disgruntled patient who demanded a certain procedure but did not receive the particular surgery. The article, published on the *Israel National News* Web site, states that a nurse was attacked 2 weeks prior and that an additional, similar incident had occurred within the past 2 months. Dr. Ricardo Alfisi, head of surgery at Hillel Yaffe Hospital, alluded to the problem as one that has been created by a lack of surgeons in Israel, causing increased waiting times for surgery, high tensions, and aggression among patients. The strike was staged to demand increased public awareness of hospital danger from violence and to forewarn the public of an increase in police presence in hospitals (Fendel, 2007).

Japanese nurses, too, have experienced much patient abuse and violence in hospitals. In 2006, more than 250 hospital employees—all employed by the Tokyo Metropolitan Hospital Association, which represents a large number of national, public, and private hospitals—quit their jobs after being physically and/or verbally abused by patients "in the course of their work" (Shimbun, 2008). Much of the reason determined to be at the root of patient abuse in Japan is the startling lack of physicians and nurses to care for hospitalized patients. Staff complained that their employers were not being proactive enough to engage in solutions. Seventy percent of hospitals in another health care association, the Aichi Medical Association, report incidents of violence. The Shizuoka Hospital Association has taken a positive stance by holding the country's first symposium in a search for answers to the growing epidemic of violence in Japan (Shimbun, 2008).

While clearly older data, a 2001 scientific study conducted in British Columbia concluded that violent episodes are frequent in the emergency department and that those violent episodes, including physical assault, adversely affected the ED staff. Furthermore, the same report determined that educational programs, while a temporary solution to reducing the number of violent events, do not diminish violence in the long term (Fernandez, 2002, p. 53).

CASE STUDY

BRITISH COLUMBIA NURSES ARE REGULAR TARGETS OF VIOLENCE

An Emergency Department RN with 12 years of experience thought she would have a typical day in the ED, but this day was her last one at work. The nurse was the victim of a violent assault when she was kicked very hard in the back by a patient who was a drug abuser. The injury aggravated a previous injury, resulting in the nurse's permanent and chronic disability, rendering her unable to work again. The nurse charged the patient with assault and he was sentenced to 2 years incarceration.

The University of British Columbia has conducted interviews with 50 nurses, regarding their experience with violence from patients while they were at work. The results confirmed that nurses "routinely encountered verbal abuse and physical violence" and that "nursing is a physically dangerous job." Nurses typically expect abuse in normal interactions with patients and families, but the report uncovered that the nurses were "profoundly affected by the level of unnecessary abuse directed at them." Abusive acts toward the nurses have affected the productivity and the retention of nurses.

"[Abuse] is a growing problem because violence . . . is not being addressed, despite zero tolerance policies," said the president of the Canadian Federation of Nurses Unions. She added that it is difficult to focus on the issue of violence and abuse when the staffing shortages are "so acute." She states that the problem of understaffing tends to intensify other issues and increases the opportunities for aggression. All 50 nurses revealed that they had been personally threatened, and several had been assaulted, causing disability. The reports of abuse included sexual harassment and sexual assault.

(Continued)

One Emergency Department nurse was attacked by a patient who was angry because he had been kept waiting in the waiting room for evaluation of a sore throat. Another ED nurse, who had 25 years of experience, was bitten by a violent female patient who needed restraint (by six people). The patient had Hepatitis C. The nurse states that she was very disappointed that hospital/ED management was of little help and felt that she was left on her own to stand up for her rights. The president reports that slow and ineffective understanding and action by administrators was all too common. The nurses who had experienced abuse were often discouraged from reporting the abuse to either the administration or the police. One of the Emergency Department nurses who was attacked was told to discuss the circumstances with the police later but now to return to work. Another interesting contradiction the nurses reported was that violence from patients was accepted as part of the job of nursing. However, violence against physicians was unacceptable. One nurse remarked that the message to the nurses and to the public is that nurses are not valued. A large majority of the nurses expressed concern that only the nurses take threats of violence seriously. A different study uncovered that of approximately 9,000 nurses surveyed, one-half had experienced one or more violent episodes in the last five shifts they had worked.

The president stressed that hospitals must promote safety and she supported an improvement in how violence is reported and specific methods for reporting violence. Nurses must feel safe if they are to provide safety to their patients and be able to provide the support necessary to enhance their health and wellness. Administration must endeavor to understand violence and to implement programs to tout safety and intervene in violent situations should they occur.

CASE STUDY

The data in this study from the Department of Nursing at Chung-Hwa University of Medical Technology in Tainan, Taiwan, represents the growing problem of violence in all Emergency De-

(Continued)

partments worldwide. Eighty-eight percent of the nurses in Taiwan who completed the survey as part of this study have been victims of patient abuse.

Nurses in Emergency Departments are high-risk groups and are likely to experience patient violence against them. In the study, staff characteristics were compared with the rate of violent acts against the nurses, including the violent behavior of verbal and physical abuse.

Emergency Department nurses from 11 hospitals in Taiwan were surveyed about patient violence that had affected them personally. Two hundred sixty-seven nurses were surveyed. Of those surveyed, 88%, or 236, of the nurses responded to the survey, replying that they had been victims of violence. Ninety-two percent of the nurses experienced verbal abuse, and 30% experienced physical abuse from patients. The reasons that were given for the abuse were:

- Long waits in the Emergency Department (89%)
- Changes in cognition (87%)
- Lack of communication (82%)

A positive correlation was made to inexperienced nurses who encountered verbal abuse, but there was no correlation between inexperienced nurses and the occurrence of physical abuse. There was noted to be a significant correlation between the occurrences of verbal and/or physical abuse and the amount of training the nurses received in learning to cope with violence (Tang, 2007).

There is no solid explanation for the limited news reports of violence in U.S. EDs. One RN particularly close to the action in the Emergency Department has stated that multiple weapons are taken off patients and visitors weekly and that nurses are consistently subjected to verbal and physical abuse (Reavy, 2007). One reason that news reports may be deficient or hospital sources are or have become less than forthcoming may be to protect the image of particular hospitals as safe and friendly so that patients will not fear coming to the ED for care in the event of a medical emergency.

There appears to be no shortage in the news regarding mass shootings in the U.S.—nine incidents in 2009 alone. The increase

(Continued)

of violence in the United States is gaining the attention of the nation's mayors. The recent U.S. Conference of Mayors is aware of the monumental increase in fatal shootings and has scheduled a "national conversation" (Johnston, 2009) for June 2009 to explore the topic of violence and the expanding occurrence of aggressive events. Several members of the conference have expressed concern that the U.S. public has become "numb to the mounting body count" or that we have "lost the ability to get shocked and angry" (Johnston, 2009). According to James Alan Fox of Northeastern University in Boston, an average of 18 mass fatal shootings has occurred in the U.S. annually, resulting in the death of nearly 3,000 people since 1976. Fox further comments that the nine incidents this year represent an "increased pace" in mass murder activity (Johnston, 2009). Fox explains that mass killings "tend to occur in clusters" but is unable to predict if the mass killings will continue in the U.S. this year. He is unsure about classifying the recent incidents as a "random cluster," saying that often mass killings are generated from bad economic times. This year, he explains, "more people are struggling with the economy and are angry about the perceived inequities related to the government's bailout of the big corporations" (Johnston, 2009).

NOTES

1. Anoxia refers to a lack of oxygen or a limited level of oxygen in the blood.
2. This phrase is equivalent to what Americans would recognize as "worked to death."
3. President George W. Bush, responding to a question regarding access to emergency care, remarked that everyone has access to health care because they can "go to the Emergency Room". According to Donna Mason, it is obvious that former President Bush is not aware of the momentous problems that simply going to the emergency room can create. If every uninsured person in the U.S. had that attitude and took the president's advice, U.S. EDs would collapse (Rollins, 2007b).

REFERENCES

AbuAlRub, R. K. (2007). Workplace violence among Iraqi hospital nurses. *Journal of Nursing Scholarship*, 39(3), 281–288.
A brief history of the original KKK, 1865–1869. (2009, January 1). Retrieved April 28, 2009, from http://www.kkklan.com/historical.htm

Bureau of Justice Assistance. (2005). *2005 national gang threat assessment.* Retrieved July 8, 2008, from http://www.knowgangs.com/gang_resources/2005_national_gang_threat_assessment.pdf

Butler, E. (2002, November 11). Violence in the workplace: Volatile patients inflict multimillion-dollar pain on hospitals. *New Orleans City Business.*

Cardiff University Violence and Society Research Group. (2007, April 9). *Violence linked to the price of beer.* Retrieved May 19, 2008.

Carmiel, O. (2007). *ER needs help with violent patients.* Retrieved May 25, 2008, from http://www.northjersey.com/page.php?qstr=eXJpcnk3ZjczN2Y3dnF1ZUVF3Xk2M DYmZm

Cooper, J. R. (2005). *Letters to the editor.* Retrieved May 19, 2008, from http://www.nursingworld.org/MainMenuCategories/ANAMarketplace/ANAPeriodicals

Emergency Department violence. (n.d.). Retrieved October 12, 2006, from http://www.acep.org/advocacy.aspx?id=21830

Fendel, H. (2007, April). *Brief hospital strike protests violence.* Retrieved February 2008, from www.israelnationalnews.com/News/News.aspx/126369

Fernandez, C. R. (2002). The effect of an education program on violence in the emergency department. *Annals of Emergency Medicine, 39*(1), 47–55.

Grossman, V. M. (2003). Gang members in the ED: Don't 'dis' their 'rep': A primer on safety. *American Journal of Nursing, 103*(2), 52–53.

Grunberg, F. K. (2007, April). *Treatment advocacy center briefing paper.* Retrieved November 17, 2007, from www.treatmentadvocacycenter.org/BriefingPapers/BP8.htm

Guidelines for preventing workplace violence. (n.d.). Retrieved July 2, 2008, from http://www.osha.gov/Publications/OSHA3148/osha3148.html

Gun control. Showdown. Gun owners are becoming emboldened. That may be premature. (2008, July 5–11). *The Economist,* pp. 38–39.

Harasim, P. (2005). *Concern from healthcare workers over hospital violence.* Retrieved June 1, 2007, from http://www.securityinfowatch.com/article/printer.jsp?id=3381

Harris, M. (2006, July 17). *Hospitals face intrusion of violent world into facilities.* Retrieved July 18, 2007, from http://www.baltimoresun.com/news/health/bal-m.o.hospital17jul06,4286517.story?col

Johnston, K. (2009, April 9). Mayors to explore roots of violence. *USA Today,* p. 3A.

Kohl, G. (2006, February 2). *Preventing violence in today's workplace.* Retrieved October 24, 2007, from http://www.securityinfoinfo.com/article/article.jsp?siteSection=356&id=7175

Kuhn, W. (1999, January). Violence in the Emergency Department. *Postgraduate Medicine, 105*(1).

Lewis, J. (2008). *Resources.* Retrieved August 15, 2008, from http://www.knowgangs.com/gang_resources/menu.php

Luck, L. J. (2007). STAMP: Components of obseravable behaviour that indicate potential for patient violene in emergency departments; Violence against nurses. *Journal of Advanced Nursing; Emergency Nurse, 15*(4), 4.

McAdams, K. (2004, August 2). *Gangstas: Not in my hospital!* Retrieved August 11, 2008, from www.findarticles.com/p/articles/mi_qa3689/is_200409/ai_n9424681/print?tag=artBody;col1

Moffatt, G. K. (2002). *A violent heart: Understanding aggressive individuals.* Westport, CT: Greenwood Publishing Group.

Pugh, A. (2005–2006, winter). *Lateral violence/horizontal hostility/workplace violence— it's all the same: Building a culture of respect combats lateral violence.* Retrieved June 22, 2007, from www.reseaufranco.com/en/best_of_crosscurrents/bullying_in_ nursing.html

Ray, M. (2007). The dark side of the job: Violence in the emergency department. *Journal of Emergency Nursing, 33*(3), 257–261.

Reavy, P. (2007, October 1). *ER nurses fall victim to increasing violence.* Retrieved September 30, 2008, from http://www.deseretnews.comarticle/1.5143.695214458.00. html

Redfern, R.R.-T. (2006, March). *Massachusetts nurse letter.* Retrieved November 2007, from www.massachusettsnurse.org/massachusetts nurse letter

Rollins, J. (2007a, March 1). Tension in the waiting room: 86% of ED nurses report recent violence. *ED Nursing.*

Rollins, J.A.P. (2007b). A statement from Donna L. Mason, MS, RN, CEN President of the Emergency Nurses Association. *Pediatric Nursing, 373*(1).

Shimbun, Y. (2008). *Violence drives medics to quit.* Retrieved July 11, 2008, from www. yomiuri.com.pf/dy/national/20080608TDY02302.htm

Survey: Most ED staff victimized by violence never report incident. (2007, October 1). Atlanta, GA: Gale Group.

Tang, J. C. (2007). Incidence and related factors of violence in emergency departments: A study of nurses in southern Taiwan. *Journal of Formosan Medical Association, 106*(9), 748–758.

Thrall, T. H. (2006, September). *Stopping ED violence before it happens.* Retrieved November 14, 2007, from http://www.hhnmag.com/hhnmag_app/jsp/articledisplay. jsp?dcrpath=HHNMAG/PubsNewsArticle/data/2006September/0609HHN_FEA_ Safety&domain=HHNMAG

U.S. Department of Justice. (2003). *Violence by gang members, 1993–2003.* Washington, DC: U.S. Government.

Worley, M. (2007). *Hospital violence shock.* Retrieved May 19, 2008, from http://www. News.com/au/mercury/story/1,22884,23782305-3462,00.html

7

Assessment of Your ED Patients: Recognizing Your Patients as Victims of Violence

It is critical to recognize these patients so as to provide information to the patient and perhaps to the appropriate authorities, to prevent subsequent injury to this patient.

INTIMATE PARTNER VIOLENCE (IPV)/DOMESTIC ABUSE

Domestic abuse now has a new name: IPV. The term may be different, but the warning signs and outcomes are the same, and the incidence is rising dramatically. Nearly 24% of all violent crime is directly caused by IPV or domestic violence (Kohl, 2006).

IPV is defined as physical, sexual, or psychological abuse to a woman or a man by a current or former partner or spouse, and it affects more than 32 million Americans—10% of the U.S. population—each year (Schneider, 2005). A 2005 statistic reports that 1.5 million women and 800,000 men annually are raped or physically assaulted by an intimate partner (Tjaden, 2000).

IPV takes the form of sexual abuse, emotional abuse, intimidation, economic deprivation, threats of violence, and assault. IPV is characterized by the misuse of power or by the physical or psychological control of one partner over another (*Domestic Violence*, 2009). IPV occurs in all culture, races, ethnicities, religions, genders, and classes and is perpetrated by both men and women.

Women experience IPV to a greater extent than men do, and female IPV leads to more Emergency Department visits than does violence against men. In any given year, 5 million U.S. women experience IPV, and up to 20% of all Emergency Department visits by women are related to IPV (Sullivan, 2004). The trauma that women experience is not only the physical and psychological effects from IPV but also financial harm. A statistic reveals that 32% of all female homicide victims were murdered by an intimate partner (Rennison, 2000). While it may be difficult to accept, one study exposes the unbelievable fact that 7.8% of pregnant women in the U.S. are abused at least once during their pregnancy as determined in a very small sample-size study comprised of 10 cities and 437 individuals (McFarlane, 2002). The study by McFarlane concludes that this is the "first report of a definite link between abuse during pregnancy and attempted/completed femicide." The researchers urge immediate implementation of a "universal abuse assessment of all pregnant women" (McFarlane, 2002).

Two-thirds of all U.S. women report being raped, physically assaulted, and/or stalked since the age of 18 by a current or former husband, cohabiting partner, boyfriend, or date, while 29% of all women and 22%–23% of all men experience physical, sexual, or psychological IPV in a lifetime (Tjaden, 2000).

While IPV may be recognized as primarily a crime against women, the statistics of male IPV are also alarming, with 800,000 or more men experiencing IPV annually in the U.S. Comprehensive staff education must include the statistics and identifiers to recognize male victimization. Men's rights groups and some scholars believe that there are as many male victims of violence as there are female victims (*Domestic Violence,* 2008).

Although there is evidence that the numbers of males reporting victimization by IPV increased from 2004 to 2008, there are seemingly logical reasons why males are reluctant to report IPV more frequently that can be attributed to several factors:

1. Male victims of IPV may be ashamed that others may perceive them as weak or less of a man.
2. The belief that police or law enforcement personnel may not take the allegations or accusations seriously or concern that the man will be arrested because people assume that only men are abusers.
3. Shame due to the nature of a homosexual relationship.

It is essential for all Emergency Department personnel to recognize the symptoms of IPV because this malady will show up in Emergency Departments frequently, increasingly, and in alarming numbers. A 2005 article in *Family Practice News* reports that Emergency Department physicians may be overlooking the signs and symptoms of IPV in their Emergency Departments (Rhodes, 2005).

In a retrospective chart review study, conducted by two University of Chicago Emergency Department physicians, they identified 986 women who were documented victims of IPV and were from one specific county in Michigan. Ninety-four percent of these women had been seen in at least one of eight Emergency Departments in the county, but only 5.8% of the victims had an ED visit that correlated—by documentation—to the IPV assault. Sixty percent of the victims had filed a police report that detailed specifics about the injury. The Emergency Department screened less than 30% of this female cohort for IPV and found that 24 .4% of the women had a negative IPV screen. This evidence suggests that EDs and health care facilities do not have information that could be critical to identifying victims in need of counseling or intervention and that those Emergency Department personnel may not have the training or skills to correctly recognize patients as victims of IPV. The findings of this study point to one important thing: the victims of IPV may be reluctant or fearful to self-report abuse when visiting the emergency room. The American College of Obstetricians and Gynecologists believe that 100% of women should be screened for IPV and that ED personnel need training to acknowledge specific physical indicators that would alert to suspicion of abuse (McFarlane, 2002). Once a victim of IPV is recognized and identified, the ED can provide valuable and often life-saving alternatives for the victim. Ninety percent of female victims of IPV do believe that their physician could facilitate a solution for them (Sullivan, 2004).

Several presenting traumatic injuries that may not correlate with the patient's explanation for these injuries should alert Emergency Department staff to the possibility of abuse. Somatic complaints such as depression, anxiety, panic disorder, difficulty sleeping, and unexplained pain may be symptoms underlying the true explanation for these conditions (Sullivan, 2004). Some of the data are replicated in Exhibit 7.1, a guide to pre-hospital conditions of violence.

Your patient may be prepared and even willing to admit to IPV. If the patient does admit that IPV is a concern or is actually occurring and he or she is ready to seek assistance, encourage the victim to take

Exhibit 7.1

GUIDE FOR ED PERSONNEL TO IDENTIFY PREHOSPITAL VIOLENT CONDITIONS IN ED PATIENTS TOOL

THERE ARE FOUR CATEGORIES OF VICTIMS OF VIOLENCE THAT MAY PRESENT TO YOUR EMERGENCY DEPARTMENT FOR CARE:

1. Intimate partner violence (IPV)/domestic abuse
2. Dating abuse
3. Elder abuse
4. Child abuse

action now. Provide information, which may be available from the hospital social worker or social services department, about local shelters, legal assistance, and/or the local police. Emergency Department staff cannot force individuals to report personal violence, but providing assistance or encouragement may empower them to take action. Action today may prevent an assault or homicide tomorrow.

If the patient is not ready to fully accept assistance, strongly urge him or her to create an exit plan over the next few days and to assign a date to leave the abusive relationship. Important components of an exit plan will include suggestions to pack and conceal a suitcase of clothing for him/herself and any children who may be involved. Other essentials to have readily available are cash, checks, a credit card, copies of important documents and prescription medication. Remind the victim to prepare in advance for his/her *permanent* departure from the relationship. Provide the name and telephone number of a resource who can answer questions and provide support during the transition, if at all possible.

Several IPV screening tools have been developed specifically for use with all female patients in the emergency room but can also be used for male patients. Initiating a routine IPV screening as an operating procedure for every patient will help identify IPV victims. The abusing partner will not be suspicious that the ED personnel have recognized IPV in his injured/ill partner who has come to the ED for care. Screening can be a relatively simple procedure to implement and use during a patient history and can lead to important clues or to critical red flags.

For a screening tool to be successful and to increase the probability that it will be used consistently, the tool should be short and easily applied in clinical situations—especially in the ED. Accurate and thorough documentation is of utmost importance, using quotes from the patient whenever possible. Include photography of the injury if at all possible. Any medical documentation can be used by the victim to substantiate allegations during court proceedings and may benefit the victim relative to compensation or other judgments against the aggressor.

One screening tool developed by the American College of Obstetricians and Gynecologists is recommended for every female Emergency Department patient. The screening should be conducted in a private area, making certain that the partner is not in the room with the woman during the screening. Ask the screening questions in a nonaccusatory manner, avoiding the use of words such as "abuse" or "violence." It is important to take time to develop an initial relationship with the patient because laying the groundwork will distinguish you as a knowledgeable and trustworthy porfessional who can offer assistance and provide ways to help the victim take that important first step away from an abusive relationship (Sullivan, 2004).

The Hurt-Insult-Threaten-Scream (HITS) Screening Tool is a four-question tool that has been developed for use in the Emergency Department to allow for screening of either male or female patients to identify victims of IPV. The CTS tool is widely accepted as a valid tool, but because the CTS tool has 19 questions it requires substantial time to administer, and therefore the CTS tool is difficult to integrate into an Emergency Department setting, where time is often lacking. The research conducted by Shakil, Donald, Sinacore, and Krepcho (2005) established the HITS Screening Tool as an acceptable and predictive tool to use in the Emergency Department for both sexes. The recommendation is to implement the tool as a questionnaire to be self-completed by the patient because the questionnaire method is more predictive when completed by the patient than when using the direct interview method. As with any screening tool, the tool should not replace sound clinical judgment but should be used as an adjunct to clinical evidence (Shakil, 2005).

A screening tool has also been developed in the University of Chicago Hospital's ED to identify IPV in patients coming to the Emergency Department for care. The tool is a quick and effective tool that "may increase the odds that a woman at risk for domestic violence will talk to a health care professional in the ED" (Rhodes, 2006). The ease of administration of a one-question screen is certainly beneficial. Each female patient is asked to answer one computer-based question: "Have you been hit, kicked, or abused in any way?" If the screen is positive, or generates a "yes" response to the question, the patient record is flagged by the appearance of a special icon so that social services will conduct a social services consultation before the patient departs the Emergency Department. If the social services consultant uncovers a serious level of abuse or if the screening or clinical examination points to other IPV indicators, the social service department will allow the patient to agree for the ED to contact the police department for further intervention (Rhodes, 2006).

Hospital EDs wishing to employ this screening method could do so manually by integrating a process whereby social services is notified of the need of a consultation. A key point is to assure that there are adequate social services staff available to respond to the needs of the Emergency Department when a potential victim of IPV/domestic abuse is identified. The question must *not* be asked if any other person is in the treatment room with the patient, as is the recommendation of other screening instruments. The University of Chicago Hospital reports that their urban Emergency Department sees a majority of African American patients. The study partner hospital is primarily a suburban ED that sees mainly White, upper-middle-class patients. The outcomes for the two groups, relative to IPV or domestic abuse, is very similar: 26% of urban ED patients and 21% of suburban ED patients report—through the screening tool—that they were at risk for domestic abuse.

Licensed health care professionals are required to report any confirmed or suspected IPV, and several states now require mandatory reporting of suspected IPV. However, to date, no standardized reporting or collecting mechanism for statistics exists in the U.S. (Frieden, 2005). It is critical for each Emergency Department to know the reporting requirements for their state.

The College of Obstetricians and Gynecologists recommends the placement of gender-specific IPV educational brochures in both male and female restrooms that contain hotline numbers and other information to help the victim take the important first step in seeking assistance. The college further suggests attaching a small card, designed to be hidden in a shoe, that contains key information and contact numbers for victim assistance so that information can be secretly taken with the patient.

As an Emergency Department nurse, physician, or staff member, you are in the best position to make what could be a significant difference in someone's life. Trust your gut instinct in situations that make you uncomfortable. Take action. It is the right thing to do and may possibly prevent the meaningless loss of life. See Exhibit 7.2 for the tool: HITS IPV screening for the ED. IPV is never OK.

Exhibit 7.2

HITS (HURT-INSULT-THREATEN-SCREAM) INSTRUMENT TO SCREEN FOR IPV

	IN THE PAST 12 MONTHS, HOW OFTEN DID YOUR PARTNER	SCORE
1	Physically hurt you?	
2	Insult you?	
3	Threaten you with physical harm?	
4	Scream or curse at you?	
		Total

Key	Never	Score 1 point
	Rarely	Score 2 points
	Sometimes	Score 3 points
	Fairly often	Score 4 points
	Frequently	Score 5 points

ANALYSIS

Females scoring greater than 10 and males scoring greater than 11 need to be assessed further by social services as a potential victim of abuse.

From "Validation of the HITS Domestic Violence Screening Tool with Males," by A. Shakil, D. Smith, J. Sinacore, & M. Krepcho, 2005. *Family Medicine, 37*(3), 193–198.

CASE STUDY

I have been the unwitting observer of an episode of IPV. Over 15 years ago, I was the occupational health/wellness nurse for a large organization. I had frequent contact with all employees. One

(Continued)

employee confided in me that she had recently separated from her husband because of his aggression with her and with the children. She was concerned because he continued to threaten her and often told her that he would kidnap their three daughters and harm her. As she spoke to me, it was apparent that she was visibly fearful. I encouraged her to discuss her circumstances with the police in her community so that they could monitor any activity that might possibly escalate into an untenable situation. I discussed the conversation with my immediate supervisor, who asked me to relay my concerns to the CEO.

Several days after the woman had spoken with me, her former spouse arrived at our workplace. He was excitable and angry and required the use of force—the local police—to be escorted out of the warehouse. This was in the days prior to the use of security guards or controlled access doors; in today's secure environment, the man would not have had access to the building or to his wife's workstation, but the episode should have alerted us to an imminent situation. We again encouraged the woman to seek the assistance of the local law enforcement authorities.

None of us will ever know whether she took our advice. Later that same week, we received the news that our employee had been found shot to death in the home she had vacated just weeks before. Our employee's former husband had been arrested on suspicion of first-degree criminal homicide.

DATING VIOLENCE (DV)

The factor that differentiates dating violence (DV) from IPV is simply the age group in which the violence occurs. DV is IPV; it simply occurs earlier in the saga of abuse.

DV is defined as the physical, sexual, or psychological/emotional violence that occurs within a dating relationship. The majority of teenage DV occurs in the home of one of the partners. One in three teenagers has experienced violence in a dating relationship (*Teen Dating Violence,* 2008). Adolescents and teens aged 11 to 14 years are the most prevalent victims of DV, while young adults aged 16 to 24 years experience the greatest per capita rate of DV at 20 DV victims per 1,000 individuals (Silverman, 2006).

There is significant underreporting of the occurrence of DV, but data and educational Web sites are more available now than even 6 months ago. Statistics support the fact that DV is a serious and growing concern for the youth of the U.S.

The Centers for Disease Control (CDC) report that one in four teens in high school has experienced DV or knows someone who has been the victim of DV. One in five college females will experience some type of abuse while dating.

The risk of DV is equal among boys and girls and is statistically greater for adolescents of the African American and Hispanic ethnic groups. Adolescents with low academic achievement appear to be at greater risk for DV.

Evidence that an adolescent may be involved in an abusive relationship:

1. Physical signs of injury (bruising)
2. Truancy or dropping out of school
3. Failing grades
4. Changes in mood or personality
5. Use of drugs/alcohol when there has not been prior use
6. Emotional outbursts
7. Isolation from friends and/or family

Several studies have concluded that DV in adolescence is a risk factor for the continuation of abuse or violence in adulthood. And, as with IPV, DV tends to escalate over time and is characterized by promises from the offender that the abuse will not occur again. Risk to the abused person can increase when the individual attempts to escape from his or her circumstances. Sixty-eight percent of young women reporting rape identify their rapist as a boyfriend, friend, or casual acquaintance and not only within the context of dating. Seven percent of all murder victims were young women who were killed by their boyfriends (*Teen Dating Violence,* 2008).

While there is not a large amount of literature about DV, risk factors have been identified that may promote the incidence of DV:

1. Living in a broken home
2. Living in a rural area
3. Inadequate parental supervision
4. The belief that violence or abuse is tolerable

5. Substance abuse (alcohol or drugs)
6. Risky sexual behavior
7. Prior abuse, as a victim
8. Dropping out of high school (St. Mars, 2007)

The 2008 CDC factsheet about dating violence includes additional risk factors of:

* Peers who live with and/or condone violence

* The use of threats or violence to solve problems

* The inability to manage anger or frustration

* Poor social skills

* The association with violent friends

* Problems in school

* Witnessing abuse or violence at home ("Understanding Teen Dating Violence," 2008)

DV is a topic that is growing in popularity. Web sites offering information and support—and those discussing personal experiences—are becoming more prevalent. Love Is Respect (http://www.loveisrespect.org) and Love Is Not Abuse (http://www.loveisnotabuse.com) are two DV informational Web sites that have great appeal and contain many interactive tools, such as a chat line and the National Dating Abuse Hotline, which are communication strategies that are in wide acceptance by teenagers. The sites are typically staffed by teen and adult advocates. The sites promote "recognize, respond, refer" and encourage teens and parents to "Break the silence. Be part of the solution" (Media Center, 2009).

The Teen Dating Bill of Rights and Pledge are prominently displayed on the Web site Love is Respect (Teen Dating Bill of Rights, 2009). Curriculum that can be integrated into regular school courses or as a stand-alone course is available free of charge. The program has been in use for several years and is currently offered in high schools in 39 states. Using the curriculum in mainstream school academics helps deliver the message that teen DV is a serious problem and provides awareness and working strategies for teens to avoid potential DV situations. The organization has made significant efforts to reach its target audience, to communicate

Exhibit 7.3

TEEN DATING BILL OF RIGHTS

I HAVE THE RIGHT:

- To always be treated with respect.
- In a respectful relationship, you should be treated as an equal.
- To be in a healthy relationship.
- A healthy relationship is not controlling, manipulative, or jealous. A healthy relationship involves honesty, trust, and communication.
- To not be hurt physically or emotionally.
- You should feel safe in your relationship at all times. Abuse is never deserved and is never your fault. Conflicts should be resolved in a peaceful and rational way.
- To refuse sex or affection at anytime.
- To end a relationship.
- A healthy relationship involves making consensual sexual decisions. You have the right to not have sex. Even if you have had sex before, you have the right to refuse sex for any reason.
- To have friends and activities apart from my boyfriend or girlfriend.
- Spending time by yourself with male or female friends or with family is normal and healthy.
- You should not be harassed, threatened, or made to feel guilty for ending an unhealthy or healthy relationship. You have the right to end a relationship for any reason you choose.

Note. From Love is Respect.org.

the problem, and to offer solutions by providing valuable information, slogans, and multiple opportunities to discuss problems immediately. Both Web sites are sponsored by the fashion designer Liz Claiborne. See Exhibit 7.3 for the Teen Dating Bill of Rights and Exhibit 7.4 for the Teen Dating Pledge.

Jennifer Ann (http://www.jenniferann.org) is a Web site/foundation founded by the father of a teenage girl who was murdered by a teen dating partner. The Web site offers information and provides complimentary educational wallet cards that list the 10 warning signs of an abusive relationship with a message on the reverse listing telephone numbers to

Exhibit 7.4

TEEN DATING PLEDGE

I PLEDGE TO:

- Always treat my boyfriend or girlfriend with respect.
- Never hurt my boyfriend or girlfriend physically, verbally, or emotionally.
- Respect my girlfriend's or boyfriend's decisions concerning sex and affection.
- Not be controlling or manipulative in my relationship.
- Accept responsibility for myself and my actions.

Note. From Love is Respect.org.

call and instructions about how to create a safety plan. Ten signs of an abusive relationship are displayed in Exhibit 7.5.

Cool Nurse (http://www.coolnurse.com/dating_violence.htm) is a different Web site supplying information and statistics about teen DV, including a dating safety plan. One particularly informative section educates the reader about the influence of "perception"—how teens view themselves and their beliefs regarding "masculinity" or the "romanticizing of a boyfriend's jealousy" (*Teen Dating Violence*, 2009).

Choose Respect (http://www.chooserespect.org), a Web site created by the CDC as an initiative for providing information about resolving conflicts and for the development of positive social skills, is designed as a tool for adolescents and teens to help prevent DV. The Web site advocates teaching children early about the potential perils of dating and relationships and advises communicating with young dating-aged and pre-dating-aged teens about the hallmark signs of an individual who may become a dating abuser.

The signs that may indicate a dating partner could be, or become, a potential abuser are:

1. Displays of extreme jealousy
2. The presence of controlling behavior
3. The desire for quick involvement
4. Unpredictable mood swings
5. The use of alcohol and/or drugs

Exhibit 7.5

DATING VIOLENCE: TEN WARNING SIGNS OF AN ABUSIVE RELATIONSHIP

- History of legal or discipline problems
- Blames you for his/her anger
- Serious drug or alcohol use
- History of violent behavior
- Threatens others regularly
- Insults you or calls you names
- Trouble controlling feelings like anger
- Tells you what to wear, what to do, or how to act
- Threatens or intimidates you in order to get his/her way
- Prevents you from spending time with your friends or family

Note. From www.jenniferann.org.

6. Demonstrations of explosive anger
7. Either dating partner's growing isolation from family and/or friends
8. The use of force during an argument
9. Evidence of hypersensitivity
10. The belief in rigid gender roles
11. The tendency to blame others for problems or feelings

IPV and DV can negatively affect health. Both groups are at high risk for substance abuse, depression, and suicide, while DV includes symptoms of weight control problems, sexually transmitted diseases, and teen pregnancy. St. Mars (2007) reports that 8.5% of the DV study participants had attempted suicide.

DV IN THE EMERGENCY DEPARTMENT

It is imperative that Emergency Department staff become alert to the growing issue of DV. Training and education may be necessary to provide

Exhibit 7.6

DATING VIOLENCE (DV) SCREENING CHECKLIST TOOL

Dating violence victimization is determined by a positive ("yes") response to the following question:

1. During the past 12 months, did your boyfriend or girlfriend ever hit, slap, or physically hurt you on purpose?

The Emergency Department goal with dating violence screening is to:

• *Document occurrence of any IPV*

• *Create a record*

• *Provide information to authorities, if appropriate*

• *Provide resources to the victim*

competency in identifying signs and symptoms of DV in adolescents and teens, aged 11 years and older who may present for care. This may be the only opportunity to provide life-changing support to this group of victims. There is evidence that DV and IPV are rarely self-reported. See Exhibit 7.6 for the dating violence screening in the ED tool. DV is never OK.

CASE STUDY

The following case study was written by Drew Crecente, the father of murdered 18-year-old Jennifer Crecente. Jennifer, a victim of DV, was murdered by her boyfriend. Jennifer's father started the JenniferAnn.org Web site to honor his daughter by providing information about dating abuse for vulnerable teens. Through Mr. Crecente's advocacy against DV, he hopes to alert young people to the reality of DV.

Jennifer Ann Crecente was a high school honors student [who] was murdered by an ex-boyfriend on February 15, 2006. Our group will keep Jennifer Crecente's memory alive through good works and by fighting Teen Dating Violence.

My daughter, Jennifer Crecente, died the day after Valentine's Day, 2006.

(Continued)

She didn't die from a childhood disease and wasn't killed in a car accident.

She was murdered by a classmate. Somebody that she'd grown to know, trust and eventually date. She was murdered by somebody that had problems. Problems that at the invincible age of 18, Jennifer thought that she could overcome.

Don't you remember? In high school we are *immortal.*

But for Jennifer Crecente and those that love her we know all too well how very painfully mortal we are. Abuse isn't a "very special episode" of our favorite television show. Problems don't disappear during the commercial break.

Good, decent people that want to help out a friend are sometimes murdered in cold blood. And the bogeyman isn't always under the bed. Sometimes he's the kid that lives down the street.

Our organization is going to do everything that it can to ensure that no other parent has to be awakened in the middle of the night by friends pounding on the door. No more groggy-eyed astonishment. No more shocked out-of-body emptiness. No more realization that nothing will ever be the same again. *Nothing.*

We will educate young people about danger signs. About warning signals. About indications that they are *in above their heads and not immortal.* And then we'll point them in the right direction—toward the many groups that offer assistance, counseling and protection. We will not rest until **every** young person has been educated about an epidemic that impacts over 20% of our teenage population.

Ignorance will not be an excuse. We won't stop until this knowledge is as fundamental as looking both ways when you cross the street.

I can't bring my baby back. Jennifer is gone, and as powerless as I may be about that, I refuse to allow this to continue unabated. Please join our forum on Teen Dating Violence so that you can join in conversations about this worldwide problem. We are a young organization but have ambition, passion and an energy borne of desperation.

Please keep Jennifer in your hearts and prayers. I sincerely wish you could have known her. (Crecente, 2008)

ELDER ABUSE

Child abuse, animal abuse, and elder abuse are the most unconscionable types of abuse because the victims are powerless to defend themselves or to escape their situations.

Elder abuse is sometimes referred to as the "violation of an individual's human and civil rights by any other person or persons" (Hutson, 2007) or the "physical, sexual, or emotional abuse of an elderly person, usually one who is disabled or frail" (*Definition of Elder Abuse*, 2004). The British journal *Age and Ageing* shares the World Health Organization's definition as a "single or repeated act or lack of appropriate action occurring within any relationship where there is an expectation of trust, which causes harm or distress to an older person" (McAlpine, 2008). Elder abuse is underreported and often goes unreported. Part of the difficulty is the assessment of the individual for the presence of abuse or neglect.

Elder abuse, according to Kathleen Loeffler, is a "burgeoning epidemic" (Loeffler, 2003, p. 1). A recent study by the CDC indicates that Emergency Departments are treating increasing numbers of neglected or abused elderly Americans. There are more adults over the age of 60 in the U.S. and in the world today and the number is growing (*Morbidity and Mortality Weekly Report*, 2008).

Public opinion and attitude toward the elderly has changed. Elderly Americans no longer live in the households with their grown children, as early immigrant families lived; elders are not revered as are the older family members in other cultures; elders are living longer and often require being cared for by adult children, which creates stress, conflict, and financial burden for the adult caregivers.

Risk factors have been used to aid Emergency Department personnel in the identification of high-risk patients who are or who may become victims of elder abuse. If any of your elderly patients exhibit two or more of the following risk factors, be alert to the potential of elder abuse or neglect:

- Elder's age is older than 75
- Elder is dependent on a caregiver
- Caregiver exhibits alcohol or substance abuse
- Caregiver is inexperienced in the care of the elderly
- Caregiver has a history of mental illness
- Elder has financial problems
- Elder has a lack of assistance or limited support systems
- Elder lives in cramped living quarters
- There is a recent change in the elder's level of functioning

The Emergency Department may be the only place that elders have to rely on to rescue them from abuse. Abused elders may be fearful of having the abuse discovered because they are reliant on their caregivers for activities of daily living or they may be financially dependent on those individuals. Although statistics strongly support that caregivers most often are the abusers, other individuals must also be considered (McAlpine, 2008).

Emergency Department personnel must learn to recognize the signs of physical, psychological, and/or sexual abuse. Training may be required to help ED personnel gain knowledge of the signs of elder abuse. Elderly patients have the right to be screened for abuse, and the source of the abuse or neglect must be identified and reported when detected.

Recognizing abuse is a difficult task because the elder may be a patient for the first time and/or the demands of the Emergency Department may preclude close inspection of potential abuse or listening for the clues that an individual is giving. Be assured of one thing: the probability is great that the elder will not report that abuse is occurring, so it is the obligation of personnel in the Emergency Department to elicit any evidence.

SIGNS AND SYMPTOMS OF ELDER ABUSE

The signs of physical abuse can include:

- Old and new bruises
- Untreated injuries or injuries in various phases of healing, including cuts; lacerations; punctures or open wounds
- Evidence of being restrained
- Poor skin condition
- Soiled clothing or bed linens
- Burns or cigarette burns
- Fractures
- Alopecia (in patches, due to trauma from pulled hair)
- A pattern injury caused from being struck by cords or objects
- Eye trauma
- Whiplash injury
- Reports of having been mistreated
- Evidence of broken eyeglasses or dentures
- Elders who are undermedicated
- Elders who are overmedicated
- Always consider the possibility of sexual abuse when physical abuse is detected, such as bruising of the breast tissue or genital area; unexplained vaginal or anal bleeding; torn, stained, or

Exhibit 7.7

SIGNS OF PHYSICAL ABUSE CHECKLIST TOOL

- Old and new bruises
- Untreated injuries or injuries in various phases of healing, including cuts, lacerations, punctures, or open wounds
- Evidence of being restrained
- Poor skin condition
- Soiled clothing or bed linens
- Burns or cigarette burns
- Fractures
- Alopecia (in patches, due to trauma from pulled hair)
- A pattern injury caused from being struck by cords or objects
- Eye trauma
- Whiplash injury
- Reports of having been mistreated
- Evidence of broken eyeglasses or dentures
- Elders who are undermedicated *or* overmedicated
- Consider the possibility of sexual abuse in the following signs bruising of the breast tissue or genital area; unexplained vaginal or anal bleeding; torn, stained, or blood-stained underclothing; and unexplained venereal diseases or genital infections.

Note. CDC, 2006.

blood-stained underclothing; and unexplained venereal diseases or genital infections. See Exhibit 7.7 for the signs of physical abuse in the elderly.

NEGLECT IS THE MOST COMMON FORM OF ELDER ABUSE

The signs of neglect can include:

- Dehydration
- Malnutrition

- Rashes or lice
- Decubitus ulcers or sores
- Poor hygiene
- Unsanitary or unclean living conditions
- Overt odor of urine or feces
- Inadequate clothing
- Untreated medical conditions
- Lack of assistance in preparation of meals or when eating or drinking
- Medication noncompliance

The signs of psychological abuse in the elderly can include:

- Elder is verbally berated
- Elder is harassed or intimidated
- Elder is chided
- Elder is treated like a child
- Elder shows signs of helplessness
- Elder exhibits confusion/disorientation or emotional upset or agitation (the possibility of an underlying medical condition may account for these symptoms)
- Elder demonstrates unexplained fear or anger without apparent cause
- Elder has social isolation
- Elder is ignored
- Elder is denied companionship
- Elder is threatened with punishment or deprivation
- Elder claims verbal or emotional abuse
- Elder displays unusual behavior including sucking, biting, or rocking
- Elder denies situations, gives implausible excuses, tells unrealistic stories, or provides accounts of incidents that are different from those provided by caregiver or family
- Elder hesitates to talk openly
- Elder has symptoms of extreme withdrawal, a lack of appropriate response, or retarded communication

The signs of financial abuse in the elderly can include:

- Signatures on elder's checks differ from the elder's signature
- Signatures are present when the elder cannot write

Exhibit 7.8

ELDER VIOLENCE—SIGNS OF NEGLECT CHECKLIST TOOL

- Dehydration
- Malnutrition
- Rashes or lice
- Decubitus ulcers or sores
- Poor hygiene
- Unsanitary or unclean living conditions
- Overt odor of urine or feces
- Inadequate clothing
- Untreated medical conditions
- Lack of assistance in preparation of meals or when eating or drinking
- Medication noncompliance
- **Neglect is the most common form of elder violence/abuse**

Note. CDC, 2006.

■ There is a sudden change in the elder's bank account, including unexplained withdrawals, the addition of another name to the account, or transfer of assets to others
■ There is an unexplained disappearance of the elder's funds or valuable possessions
■ There is an abrupt change to the elder's will or the sudden establishment of a will
■ The sudden arrival/appearance of previously uninvolved relatives who claim to have an unusual interest in the elder person's affairs
■ Concern expressed by family members or others in the amount being spent to care for the elder individual
■ Elder has numerous unpaid bills or overdue bills when they are to have been paid by others
■ Elder lacks the amenities of daily living such as grooming items or appropriate clothing
■ Elder is experiencing deliberate isolation from friends, giving the caregiver complete control over all circumstances (Loeffler, 2003)

See Exhibit 7.8 for the signs of neglect in the elderly.

Exhibit 7.9

ELDER VIOLENCE OR ABUSE SCREENING CHECKLIST TOOL

ELDER VIOLENCE OR ABUSE VICTIMIZATION IS DETERMINED BY ANY OF THE FOLLOWING:

1. Any evidence of mistreatment without sufficient clinical explanation
2. Whenever there is a subjective complaint of elder mistreatment made by the elder
3. Whenever clinician believes there is a high risk of probable violence, abuse, neglect, exploitation, or abandonment

THE EMERGENCY DEPARTMENT GOAL WITH ELDER VIOLENCE OR ABUSE SCREENING IS TO:

- *Refer to social services if any of the above (1–3) exist*
- *Document occurrence of any elder violence or abuse*
- *Create a record*
- *Provide information to authorities, if appropriate*
- *Provide resources to victim*

The most effective tool that ED personnel have is their skill of observation and listening. Even at best, the task of separating normal circumstances from those that indicate a reportable violent incident is enormous. "Exhaust all resources before you risk discharging an elderly person back to an abusive environment" urges Linda Hutson, an assistant nurse manager in the ED and a SANE RN.[1]

If abuse is suspected, ED personnel have a legal and moral obligation to report findings to the local adult protective services agency (Hutson, 2007). See Exhibit 7.9 for the elder violence or abuse screening in the ED tool. Elder Abuse is never OK.

CASE STUDY

"Elder mistreatment is a hidden and often ignored problem in society," according to the British journal Age and Ageing *(McAlpine, 2008). In the UK, the term "Granny Battering" dates to 1975 but*

(Continued)

demonstrates that the general public knows little else about elder abuse. The article highlights the slow response in the UK to educate the public about elder abuse and points to the fact that the country is resistant to admit that a problem so heinous could exist.

The article states that a major force in creating awareness in Britain has been the British Geriatrics Society Conference, titled the "Abuse of Elderly People: An Unnecessary and Preventable Problem." In 1990 Age and Ageing published an article describing the problem of elder abuse by caregivers that led to the founding of the charity Action on Elder Abuse 3 years later. It has been determined that more than 4% of "older people" were being abused by family members or acquaintances (McAlpine, 2008, p. 132). The types of abuse and neglect and their prevalence appear to be level across Western societies according to the article. Since the lack of awareness was first recognized, much has been done in England to increase awareness and combat the growth of elder abuse. Current emphasis is to educate physicians who work with the elderly to be alert to the potential of elder abuse (McAlpine, 2008).

CHILD VIOLENCE AND ABUSE OR PEDIATRIC ABUSE

Child violence and abuse, or pediatric violence and abuse, is the type of abuse that is the more widely known among the four forms of violence against patients who will arrive for treatment in the Emergency Department. The atrocities of child violence and abuse have been around a very long time. For many years, people have heard about child violence and abuse; there are many organizations and resources to educate about, report on, and help diffuse this despicable societal problem.

Child violence and abuse is characterized as doing something or failing to do something that causes harm to a child or puts a child at risk of harm. The long-term danger of child violence and abuse is the emotional trauma that children experience from the physical abuse or neglect. Depression, withdrawal, suicidal ideation, drug or alcohol use or abuse, isolation, maltreatment or abuse of others, and violence are not uncommon adult manifestations of child violence and abuse (*Child Abuse*, 1999).

According to the American Academy of Child and Adolescent Psychiatry, hundreds of thousands of children are abused annually by a parent or close relative. Of the numbers of abused children, thousands die from the acts of abuse or neglect. One of the key components of helping children heal and recover from physical abuse and the side effects of accompanying psychological scarring is early intervention. For this reason, prompt and early recognition of child violence and abuse is critical so that the child can receive comprehensive and adequate treatment. The academy stresses that whenever a child says he/she has been abused—and understands what abuse means—that the statement must be regarded as fact and thoroughly investigated (*Facts for Families: Child Abuse*, 2008). There are four categories of child violence and abuse:

1. Child neglect. Types of neglect consist of:
   - Physical neglect. Physical neglect is identified when the child lacks appropriate clothing or hygiene.
   - Educational neglect. Educational neglect is defined as the failure to facilitate education for the child when the child is not enrolled in school or provided an education through homeschooling or other channels.
   - Psychological/emotional neglect. Emotional neglect is generally thought to be an attack on the emotional or psychological well-being of a child through many means, including the withholding of affection, inadequate nurturing, ignoring, terrorizing, or isolating the child.
2. Child physical abuse. Physical abuse includes hitting, shaking, pinching, pulling hair, or radically cutting off a child's hair despite the child's wishes.
3. Child psychological or emotional abuse. Psychological abuse has a wide variety of meanings and includes nonphysical maltreatment or belittling, verbal threats, criticism, put downs, or the exertion of power or intimidation.
4. Child sexual abuse. Sexual abuse is characterized as contacts or interactions between a child and an adult when the child is being used for the sexual stimulation of the perpetrator or another person who is in a position of power or control over the child victim. This form of child abuse is routinely underreported due to the secrecy or "conspiracy of silence" to cover up the acts against the child (*Child Abuse*, 1999).

Government agencies around the country that are in the business of investigating the many reports of child violence and abuse report that child protective services (CPS) in the U.S. receive 50,000 reports of child violence and abuse every week. In 2002, the most current data available, cases from 4.5 million children were investigated, and of this number, 67% were found to be victims of child violence and abuse or neglect. This number averages to approximately 2,450 children every day who are found to be victims of violence and abuse or neglect (Iannelli, 2007).

Sixty percent of the children were found to be victims of neglect; the investigators found that these children were not receiving the basic necessities of life. Twenty percent of the children were being physically abused. Ten percent of the cases were victims of sexual abuse, and 7% were experiencing emotional abuse. A staggering and disturbing statistic from 2002 reveals that an average of four children die every day in the U.S. as a result of child violence, abuse, or neglect. In 2002, there was 1,400 documented deaths due to child violence and abuse (Iannelli, 2007).

STATISTICS RELATED TO CHILD AND NEGLECT

There appears to be no correlation between race or gender and the prevalence of violence or abuse and neglect of children. Statistics from 2002 reveal:

- 54% of the victims were White children
- 26% were African American children
- 11% were Hispanic children
- 2% were American Indian or Alaska Native children
- 1% were children of Asian-Pacific Island descent

In 2002, children aged less than 1 year old accounted for 41% of all abuse-related deaths; 76% of the children who died from child violence and abuse were aged less than 4 years old (Iannelli, 2007).

How Is Child Violence and Abuse Discovered and Reported?

In 2002, 57% of all reports received from child protective agencies were made by professionals who had contact with the child:

- 16% were from teachers
- 16% were from law enforcement, legal professionals, or criminal justice professionals
- 13% were from social workers
- 8% were from medical professionals
- 44% were from nonprofessionals (parents, relatives, neighbors, friends)
- 10% were from anonymous sources (Iannelli, 2007)

What Does Child Violence and Abuse Look Like?

When a child is a patient in the Emergency Department, there is not much time or opportunity to develop rapport or become a trusted ally. It is critical to search for any symptoms that may provide clues as to the possibility of child violence and abuse or neglect. Some of the symptoms to look for as advocated by the Child Welfare Gateway in 2007 are listed here.

The Child . . .

- Shows sudden changes in behavior or school performance
- Arrives very early to school, or stays very late; this may indicate that he does not wish to go home
- Has not received help for physical or medical problems that were brought to the parents' attention
- Has learning difficulties or difficulties with concentration that are unexplained by physical or psychological causes
- Exhibits paranoia or seems to be concerned that something bad may happen
- Has limited or nonexistent parental or adult supervision
- Exhibits passive or withdrawn demeanor, is overly compliant, or is trying too hard to please

The Parent . . .

- Has or demonstrates little concern for the child
- Does not share responsibility for the child's problems at school or at home
- Demands that teachers or caregivers punish the child with harsh discipline for any misbehavior

Exhibit 7.10

CHILD VIOLENCE OR ABUSE SCREENING CHECKLIST TOOL

Child violence or abuse victimization is determined by any of the following:

1. *Physical abuse*: Any evidence of physical injury that is not accidental, such as bruising, welts, burns, cuts, or broken bones without sufficient clinical explanation

2. *Neglect*: Any evidence of lack of care that risks or causes harm to a child including lack of food, lack of clothing, lack of supervision, denial of medical attention

3. *Emotional or psychological abuse*: Any evidence of harm to a child's ability to think, reason, or to have feelings, such as cruel acts or statements, intimidation, rejection, noninclusion, or indifference

4. *Sexual abuse*: Any evidence of sexual contact including rape, sodomy, fondling, or sexual exploitation, including the use of children for pornography, prostitution, or personal pleasure

5. *Threats of harm*: Any evidence of activities, conditions, or persons that place a child at risk of abuse or danger, including threats, domestic violence, drug/alcohol abuse

The Emergency Department goal with child violence or abuse screening is to:

- *Refer to social services if any of the above exist*

- *Document occurrence of any child violence or abuse*

- *Create a record*

- *Provide information to authorities, if appropriate*

- Indicates that the child is bad, worthless, or burdensome
- Demands overachievement in academic or athletic pursuits that are unreasonable and often unattainable
- Demands care, attention, and emotional support from the child

The Parent and Child . . .

- Appear to have no affection for each other, rarely having interpersonal communication
- Have nothing positive to say about their relationship when asked
- Remark that they do not like each other (*Recognizing Signs and Symptoms of Child Abuse and Neglect,* 2003)

Many of the symptoms of child violence and abuse or neglect would be difficult to discern during the course of an Emergency Department visit, but an astute practitioner might be able to get a clue from some of the interactions between the child and parents or remarks the child makes. Evidence of physical signs, such as bruising or fractures, would be the most apparent sign of possible physical abuse. It is the responsibility of ED professionals to identify and report clinical findings that verify the existence of child abuse. See Exhibit 7.10 for the child violence or abuse screening in the ED tool. Child abuse is never OK.

CASE STUDY

WHERE IS CAYLEE?

Recently, the tragic story of the missing Florida toddler Caylee Anthony has captured the interest of many individuals worldwide.

Caylee is a beautiful 3-year-old child whose only crime was being born to a too-young mother who apparently did not wish to give up her girls-gone-wild lifestyle to commit to the obligation of raising a child. There is evidence that Caylee's mother had wished to give her child up for adoption at the time of Caylee's birth but for unknown reasons did not follow through with her plan. I am certain that many of us wish that she had found a loving couple to adopt this beautiful child.

The unfortunate thing is that Caylee's story is probably more typical than we may know; the only reason that the U.S. public heard Caylee's story is that her grandmother reported her missing. Although Caylee and her mother lived with the grandparents, Caylee's grandparents had not seen Caylee—or her mother—in over a month. The grandmother happened to find the mother's car parked on a street, near their home, and was concerned about the odor of human decomposition. The grandmother was inconsolable in her concern and her grief as the news stations replayed the conversation that she had with the police department that day. She believed, I am sure, that Caylee and/or Caylee's mother had been murdered.

We don't know whether Caylee has been the victim of abuse, or worse. I speculate that although the mother has made a lot of very

(Continued)

bad choices, she does not seem likely to have murdered her child. The police prediction that Caylee may have accidentally died or been killed is, I believe, a logical conclusion. I am not sure we will ever know the entire truth.

The exploitation of children—in this case, little Caylee Anthony—is child abuse, child violence, child neglect. This mother has been officially accused with child neglect for failing to report her child missing and recently was indicted for the murder of the child.

Child abuse occurs all of the time. Our challenge is to recognize the symptoms in children who come to the Emergency Department for care. It is critical that we identify the signs and intervene to give the child a chance to thwart the abuse or neglect he or she is confronted with every day.

It is tragically too late for us to save Caylee.

Child abuse is an appalling societal ill. It is difficult to imagine how anyone could harm a child, especially the act of physically abusing an innocent being. Inexperienced, youthful parents may not have the emotional maturity to understand the needs of a young child, and when typical demands of an infant or child are encountered, the immature parents react with frustration and rage. Other individuals may blame the child for their limited economic conditions and withhold necessities of life. Occasionally there is the rare circumstance of Munchausen syndrome by proxy (MSBP), the mental health malady of a parent in which the parent, or caregiver, creates a cause for disease symptoms in the child. Because this disorder is violence against a child, MSBP is considered child abuse.[2] Additionally, parents or other recurrent caregivers may have a serious mental deficit or illness, such as schizophrenia or psychosis, that prohibits an individual from understanding what is necessary to care for a child. Whatever the reason, child abuse is unacceptable; any measure that Emergency Department personnel can take to stop injury and to prevent the impact of further injury must be done (Understanding and Dealing With Child Abuse, 2007).

NOTES

1. SANE stands for Sexual Abuse Nurse Examiner. SANE is a program promoting the special training of RNs to collect forensic evidence from alleged victims and providing support and follow-up care.

2. MSBP is a mental health disorder in which a person falsely reports or causes symptoms in another person who is under his or her care. The caregiver almost always is a mother, and the victim her child.

REFERENCES

Child abuse. (1999). Retrieved August 22, 2008, from http://www.medterms.com/script/main/art.asp?articlekey=8452

Crecente, D. (2008). *About Jennifer.* Retrieved from http://www.jenniferann.org

Definition of elder abuse. (2004, October 1). Retrieved April 26, 2009, from http://www.medterms.com/script/main/art.asp?articlekey=11196

Facts for families: Child abuse: The hidden bruises. (2008, May). Retrieved April 26, 2009, from http://www.aacap.org/cs/root/facts_for_families/child_abuse_the_hidden_bruises

Frieden, J. (2005). More screening for violence needed in EDs. *Clinical Psychiatry News, 34*(1).

Hutson, L. (2007). Elder abuse: The same old story? *Emergency Nurse, 15*(3).

Iannelli, V. (2007). *Child abuse statistics.* Retrieved August 13, 2008, from http://pediatrics.about.com/od/childabuse/a/05_abuse_stats.htm

Kohl, G. (2006). *Preventing violence in today's workplace* (G. Kohl, Ed.). Retrieved October 24, 2007, from http://www.securitywatchinfo.com

Loeffler, K. (2003). Elder abuse increasing: Can you recognize it? *ED Nursing, 16*(3).

McAlpine, C. (2008). Elder abuse and neglect. *Age and Ageing, 37*(2), 132–133.

McFarlane, J. C. (2002, July). Abuse during pregnancy and femicide: Urgent implications for women's health. *Obstetrics and Gynecology.* Retrieved from http://journals.lww.com/greenjournal/pages/results.aspx?k=women%20murdered%20by%20intimate%20partner&Scope=AllIssues&txtKeywords=women%20murdered%20by%20intimate%20partner

Media Center. (2009). Retrieved April 26, 2009, from http://www.loveisnotabuse.com/rrr.htm

Morbidity and Mortality Weekly Report (MMWR). (2008, June 11). Retrieved April 26, 2009, from http://www.cdc.gov/mmwr/preview/mmwrhtml/mm5723a5.htm

Recognizing signs and symptoms of child abuse and neglect. (2003). Retrieved August 22, 2008, from http://www.childwelfare.gov/can/identifying/recog_signs.cfm

Rennison, C. W. (2000, July). *Intimate partner violence.* Retrieved April 17, 2009, from http://ojp.usdoj.gov/bjs/pub/ascii/ipv.txt

Rhodes, K. (2005, December 15). Intimate partner violence missed in ED. *Family Practice News,* p. 40.

Rhodes, K. (2006, August 1). *Computers aid EDs in violence screening: Staff, patients discuss sensitive issues.* Retrieved November 5, 2007, from www.find.galegroup.com/itx/start.do?prodId=ITOF

Schneider, M. E. (2005, December 1). Costs of intimate partner violence. *OB GYN News,* p. 31.

Shakil, D. S. (2005). Validation of the HITS Domestic Violence Screening Tool with males. *Family Medicine, 37*(3), 193–198.

Shakil, A., Smith, D., Sinacore, J., & Krepcho, M. (2005). Validation of the HITS domestic violence screening tool with males. *Family Medicine, 37*(3), 193–198.

Silverman, J. (2006). *National teen dating prevention initiative: Teen dating violence facts.* Harvard University, School of Public Health. Chicago: American Bar Association.

St. Mars, T. V. (2007). Adolescent dating violence: Understanding what is "at risk." *Journal of Emergency Nursing, 33*(5), 492–494.

Sullivan, M. G. (2004, April 1). Domestic violence screening. *OB GYN News,* p. 22.

Teen dating bill of rights. (2009). Retrieved April 26, 2009, from http://www.loveis respect.org/resource-center/teen-dating-bill-of-rights/

Teen dating violence. (2009). Retrieved April 26, 2009, from http://www.livestrong.com/article/13801-teen-dating-violence/

Tjaden, P. T. (2000). *Full report of the prevalence and consequences of violence against women.* Washington, DC: CSC.

Understanding and dealing with child abuse. (2007). Retrieved August 23, 2008, from http://www.scf.hr.state.or.us/reprtlaw.htm

Understanding teen dating violence: 2008 fact sheet. (2008). Retrieved April 26, 2009, from http://www.cdc.gov/ViolencePrevention/pdf/DatingAbuseFactSheet-a.pdf

Intervention in the ED: Tools and Strategies for a Violence-Free ED

We can't solve problems by using the same kind of thinking we used when we created them.

—*Albert Einstein*

8

Initiating Change for ED Violence Prevention

INTRODUCTION TO DEFENSE STRATEGIES FOR A VIOLENCE-FREE ED

The number of Emergency Department (ED) visits are at record high and growing substantially every year. On average, each U.S. ED sees 30,000 patients every year, and the Medicaid or State Children's Health Insurance Program (SCHIP) population represents the highest rate of Emergency Department visits, 82 out of 100 persons. In 2005, 13.9% of the 115.3 million people (over 16 million) who visited an Emergency Department, and 14.5% of the 119.2 million people (over 14 million) who visited EDs in 2006, were *low acuity* patients. The delivery of care to those patients who truly need emergency care is at serious risk (Nawar, Niska, & Xu, 2007; Pitts, Niska, Xu, & Burt, 2008).

Coupled with increasing numbers of patient visits and fewer physicians to see and care for the ill or injured patient, the risk for violence increases radically as more Americans who have access to weapons and violence in our society intensifies. Added to that, many hospital Emergency Departments are closing.

Hospital administrators have been reluctant to commit resources to Emergency Department violence since it is a problem that is ill-defined and not well understood by administration. It is critical that hospital leaders become educated about the serious nature of emergency department violence. The hospital leaders must confront the reality that there is significant potential for violence within any ED environment. Investing in a plan to safeguard all employees and patients against violence, engineered to the hospital's specific needs, is a future-forward formula for enhancing business, for cultivating patient and community relations, and for guaranteeing revenue growth for the future. This is a very difficult period for Emergency Departments, and it is time for radical change. "Pleasantville" community hospital has vanished.

MAKING SECURITY IMPROVEMENT CHANGES TO THE ED WAITING ROOM

Making improvements to the waiting room in the Emergency Department can enhance value for your hospital because the waiting room is the first point of contact for your customers/patients and the place that they will be spending time. It is important to consider changes that will encourage your patients to want to visit your Emergency Department again. Strategies for enhancing the look, feel, and welcoming appearance and atmosphere of your Emergency Department waiting room will be discussed later in this section.

Before you can present a welcoming environment for the patients, families, and visitors, it is essential to have the elements in place that will keep the patients and the staff safe. The schematic of a safe ED waiting room (Figure 8.1) is a visual depiction of the essential elements required for a safe waiting room.

Before letting anyone into the Emergency Department or into the waiting room, there are several *strategies* to consider implementing that will contribute to promoting increased safety within the ED environment. These strategies are discussed in detail later in this chapter. They include the following:

1. *Public awareness* of your Emergency Department's attentiveness to and approach to preventing violence, including strict policy and signage to support zero tolerance for aggression, violence, and abuse in the Emergency Department, complete with a statement of consequences for violations to the zero tolerance policy.

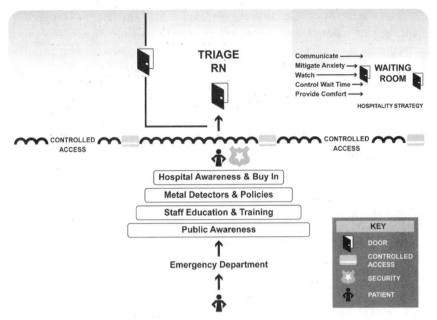

Figure 8.1 Model for violence prevention in the Emergency Department.

2. *ED Staff education and training* in de-escalation tactics/aggression management, policies to support violence prevention, panic/duress alarm training, enhancement of the triage staff, policies for use of the secure room and restraints, and consistent use of metal detectors.

3. *Contraband* definitions and policy to stop guns, knives, blades, and/or chemical weapons from making their way into the Emergency Department; contraband locker policy to support the storage and return of contraband.

4. *Enterprise awareness and buy-in* represents the hospital's commitment to support violence-prevention activities for the hospital and Emergency Department.

Controlled Access

One of the most important strategies to implement with regard to improving a safe environment is to prevent the free access of unauthorized individuals in the waiting room or ED. Control access to all doors, both exterior and interior, leading into the Emergency Department, including control of the ambulatory and EMS entrances. Implement a locking or electronically controlled apparatus that can be triggered by security and certain other individuals. The presence of a security guard/staff in the waiting room, at the ambulatory entrance to the Emergency Department, to function as a visible control, is very effective. The final key to controlling access to the ambulatory entrance is the installation of metal detectors, both walk-through detectors to halt the entry of weapons brought in by ambulatory patients, and the use of hand-held detectors for monitoring the entry of weapons via EMS/ambulance patients.

Triage Nurse

The use of the triage nurse is another key strategy to securing a safe ED environment. The triage nurse is the critical point person for evaluating patient condition and monitoring the potential for aggression or violence that may occur in the ED waiting room. The critical nature of the triage nurse and the important functions that the triage nurse performs are addressed in detail in the section headed "Strategy 7."

The final point represented in the schematic overview of a safe ED is that whenever possible, a back door should be provided to exit from any of the enclosed triage areas/rooms so that triage personnel have a ready escape from the area in the event that a threatening situation or perceived risk to safety develops.

The triage nurse is the flow czar for the patients in the waiting room and is responsible for communication and for making the patients and families aware of queuing and potential delays, to help prevent anger and violent outbursts. It is the role of the triage nurse to eliminate any potential for violence occurring in the waiting room of the ED.

The triage nurse must also have a quiet space or area to privately evaluate and communicate with patients and families. The triage nurse must manage all aspects of the patients and families occupying the waiting room while overseeing the potential for patients to become frustrated or angered. One method for providing a private space for the triage nurse yet allowing the nurse a full view of the waiting room is to have shatter-resistant glass installed into one wall of the room or space that allows viewing from inside the triage room. The triage nurse can then watch all patient, family, and visitor activities and interactions and can step out to evaluate, troubleshoot, or control any situation.

SAFETY ELEMENTS THAT CAN BE INTEGRATED INTO AN ED DESIGN

If you have the opportunity to design a new Emergency Department or are developing a new space for your ED, there are three major strategic design approaches to consider:

1. Place security staff at the entrance to the Emergency Department. The location of the security staff is a critical strategy. The security staff needs to be as visible as possible to individuals who are entering your ED. The visible presence of security may be a successful deterrent especially when used in conjunction with closed-circuit television (CCTV), metal detectors, and the restricted access to the ED.

2. Utilize less obtrusive barriers and increase the comfort of the environment. This very logical approach improves the aesthetics of the area. When patients and families feel welcome and comfortable, there is less rationale for anger or frustration. This is a particularly good strategy to use with mentally ill patients who respond well to calm, less chaotic environments. Barriers—represented by the security staff and metal detectors—can be a physical and a psychological deterrent to irrational behavior. If the hospital is located in an area that is rampant with gang crime or is prone to other violent incidents, several layers of security and protection for the triage staff will be necessary. In other instances, glass and protective (bullet-proof) barriers can and should be used to protect the triage staff from an unauthorized approach in the event that security is not present. As long as the glass barrier is easily accessible—can be walked around, for example—and the triage nurse does not talk *through* the barrier to the patient, a protective area is an acceptable approach.

3. The first point of contact with hospital staff will most likely be with the security guard/staff. Position a video monitor so that the individual can see himself on the monitor. This method has been used effectively in banks to communicate to the individual that he is being watched and his behavior is being monitored. The view of the individual's own image gives a subliminal but effective message for the individual to behave appropriately in the Emergency Department (Thrall, 2006).

The ideal layout of an Emergency Department waiting room and treatment areas depends on a great many variables, including the average number of patient visits, the length of stay (LOS) of patients' from arrival to discharge, average patient surge experience, available space in the waiting room, and process and procedure. Many EDs are faced with the retrofit of a 20-year-old structure with a great many limitations, such as the small size of the waiting room, too few restrooms, or the lack of an area in the waiting room that can function as a triage area. Additionally, the complexity of security, including metal detectors, requires the expertise of a keen creative eye and flow specialist so as to enhance the opportunity for patients to move easily through the various required patient functions such as triage and registration. Most EDs have improved the registration process so that patient registration can be done at bedside. Registration clerks can now come to the patient instead of the patient having to sit and register at a window in the waiting room. This new capability improves the time and efficiency of registration.

It is important to keep the needs of the patient in mind, including his comfort and the necessity for rapid evaluation of his chief complaint. It is also critical for the triage nurse to have a full view of the waiting room at all times so that he/she can assess any potential problem such as a change in patient status or a potential for an increase in anxiety or frustration that may potentially lead to a violent reaction.

Security staff roles need to be reevaluated, and new personnel need to be trained to take an active role in customer service, providing a smooth and efficient flow for the patient and family as they enter the Emergency Department and progress through the metal detector into the waiting room.

10 STRATEGIES FOR VIOLENCE PREVENTION

What Would You Do Differently Tomorrow if You Had a Violent Incident Today? (Thrall, 2006)

Many facilities do not have a plan to control violence in the Emergency Department until an incident occurs and changes everyone's impressions and priorities about violence. Violence can happen in your Emergency Department, and the best method to control injury, loss, chaos, and even death is to have a violence-prevention plan in place before it is needed. The following 10 strategies can help prevent violence in your hospital. The 10 strategies are in broad categories and contain important tactics within each strategy. See Exhibit 8.1 for cost projections for the strategies presented.

Strategy 1: Assess the Risk for Violence in Your ED

Determine your hospital's risk for violence by completing the 12-question violence risk self-assessment that appears in Exhibit 8.2. Depending on the culture of your hospital and the support or lack of support that you have from hospital administration, you may want to complete the violence risk self-assessment before discussing the need to implement a violence prevention strategy for the ED with hospital administration so that you will have established the case for making recommended changes.

Tips for Administering the Violence Risk Self-Assessment Questionnaire

- Ask yourself the 12 strategic questions on the violence risk self-assessment questionnaire to assess the exposure that your hospital and Emergency Department have to violence.
- Answer the questions honestly.
- Use your responses to evaluate some of the vulnerable areas you may have in your Emergency Department.
- Determine if more resources are required to prevent violence from occurring in your ED and/or hospital.
- Determine the level of internal and geographic risk to your Emergency Department.
- Determine the breadth of violence-prevention strategies to control violence or to correct deficiencies.
- Develop the case for defining your incursion risk.
- Communicate your findings to the hospital administration.

Follow-Up Strategies Based on the Results of Your Violence Risk Self-Assessment Questionnaire

- If you determine that your ED is at *high risk*, implement all 10 strategies. If the self-assessment scores 50 points or more, consider your facility at high risk.
- If you determine that your ED is *not at high risk*, choose and implement the strategies that remedy the deficiencies you have in

Exhibit 8.1

COST OF IMPLEMENTING 10 STRATEGIES FOR VIOLENCE PREVENTION

ACTIVITY	COST PROJECTIONS (IN USD)
1. Conduct violence risk self-assessment	Administering self-assessment = $0, CAP-index online report = $199
2. Initiate zero tolerance policy	Signage = $25/sign, Professional time to write and communicate policies = $300
3. Control free access	Security personnel for visitor management = approx 1.5 FTE[a] @ $30/hr (×2080) × number of visitor management stations, Signage = $25 per sign, Security staff training time = $2,500–$4,000
4. Implement panic/duress alarms	Foundation equipment = $2,500–$3,000 User fob or page = $210–375 per unit
5. Train all staff in de-escalation management	1-day seminar for up to 40 individuals = $400, 2-day seminar for up to 40 individuals = $780, 4-day seminar certification program = $1,239
6. Establish a secure room	Retrofitting of room, quilted surfaces; door and lock; locks for cabinets; two-way communication device; window; securing/padding of treatment bed; CCTV; approximately $6,000–$10,000
7. Reinforce and re-educate triage staff	Additional RN triage staff - $35- 50/hour/ RN, Add nonlicensed staff (if necessary) = $14–18/hour/staff, Signage = $25 per sign, Shatter-resistant glass = $100/square foot + installation (to enclose triage area and/or open registration area), Hospital strategy = $500–$5,000—cost of pillows and blankets, upgrade or add TVs, creation of a children's corner (toys/supplies), coffee station, upgrade/add furniture, painting/ redecoration, Wi-Fi connection and laptops (optional), small gift kiosk or cart, Comfort Bag = $4–$5 per bag (depending on contents of bag)
8. Install metal detectors	Walk-through metal detectors - $1,600-6,000, Hand-held wand/metal scanner - $100, Contraband locker/gun safe: $114–$600 + CCTV system = $500–$1,500 dependent on number of cameras and optional preferences

(Continued)

Exhibit 8.1

COST OF IMPLEMENTING 10 STRATEGIES
FOR VIOLENCE PREVENTION (*Continued*)

ACTIVITY	COST PROJECTIONS (IN USD)
9. Add security officers and staff	Additional security officer = $30–$40/hour Training time = $30–$40/hour dependent on the number of officers and level of training needed
10. Initiate Violence Awareness & Prevention Plan	80-100 personnel hours = estimated $40-$65/hour

Note. [a]FTE is defined as full-time equivalent, or the measure of time of a full-time position (2,080 hours/annum).

your ED or hospital. If the self-assessment scores 50 points or less, you may consider your facility at lower risk.

■ One strategic tool to determine your hospital's geographic risk of crime is the CAP Index.[1] This low-cost crime forecasting service provides an accurate Internet-based report derived from the zip code and street address of the hospital. The CAP Index tool provides statistics for your hospital location for the current date and projects crime data 5 and 10 years from now. The CAP Index will help pinpoint if your hospital is in a high-risk location. The crime index statistics that are available on the CAP Index report can assist your hospital in making key planning decisions about the risk and vulnerability of your hospital to crime (see http://www. capindex.com).

■ Reassess your ED risk every 6 months or each time that a violent or a near-miss violent event occurs in your ED or in your city in the vicinity of your ED.

■ *Tip: Things change! Be certain that your ED has not become at risk in the past 6 months. Enter calendar alerts to reassess your ED risk every 6 months whether there has been an incident or not. The best defense is to be prepared!*

Once you've evaluated the results of the questionnaire, discuss the results with the ED medical director and then with hospital administration. Recognize that implementing changes of the magnitude and importance of a violence protection plan can be overwhelming.

Exhibit 8.2

12-QUESTION VIOLENCE RISK SELF-ASSESSMENT CHECKLIST TOOL

1. Has your Emergency Department *ever* had a violent episode or a near-miss episode of violence requiring intervention by the local police department?

   Assess 10 points for a "yes" to each question.

2. Has your ED ever found a weapon (gun, knife or blade, brass knuckles, chemical weapon, or any potential weapon) in the possession of an EMS/trauma patient brought to your hospital for care?

   Assess 10 points for even one weapon found in the past 1 year.

3. Does your hospital have any unlighted or unpatrolled parking lots or parking structures near the entrance to your Emergency Department?

   Assess 10 points for a "yes" response.

4. Have *all* of your ED staff been trained in violence or aggression/de-escalation techniques or have all received formal training in methods to control a violent patient, visitor, or gangs? Training must include initial orientation plus annual refresher training for all staff, including physicians, and PRN and agency staff.

   Assess 10 points if even one individual on your staff does not have training.

5. Does your Emergency Department have a secure room in which to place individuals who exhibit violent tendencies, to prevent harm to themselves or others?

   Assess 10 points for a "no" response.

6. Does your Emergency Department have and consistently use a visitor control system?

   Assess 10 points for a "no" response.

7. Do you have security personnel or off-duty police officers in your Emergency Department 24/7?

   Assess 10 points for a "no" response.

8. Is your hospital in a high-risk area of your city?

   Assess 10 points for a "yes" response.

9. What happens when a patient or visitor enters your Emergency Department with a weapon? Are you aware—100% of the time—that the individual has a weapon? Do you have a policy regarding weapon possession in your ED? Do you have a contraband locker and policies regarding its use?

(Continued)

Exhibit 8.2

12-QUESTION VIOLENCE RISK SELF-ASSESSMENT CHECKLIST TOOL (*Continued*)

Assess 10 points if your ED has not addressed the issue of weapons that are brought into your ED. Assess an additional 10 points if your ED does not have a contraband locker. Assess an additional 10 points if there are no formal, written policies regarding weapon screening and possession and the use of contraband lockers.

10. How many of your staff, including the physicians, feel unsafe or at risk while working in your Emergency Department?

    Assess 20 points if even one of your staff feels unsafe or at risk while working in your ED.

11. Does your ED have one or more duress/panic alarms or personal alarms, and is the use of the alarms governed by policy?

    Assess 10 points for a "no" response.

12. Do you consider your ED open access? Open access consists of the following:

    - Aside from the patient ambulatory entrance, one or more doors from the outside or from other areas of the hospital, without card access or keypad, leads directly into the ED (include EMS entrance).
    - No visitor management system is used to identify visitors or track their movement within your ED and hospital.
    - The ED has no formal process that requires every employee to have and *wear* a hospital-provided name badge (include physicians and PRN and agency staff).
    - There is no video camera or other surveillance system scanning the entrance to the Emergency Department.
    - The registration and/or triage area is located in an open area (no bulletproof glass or walls) within the waiting room.
    - The ED has no method to identify when weapons are brought into the ED.

    Assess 25 points if your ED meets even one of the criteria for an open access ED.

What would you do differently tomorrow if you had a violence incident today?

Determining your risk score:
Add the assessed points.
A score *greater than 50 points* indicates that your ED is at significant risk for violence.

Project Planning

The key to a successful project outcome lies in the planning. The project plan can be as detailed or as informal a plan as is appropriate for the circumstances. A project will be implemented and executed more successfully with a dynamic, flexible plan and a project manager. Even if your Emergency Department plans to implement only two or three of the strategies, it will require time to research all options to decide the best strategy for your Emergency Department. Assign a project manager (full-time or part-time) to oversee the aspects of the project. A sample template for use in planning the project appears in Exhibit 8.3.

Arrange a strategy planning meeting with hospital administration. Include the following individuals in the strategy planning meeting: chief medical officer of the hospital, ED medical director, security director,

Exhibit 8.3

PROJECT PLAN FOR VIOLENCE PREVENTION PLANNING IN THE ED

TEMPLATE			
STRATEGY/ TACTICS	TARGET DATE TO BEGIN	TARGET DATE FOR COMPLETION	TACTIC MANAGER
Implement zero tolerance policy	10/1/2008	10/3/2008	Jane Doe
Create policy			
Send to medical executive committee (approval process)			
Order/create signs for ED and front entrance			
Communicate zero tolerance policy to all hospital personnel			
Communicate zero tolerance policy to community and police department			
Consider public service announcements			

and other key Emergency Department management and clinical staff. Involve all stakeholders in your Emergency Department. Ask questions and listen to your employees' input.

Discuss one strategy at a time, evaluating all aspects and costs involved in implementing the strategy and tactic. Define the best approach and timeline for your hospital. Use the strategies and tactics as a guideline to develop your own violence protection plan.

Once the project has been established and there is agreement about how to proceed and the strategies your stakeholders have chosen, build a project plan. Ask for project volunteers from the Emergency Department and security department to be on a task force to help implement the strategies.

Strategy 2: Initiate a Zero Tolerance Policy

- Initiate a hospital-wide zero tolerance policy against aggression, violence, or abuse and for the possession of weapons in the Emergency Department and hospital.
- Communicate to the public in the community and to the patients who arrive in your ED for care that the hospital and Emergency Department will not tolerate any acts of aggression, violence, or abuse from any individual and that weapons are not permitted.
- Post a statement of the consequences to acts of behavior that violate the policy in any manner.

Rationale: Let the public, your patients, the ED staff and physicians, and the PRN or agency staff know that violence is unacceptable behavior and that patients and/or families may be asked to leave the Emergency Department for behavior that constitutes a violation or if any behavior is considered to be aggressive, unacceptable, and/or inappropriate.

Consistently reinforce the zero tolerance policy against aggression, abuse, and violence and talk to your staff regarding the prohibition of weapons possession; communicate that *violence, abuse, and aggression are unacceptable* under any circumstances and must be reported immediately. Weapons (guns, knives, blades of any kind, and chemical weapons, such as mace, pepper spray, etc.) will be confiscated. Inform staff of consequences that the perpetrators can face. An example of a zero tolerance policy is depicted in Exhibit 8.4.

Exhibit 8.4

SAMPLE POLICY (ZERO TOLERANCE)

[Name of hospital/medical center]   Policy #
Emergency Department services   Original date: Review date:

Policy/procedure

**Zero tolerance for possession of weapons in the Emergency Department;
Scanning for weapons (ambulatory and EMS patients)**

Policy:

- [Hospital name] maintains a zero tolerance policy for the possession of weapons in the Emergency Department.
- Weapons are not permitted inside the Emergency Department or inside the hospital. [Hospital name] maintains the right to screen any patient, visitor, or other person utilizing hand or machine screening for weapons and to confiscate any weapons.
- [Hospital name] defines a weapon as any tool or implement that can kill, injure, or maim another individual. Weapons include guns, knives, box cutters or any blade that can cut or lacerate, brass knuckles, explosive devices, and chemical weapons including Mace or tear gas.
- Any weapon that is voluntarily reported, surrendered, or confiscated will be locked in a contraband locker attached by ownership documentation. The weapon will be transferred to and maintained by the local city police department. [Hospital name] will not return any weapon to the owner under any circumstance. Owners may obtain their property at the local city police department.
- [Hospital name] maintains the right to refuse entrance into the emergency room or hospital to any individual who will not relinquish control of defined weapon.
- Zero tolerance signage will be prominently displayed near entrance to the Emergency Department, near entrance to hospital, and in triage, stating: "Any individual who threatens or incites verbal or physical aggression, abuse, or violence against another individual, staff, or patient in this facility may be prosecuted."

Procedure:

1. Whenever an ambulatory patient arrives for care at the Emergency Department, the patient and all persons who accompany him and all other persons are subject to a weapons search. The search may be performed utilizing a hand-held scanner or metal detectors.

(Continued)

Exhibit 8.4

SAMPLE POLICY (ZERO TOLERANCE) (*Continued*)

2. Whenever an EMS patient is brought to the Emergency Department for care, the patient and all persons who accompany him, and all other persons, are subject to a weapons search. The search may be performed utilizing a hand-held scanner or metal detectors and may be conducted by security officers or other duly authorized individuals.

3. It is possible that weapons may be undiscovered during screening upon entrance to the Emergency Department. If a weapon is discovered or reported during evaluation, ask the patient to place the weapon on a rolling cart and move the cart away from the patient. Summon security without leaving the room by using the duress alarm. Weapons that are discovered during the course of Emergency Department evaluation will be confiscated immediately by security.

4. If a weapon is detected, surrendered, or reported, the weapon will be confiscated and placed in a contraband locker with accompanying documentation of ownership.

5. The weapons will be transferred to the possession of the local city police department for safeguard.

6. Owner may contact local city police department to request return of the weapon.

Approvals

Director, Emergency Department	Date
CNO	Date
Director, Security Department	Date
CMO / Medical Director, Emergency Department	Date
CEO / Administrator	Date

- Post the zero tolerance signage and/or policy at the entrance to your ED, in the waiting area, and at the main entrance to the hospital. (Consider posting the zero tolerance policy and consequences for aggressive action in any other high-visibility area in your hospital.)

- Establish written definitions for aggression, violence, and abuse.
- Establish written definitions for weapons to include guns, knives, blades of any kind, and chemical weapons, such as mace or pepper spray.
- Remind staff that the zero tolerance policy for aggression applies to a patient only if the patient is medically stable; however, family or visitors who exhibit inappropriate behavior may be asked to leave the Emergency Department.
- *Tip: Psychiatric aggression is a situation that will require some thought among the nurses, physicians, and staff. Psychiatric patients will be out of control frequently, and this behavior should be anticipated. Train security staff and ED staff to manage psychiatric aggression through de-escalation techniques and by using a secure room within the ED. If the ED does not have a secure room, a policy for management of this type of patient must be decided in advance and addressed through policy.*
- Provide each staff member and contracted employee with a copy of the policy "Reporting Aggression, Violence, or Abuse." Discuss the policy in staff meetings and in-service training sessions. Be open to questions and provide clarification if requested.
- Determine how the staff is to report any episodes of aggression, violence, or aggressive episodes from a patient, visitor, or from other staff and communicate the process of reporting, including forms to be used and where policy report forms can be found in both electronic and hardcopy format.
- Assure staff that it is appropriate and expected that all episodes of aggression, abuse, or violence are to be reported, no matter how minor the incident may appear.
- Reassure staff that there will be no retribution for reporting any incident of aggression, violence, or abuse.
- Weapons of any kind are not permitted in the Emergency Department and must be surrendered before coming into the ED, whether the owner is a patient, family, visitor, employee, or consulting professional. Employed or contacted security or police officers are permitted to have weapons that have been issued to them in the course of their employment.
- Weapons are to be stored in a contraband locker. Owners who wish to recover property are to contact the local police department (see security strategy).
- Any weapon discovered on a patient, family, or visitor must be surrendered immediately to security staff.

■ Determine with hospital administration the phrase that the entire hospital will use to announce a hospital-wide alert, requesting aid for an outbreak of violence. Communicate the phrase chosen with all hospital staff and educate hospital staff about how and when to initiate a Code V (or your choice of phrase/violence code). Educate all hospital staff about how to respond when a Code V is announced.

Reporting Episodes of Violence

The most important aspect of reporting violent episodes is to outline and communicate a clear policy and protocol so that every individual knows the following, in advance:

■ The definitions of aggression, violence, and abuse
■ The importance of reporting every episode
■ How to report the incident
■ *Tip: Ensure that the process to report violence is simple and streamlined and takes very little time to complete. The Australian Health Service states that incidents are unreported or underreported because of what they call system blockers. Some of the system blockers identified are complexity of forms, lack of time to complete forms, reports or systems that are not guaranteed to be confidential, negative feedback from supervisors, peer pressure or negativity, and the stigma of being a victim. The Australian Health Service also reports that often violence occurs so frequently that nurses and physicians become desensitized to the importance of reporting every occurrence (Kennedy, 2005). Ensure that the process and procedure you establish is not a system blocker.*

Strategy 3: Control the Free Access of All Ambulances, Personnel, Visitors, and the Public Into Your Emergency Department and Hospital, 24/7

Individuals—other than health care personnel—who walk into the Emergency Department for reasons other than to seek emergency care, put your facility at risk for violence. It is critical that the systems and people whose job it is to create barriers are in place every hour of the day and night. The safety of your Emergency Department depends on prohibiting the entrance of nonauthorized individuals.

Rationale: Create barriers to prevent the entry and intrusion of unauthorized or dangerous individuals into your ED.

- Adopt or enforce usage of an official hospital or health care system photo identification badge.
- Assign photo identification badges to all employees, including PRN and agency staff, all physicians on staff, consulting physicians and other professionals, all security guards, and all contracted employees.
- Establish policy for the use of photo identification badges. Communicate the policy.
- Set expectations:
  - The photo identification badges must be worn 100% of the time, without exception. Establish consequences for noncompliance and enforce the consequences.
  - The photo identification badge is to be displayed prominently on the upper torso.
  - Establish a back-up plan for employees who arrive at work without the photo identification badge. A back-up plan will prevent having to ask the employee to leave or to leave and retrieve their personal badge. A feature of the newer photo identification badge systems is that they have the ability to print a temporary badge for the employee if policy supports this plan.
  - Establish policy and protocol with the security department to detain individuals who are not wearing or do not have a photo identification badge.
- *Tip: Set the expectation that any employee has the right to question any individual who is not wearing a photo identification badge. Do not allow anyone to remain in the ED if they do not have the photo identification badge. Security must be committed to escorting individuals out of the ED and hospital for noncompliance with the policy. Security must track any incident of unauthorized entry in the daily security report of occurrences* (Exhibit 8.5).
- EMS personnel must wear the official identification badge provided by their companies. Establish a log of EMS companies that routinely bring patients to the ED. Communicate with all EMS providers regarding the necessity for compliance with the identification badge policy.

Exhibit 8.5

TEMPLATE FOR DAILY SECURITY REPORT OF OCCURRENCES

YEAR:
MONTH: FEB 2009

TEMPLATE: DAILY SECURITY REPORT OF OCCURRENCES

	DATE	TIME	DETAILS	SECURITY AUTHORIZATION
1	2/1/2009	10:16:00 AM	White male detained at entrance to waiting room by triage RN; no personal identification badge; individual identified as Henry Bendel of Green Valley and identified as employee of All-Air Oxygen Supply; I accompanied Mr. Bendel to O2 storage location in ED and accompanied him to ED exit when distribution of canisters was completed.	John Blakeford-Jones, Security Supervisor

- *Tip: Discussion point: the United States is vulnerable. U.S. EDs are particularly vulnerable. For years, health care professionals have been able to trust everyone who enters the Emergency Department. EDs are in the business of the helping people, and the natural assumption is to have confidence in people who come to the ED for care. Things have changed in the U.S. It is important for the safety of your staff to rethink how services coming into your ED are screened and hired, to be certain that you can trust them. EMS is one of those services. For as many years as EMS has been in operation, there has been a mutual trust. It is wise practice for the ED director and medical director to meet with the supervisors of EMS providers to discuss their employee screening methods so that you can ensure the safety of your ED.*
- Decide to use either radio frequency identification (RFID) technology solutions, card readers that are bar-coded to ID badges, or a code access touch pad at all exterior doors leading into the

Emergency Department and at the main public entrance to the hospital to prohibit unauthorized access.

- *RFID:* If administration chooses to implement the RFID system, the capabilities of systems can vary greatly. Some systems have the capability to supply and manage employee ID badges, which can be a cost savings in terms of time and supplies. Typically, the security department manages RFID technology systems.
- *Code access touch pad:* If administration chooses a *code access touch pad,* assign management of the codes to the security department and make the location and access to the security office as convenient as possible for all staff (for troubleshooting, for the assignment of new codes, or for the global changing of the code). Staff the office around the clock with a unit clerk who has the authority and the training to solve problems that arise.
- *Card readers:* If administration chooses card readers/barcoded name badges, information technology (IT) may be the department to oversee the administration, depending on the organization of your hospital. IT will need to coordinate with security to alert the security department of downtime procedures or timing and other issues that may arise in the management of electronic systems.
- Conduct weekly door access testing to ensure the proper functioning of the system.
- Decide on the time of day that the main hospital entrance will be closed and locked every day.
- Communicate the main hospital entrance door closing time to all stakeholders.
- Post signage at the main hospital entrance notifying hospital patients or visitors of the times that the main entrance of the hospital opens and closes. Include clear information about the location of the emergency room. Display a simple map if the route to the ED is confusing.
- Install a visitor and vendor locator/management system in your ED and if possible also install the system at the main entrance to the hospital. Do not rely on hospital volunteers to manage the visitor management system at the main entrance and/or ED entrance.
- *Tip: Discussion point: All visitors—including accreditation officials and surveyors (for example, the Joint Commission), external*

health care professionals (for example, hospice), or visiting consulting physicians and police officers—must have visitor credentials authorized by the electronic visitor management system. Each individual must have a visitor badge. Several sources report that imposters are gaining access to EDs and hospitals by alleging to be officials who would typically be welcomed into the ED for the purpose of accreditation or survey. Experts suggest staying alert to cars or individuals lingering near the ED entrance or slowly driving or walking around your hospital campus (Imposters Targeting U.S. Hospitals, 2005).

- *Tip: It will be necessary to factor in the expense for additional security staff to manage the visitor management system for optimal benefit. Consider the cost of the system and the additional personnel that will be required for planning and implementation.*

- Provide training for use of the access control system for all stakeholders.

- *Tip: Training staff on the new policies, procedures, and equipment will be the essential to success of your violence prevention plan. Providing staff training in the Emergency Department setting is very challenging because of the volume and flow of patients and the diverse hours that staff are in the ED. Training that can be conducted by the user may be an effective method. Ask the vendors of products that are purchased for your ED if they provide online or video training. Get the nursing educator involved to help plan and construct a comprehensive training plan.*

Strategy 4: Implement Panic/Duress Alarms in Key Locations Inside the ED

A simple but effective way to provide ED staff with a method for requesting emergency assistance is to install wired panic or duress alarms in strategic locations within the Emergency Department or to provide wireless, supervised panic or duress alarm fobs or medallions for all stakeholders.

The Best Solution Is to Provide a Combination of Both Types of Alarms

Rationale: Provide a method for any staff member in any location in the Emergency Department or waiting room areas to immediately summon security and other assistance in the event of patient/family/visitor aggression, abuse, or violence.

The key locations for wired panic/duress alarms are:

■ Triage nurses station
■ Strategic location(s) in the waiting room
■ Any open area in waiting room, such as the registration desk, if manned by an individual at any time during a 24-hour period
■ Several strategic locations in the hallway of the ED treatment area
■ Each treatment room or bay
■ Nurses' station. If the ED nurses' station is large, two alarms may be necessary so that all staff has access to an alarm.
■ *Tip: The location of the alarm in the treatment room/bay is important. Place the alarm in an inconspicuous site so that patients or families cannot see and/or activate the alarm but that nurses can readily access and use it.*

Key considerations for *wireless* devices:

■ Wireless panic/duress alarms have a tendency to walk or disappear over time because staff carry a wireless fob or wear a wireless medallion while at work and may forget to return the appliance before leaving the ED.
■ Batteries or charging stations are essential for most wireless devices; recharging or battery changes for devices require unconditional compliance.
■ Ensure that comprehensive testing of the wireless device function can be completed simply and quickly.
■ Select the terminology for the alarm—use *duress alarm* or *panic alarm*. Use the term consistently.
■ Establish policy for the use of the alarms. Communicate the policy governing the use of panic/duress alarms.
■ Conduct training on the appropriate use of the alarms (and the location of the alarms, if wired) for all appropriate stakeholders, including staff and physicians, PRN, agency staff, administration, and EMS. Train any individual or group of individuals who may have a need to use the alarm.
■ Conduct monthly drills to ensure the staff knows how to use the alarms (and the location of each alarm, if wired) in the Emergency Department.

- Integrate an alarm testing protocol and assess responsibility for every shift to test the alarms to be certain that the alarms are 100% operational 100% of the time. (Preferably, alarm testing should be the responsibility of the security staff.)

Strategy 5: Train All Staff in De-Escalation/ Aggression Management

Your staff must know how to manage an out-of-control patient who is threatening to inflict abuse or violence. Train your ED staff, physicians, and all internal security staff in de-escalation tactics/aggression management including when to implement the tactics.

Rationale: Empower staff with methods to control physically violent patients and to prevent injury to the patient or the staff.

- Provide training for staff so that they can recognize the signs and symptoms of impending violence in an individual.
- Provide training and de-escalation tactics/aggression management. There are several vendors who provide on-site classes for staff training.
- Conduct initial training for current ED staff, physicians, PRN and agency staff, and security staff.
- Conduct periodic, ongoing training for each stakeholder according to the recommendation of the vendor providing the training.
- Determine how to provide initial and ongoing training for employees who join the staff after the initial training has occurred.
- *Tip: Several vendors who provide de-escalation/aggression management training may offer a train-the-trainer plan option. A train-the-trainer plan provides training for one or several ED staff (or other individuals if you choose) to teach the de-escalation skills and also teaches coaching management strategies for the ED staff. A train-the-trainer option for programs, such as de-escalation training that need to be presented often, may provide a significant cost savings over time.*

Strategy 6: Establish a Secure Room and Establish Restraint Policy

Provide a secure room for protection of staff or other patients from a patient who is violent, unmanageable, or physically unable to be controlled. Consider retrofitting an existing treatment room into a secure room for the protection of the patient and the staff against intentional or unintentional harm. A patient who is out of control or who may endanger himself or his caregivers should be confined and treated in a secure room.

Rationale: provide a safe, quiet, and secure environment for patients—primarily psychiatric patients—who are violent and may injure themselves or others, including staff.

- A secure room can be retrofitted from an existing treatment space.

Secure room characteristics include:

- An environment free from utensils; equipment; and movable furniture (permanently affix treatment bed or other necessary furniture to the floor) or any object that could be used as a weapon such as bedside tables, trashcans or chairs
- CCTV video surveillance connected to charge nurse station or area
- Door that can be locked from the inside and from the outside
- Lockable cabinets
- A shatterproof window
- Soundproofing
- Cushioned, quilted elevator-type pads on floors and walls
- Two-way communication device
- Panic/duress alarm
- Durable, padded treatment bed with built-in restraints

- Secure rooms can be used for any patient who is out of control or has the potential for violence, for example, because of:
  - Severe intoxication or effects from drugs
  - Psychosis or other psychiatric crisis
  - Severe agitation with shouting or swearing
  - Potential suicide
  - Patients who are physically lashing out
  - Patients who are potentially violent or who have exhibited violent acts, such as a gang member who threatens staff with a weapon

- When a patient must be confined in a secure room, conduct a brief stand-up session with staff to review the warning signs of potential violence and to communicate the general guidelines for communication and personal safety when treating violent or potentially violent patients as follows:

- ED staff and physicians are to enter only when accompanied by another person
- Limit eye contact
- Approach the patient only from the front
- Maintain a safety zone of four times greater than normal (approximately 4 feet)
- Ask the patient where he would like you to stand, especially if the patient retreats from you
- Stand at an oblique angle to the patient
- Stand with your back to the door for easy escape if this becomes necessary
- Post security staff who have been trained in de-escalation techniques outside the door at all times
- *Tip: New restraint guidance was issued by the Centers for Medicare and Medicaid Services (CMS) on December 6, 2006. Be certain to review the guidelines, which include training requirements, other interventions, and potential harm that restraints can cause to patients. CMS/restraint Web link: (CMS Publishes Final Patients Rights, 2006).*

Strategy 7: Reinforce Triage Staff and Re-Educate Triage Nurses

The triage nurse is responsible for providing more than the initial triage/status evaluation of a patient and assigning the correct triage level.

The triage nurse must also:

1. Continuously evaluate and reevaluate any changes in a patient's condition
2. Communicate frequently and comprehensively with the patient and the family/visitors
3. Respond to simple requests
4. Answer questions
5. Manage the waiting room to ensure safety for all
6. Provide a welcoming, hospitable environment
7. Identify the potential for impending violent conditions
8. Coordinate movement of patient from the waiting room to the ED treatment area

Rationale: Establish strong front-end processes and a trained triage team to provide a core competency for a hospitality-based waiting room and in triage; enhance the ability of the triage nurse staff to recognize any potential for violence in patients, families, or visitors as depicted in Exhibit 8.6.

- Train all Emergency Department RN staff in the triage process so that any RN can step into the role of triage nurse
- Train all staff to recognize signs of impending danger or violence
- Train all staff to understand the safety focus and the hospitality focus of managing the waiting room
  - Position the triage nurse so that he/she has a full view of the waiting room but is located in an area that protects him/her against weapons and from unauthorized approach and/or impending violence
  - Install bullet-resistant or shatterproof glass in the triage area or office
- Implement a hospitality strategy including reassurance rounds (also called comfort rounds or hospitality rounds). Empower a

Exhibit 8.6

KEY STRATEGIES TO MANAGING THE WAITING ROOM

VIOLENCE PREVENTION AND SAFETY FOCUS—TRIAGE NURSE

- Identify emergency need of patient to be seen by provider
- Assign accurate triage level
- Reassess patient at least hourly to ensure patient status has not deteriorated
- Identify the early warning signs of violence and intervene to prevent injury
- Protect triage staff from violence
- Maintain communication with patients, families, and visitors

VIOLENCE PREVENTION AND HOSPITALITY FOCUS—ALL STAFF

- Greet and welcome patient and family promptly
- Maintain communication with patients, families, and visitors
- Identify the early warning signs of violence and intervene to prevent injury
- Initiate reassurance rounds
- Listen
- Answer questions
- Provide service/status updates

technician or other staff member to take responsibility for the care and comfort of the waiting room patients, with the goal of keeping the patient and family comfortable, free from agitation, and updated about the progress and timing of their place in line.

- Specifically outline what the reassurance rounds staff can and cannot do. Some options are:
  - Ask how the patient and family are doing
  - Provide pillows and/or blankets
  - Offer coffee or refreshments and snacks (triage nurse must authorize)
  - Arrange seating to provide more privacy
  - Talk to the patient and family
  - Offer reading material
  - Respond to simple requests
  - Communicate *any* change that the patient or family tells you or that you notice to the triage nurse immediately. It is understood that the individual conducting reassurance rounds probably will not have medical or first-aid training; it is the ultimate responsibility of the triage nurse to identify triage level change/deterioration of patients.
  - Example: Reassurance rounds communication with patient: "EMS just arrived with an injured patient. The doctor needs to stabilize the patient. You are fifth in line to be seen after that. I anticipate that the doctor will see you within 1 hour."
  - *Tip: Provide a comfort/welcome package for each patient. Items can be presented in a plastic bag inscribed with the hospital name and with a sincere phrase such as "Thank you for choosing (or Welcome to) Hospital Name, your community hospital." Items to include in the bag could be hand sanitizing lotion or cloths; tissues; notepad and pen with hospital name; small bottle of mouthwash; travel toothbrush and toothpaste; brochure about violence in the ED; information regarding the ED and the waiting room, including an explanation about reasons for the waiting room wait; and a hospital policy about aggression, violence, and abuse, focusing on the patient safety aspect.*

- Establish bilateral communication between the triage nurse and the staff as a key strategy in preventing individuals from becoming anxious and frustrated, an acknowledged reason for violence in Emergency Department waiting rooms.

■ Consider adding signage to welcome the highest revenue-producing patient who comes to your ED, for example, pediatric patients:

"(Hospital Name) LOVES Its Kids!"

Strategy 8: Install Metal Detectors

Install metal detectors at the main entrance to the Emergency Department and hire security personnel around the clock to manage the patients, families, visitors, consultants or other professionals, or any individual who wishes to gain entrance to the Emergency Department. Utilize a hand-held detector (wand) for scanning EMS patient arrivals. Install a contraband locker for storage of all weapons.

Metal detectors provide the highest level of protection to prevent weapons from entering the Emergency Department. Contraband lockers are used to store all weaponry that is discovered during the scanning process. Weapons are not to be returned to the individuals who bring them into the ED; instead, they may be arranged to retrieve them from the local police department. Making this arrangement is the responsibility of the Emergency Department, but arranging for weapon retrieval from the police department will prevent use of the weapon in the parking lot of the hospital as patients leave. The goal of the Emergency Department is to initiate any barrier possible to vanquish the use of weapons in or around the Emergency Department.

Rationale: Metal detectors are the ultimate in protection against weapons (guns, knives, blades, containers of chemical weapons) entering your Emergency Department.

■ Install walk-through metal detectors, which are used for ambulatory patients, families, visitors—anyone who walks into the Emergency Department.
■ Use hand-held metal detector(s) to scan EMS patients who are brought to the Emergency Department, to detect whether ambulance patients are in possession of weapons and to safely remove these weapons.
■ Install a contraband locker to store weapons found during search, surrender, or confiscation.
■ Evaluate the need for engineering or design changes including assessment of the adequate number of significant light sources

in the surrounding parking areas/structures and any area in close proximity to the ED entrance.

■ Install a digital video camera at the ambulatory entrance to the ED. A CCTV camera system is a real-time video camera and will require constant monitor surveillance.

■ If your Emergency Department waiting room and/or treatment area is large, consider installing several CCTV cameras for complete surveillance options.

■ Establish policy for the prohibition of weapons being brought into the Emergency Department or hospital.

■ Establish policy for the identification and storage of all contraband discovered or surrendered in the Emergency Department.

■ Arrange with local police to have contraband that has been collected in the Emergency Department picked up daily.

Strategy 9: Add Security Officers/Staff

The security department and its many roles will be critical to the success of the violence protection plan for the Emergency Department. If your Emergency Department is at high risk for violence, consider implementing a full-service security department. The security department for the Emergency Department should be on site in the waiting room at all times. It is important that the ED security department is a dedicated staff without responsibilities to other departments.

The items in this strategy are comprehensive tasks that can or should be functions of the security department. Select the functions and tasks that are appropriate for your needs. Security guards should have knowledge about how to perform requirements and competencies so that training should encompass how to perform the tasks based on the specific needs and polices of your Emergency Department.

Rationale: The role of the security staff in the Emergency Department is a critical function for protection of the Emergency Department against violence and for the successful implementation of a violence protection plan.

■ Develop a culture and environment of nonviolence

■ Install a CCTV video monitor so that patients, families, and visitors can view themselves upon entering the Emergency Department

■ Team-based security: developing familiarity and communication of Emergency Department policies and procedures with security staff

- Security and ED staff need to be able to identify each other by name and face
  - Hold joint staff meetings
  - Develop proactive safety and security goals
  - Build rapport
  - Ask security to participate in change of shift reports and to communicate any security issues that have occurred in the past 8–12 hours
  - Have physical and personal rounds with nursing, instead of having security sit behind a desk (this is called rounding vs. desk duty)
- Include security in debriefing sessions
- Involve security in joint hospital activities such as disease walks (e.g., Walk for the Cure) or volunteering (e.g., Habitat for Humanity)
- Joint program development
  - Hospital safety officer to design and build drills for joint response among ED staff and security
- Establish goals for quality improvement for security in the Emergency Department
  - Track and use quality data to support change for staffing surveillance or other safety goals
  - Break down departmental silos
- Train and educate the security staff in policy and security response to:
  - Code V announcements
  - De-escalation tactics/aggression management
  - Meet-and-greet strategies of successful customer service, including the appropriate welcoming and screening of patients and visitors
  - Crisis and violence prevention
  - Violence-prevention strategies and responses
  - Sounding of the duress/panic alarm
  - Responsibilities for watch patients and patients in the secure room
  - Procedure and use of the walk-through metal detector
  - Procedure and use of the hand-held metal detector scanner/wand

- *Tip: The ideal procedure would be to have a second security guard posted at the EMS/ambulance entrance. It is rare that ambulances arrive in a nonstop fashion at the Emergency Department; consider training other individuals—in addition to security officers—in use of the hand-held metal detector/ wand.*
- Procedures for restraint use and alternative methods to the use of restraints
- Procedure for discovery of and securing of contraband
  - Procedure for local police department to collect contraband daily
  - Procedure for individuals to pick up contraband at police department
  - Surveillance
  - Search and seizure methods
- Procedure for lockdown and capabilities of the system
  - Procedure for lockdown of perimeter doors, tunnels, and sky bridges to secure hospital campus in case of emergency
- Procedures for forensic patients
  - Lockdown of Emergency Department if patient arrives with penetrating wound (gunshot wound or stabbing)
  - Reporting responsibilities
- Search for graffiti in or around hospital and Emergency Department
- Procedure for family and visitors in Emergency Department

The following functions are general roles for security officers. The appropriate training and competencies/skills review and timing of competency checklists for security officers is beyond the scope of this book. Specific training for hospital and Emergency Department security officers may be required. Training is provided by law enforcement professionals and vendors.

- Procedures for traffic and crowd control relative to emergency management (large casualties) and potential decontamination; setting up decontamination and hot/warm/cold zones and maintenance of zones
- Procedures for environment of care, including the

- Understanding of policy and roles and responses required in the event of internal codes (child abduction, fire, violence) and the arrival of mass casualty victims
- Handcuff policy and use
  - Knowledge of the correct procedures and responsibilities for guarding a prisoner and so forth
  - Proficiency may require accredited law enforcement training
- Knowledge of community and regional disaster plans
- Knowledge of local and state criminal codes and standards
- Knowledge of the correct and appropriate use of PPE
- Heightened awareness of potential terrorist activities; complete weapon destruction/terrorism awareness training

Strategy 10: Initiate Violence Awareness and Prevention Campaign

The community and hospital-wide violence awareness and prevention campaign is the most important strategy to implement. The community will be made aware that positive change and improvement is occurring at the Emergency Department for the benefit of the community. Potential offenders will be warned of the consequences of committing violent acts in the Emergency Department and hospital.

The public relations outreach will reward the Emergency Department and hospital with an increase in new and repeat patient/customer business, especially with the addition of the hospitality strategy.

Rationale: To inform the public—your customers—that violence will not be tolerated and that because you care about the safety, security, and comfort of patients when they choose your Emergency Department for care, violence awareness is one focus of the ED.

Communicate the measures being implemented to ensure a safe ED for patients and tell them of the changes you have made to the waiting room to ensure their comfort.

- Partner with the local media and the police department to mutually communicate the roll-out of the public violence awareness and prevention campaign. Enlist their ideas.
- Engage the hospital marketing department to help develop a marketing campaign for violence awareness and prevention in the Emergency Department (ask a marketing representative to be on

the task force to develop the violence awareness and prevention outreach).

■ Sponsor a hospital-wide contest to choose a slogan for the campaign.

   ■ Make the prize substantial (minimum $300) to attract a large group of participants.

■ Develop external (vinyl) signs and posters for the waiting room.

■ Develop customer brochures:

   ■ Brochure to describe and explain the ED and waiting room process and why patients may have to wait

   ■ Brochure to communicate hospital marketing messages about new programs or equipment to enhance the customer experience.

■ Communicate the addition of comfort initiatives in the waiting room. Communicate that the hospital is safe for its patients—and make sure that it is.

■ Host a meeting with the local police department.

■ *Tip: Several security consultants recommend against employing off-duty police officers for PRN security staff. The security staff in your ED needs to be focused on the unique needs of your ED. However, it is critical to partner with the police department to establish a relationship between the security staff and local law enforcement.*

■ Execute the strategy to refurbish the Emergency Department waiting room. If the decision has been made to install metal detectors, order and install the detectors, then initiate training for the nurses, physicians, and for other ED and security staff.

■ Consider purchasing or creating continuous-play videos to broadcast in the waiting room to entertain, educate, and communicate messages to the patients and families. A video explaining to patients what they can expect during their Emergency Department visit can help a patient have a positive experience in the ED. Educating patients, families, and visitors about the ED experience improves their understanding and increases patient satisfaction.

Consider video communication for the following topics:

■ Emergency Department violence awareness and prevention

■ What a patient and family can expect during an Emergency Department visit at your hospital

- Health and wellness education/medical topics
- Marketing messages: what makes your hospital and Emergency Department unique and better
- *Tip: A study done in Canada in 2007 was conducted to determine whether an Emergency Department video, played for patients in the waiting room, had any significant impact on patient satisfaction and an increased understanding of the ED experience, including the potential for waits in the waiting room. The study also evaluated whether the communication/educational video changed patient perception about the length of wait times (the mean length of ED stay was 5.9 hours). Postvideo analysis revealed improved patient satisfaction, from a 58% "excellent or very good" ranking to a 65% ranking; however, the patient perception of length of time spent waiting in the waiting room did not change significantly* (Papa, 2008).

EVIDENCE-BASED STRATEGIES FOR PROTECTING AN ED FROM VIOLENCE

"Little research exists examining the effectiveness of clinical strategies in addressing violent behaviors; consequently, this lack of benchmarks results in performance variability and inadequate evidence-based practice" (McGill, 2006). What are the causes of a violent outbreak of psychiatric patients in the Emergency Department? There are a series of logical answers to this question:

1. An episode of high stress triggers a response in an individual that caregivers or family cannot manage, and they bring the individual to the Emergency Department where the violent, out-of-control response continues
2. A patient may be overstimulated by the activity and chaos in the Emergency Department
3. A patient misunderstands basic communications with others
4. There is an extended period of antisocial and/or out-of-control behavior
5. The basic psychiatric condition is causing an increase in confusion, or the effects—either positive or negative—of psychopharmaceuticals

A federal survey conducted in 2001 reveals that 68.2 per 1,000 mental health workers, versus 12.6 per 1,000 other workers in all occupations, have been victims of psychiatric patient abuse or violence (McGill, 2006, p. 41). A critical strategy for dealing with the potential for psychiatric patient abuse or violence is staff training and learning how to apply effective and the least-restrictive interventions to protect oneself and the patient. Training is recommended and consists of methods of therapeutic communication with the goal of educating staff to avoid unnecessary confrontation and to learn skills and techniques to de-escalate aggressive patient behavior (McGill, 2006, p. 41).

To train and educate staff in therapeutic communication and de-escalation techniques, adult-learning tools and learner-centered principles that are best presented via computer-based-training (CBT) because the objective, positive, and immediate feedback provided by CBT systems were preferred by the learners, as compared with instructor-led sessions (McGill, 2006, p.42).

The largest gap in the successful management of psychiatric patients appeared to be the skills of therapeutic communication for the Emergency Department nurse—or other nurses—when dealing with a potentially violent patient (McGill, 2006, p. 43). CBT, or computer-based training, for all staff was implemented, and despite an increase in factors that could contribute to an increase in assaults such as a high census and sicker patients, assaults decreased by 58% (McGill, 2006, p. 44). One hundred percent of the staff believed that the therapeutic communication skills that were learned were very practical and could be applied successfully to a clinical setting (McGill, 2006, p. 44).

CASE STUDY

FORT WALTON BEACH HOSPITAL LACKS IMPORTANT SECURITY

One of the Emergency Department physicians at Fort Walton Beach Hospital in Florida reminds everyone that the hospital administrator has always been against evaluating the need for additional

(Continued)

security in the hospital's ED. The hospital staff—especially the staff in the Emergency Department—questions the wisdom of the administrator's decision because an average of 26 mentally ill patients escape every year from the hospital. From January 1 through July 20, 2008, 21 mentally ill patients have escaped.

A former ED physician had organized a meeting 4 years ago with the administrator and the local county sheriff. The physician was interested in lobbying for additional security, wanting to add off-duty police officers in the Emergency Department, but the administrator was against it, worried that the presence of a uniformed police officer would "send the wrong message to the community" (McLaughlin, 2008).

On July 21, a Baker Act detainee escaped from the Emergency Department two times in one evening.[2] The patient/detainee shot and killed the deputy sheriff and then committed suicide during a confrontation with the sheriff following his second escape.

The former Emergency Department physician had visited the hospital just 5 days prior to the incident and remarks that he was able to enter the hospital using a short cut that let him enter the ED through an unlocked door near the back of the Emergency Department. He did not see any security staff, and no one stopped him, challenged him, or asked who he was.

The issue of ED security, especially when dealing with the mentally ill, has escalated since the episode when the detainee had a fatal shoot-out with the deputy sheriff. Finally, something may be done about the lack of security in the Emergency Department, because the chairman of the board of directors had requested answers and a report to address the situation and identify the problems of the recent past. The report, to be presented to the board, will hopefully illuminate not only the serious nature of unlimited access to the Emergency Department and the inadequate focus or presence of security but will also reveal the need for policy change and staff education (McLaughlin, 2008).

NOTES

1. CAP Index is the online crime statistics tool marketed by the company of the same name. The low-cost ($199.00) fee grants access to reports targeted to your address and zip

code, providing crime statistics for the current date, and projects crime in the future, at 5 years and 10 years. For more information, contact Cap Index at www.capindex.com.

2. The Baker Act is a Florida state mental health law that was enacted in 1971 allowing for emergency or involuntary commitment to a mental health facility if a patient has a documented mental illness. For aditional information, please see Frequently Asked Questions about reform of Florida's Baker Act, http://www.psychlaws.org/PressRoom/faqonbakeract.htm.

REFERENCES

CMS publishes final patients rights rule on use of restraints and seclusion. (2006, December 9). Retrieved April 28, 2009, from http://www.cms.hhs.gov/apps/media/press/release.asp?Counter=2057

Imposters targeting U.S. hospitals: Could terrorists come to your ED? (2005). *ED Management, 17*(6), 61–63.

Kennedy, M. (2005). Violence in Emergency Departments: Under-reported, unconstrained and unconscionable. *MJA Medical Journal of Australia, 184*(7), 362–365.

McGill, A. (2006). Evidence-based strategies to decrease psychiatric patient assaults. *Nursing Management, 37*(11), 41–44.

McLaughlin, T. (2008). *In FWB, Fort Walton Beach, FL hospital security is lacking.* Retrieved August 19, 2008, from http://www.nwfdailynews.com/common/printer/view.php?db=nwfdn&id=9802

Nawar, E. W., Niska, R. W., & Xu, J. (2007). *National Hospital Ambulatory Medical Care Survey: 2005 Emergency Department.* Hyattsville, MD: Centers for Disease Control, U.S. Department of Health and Human Services, National Center for Health Statistics.

Papa, L. S. (2008, July/August). Does a waiting room video about what to expect during an emergency department visit improve patient satisfaction? *Canadian Journal of Emergency Medicine, 10*(4), 347.

Pitts, S. R., Niska, R. W., Xu, J., & Burt, C. (2008). *National Hospital Ambulatory Medical Care Survey: 2006 Emergency Department Survey.* Hyattsville, MD: Centers for Disease Control,.

Thrall, T. (2006, September). *Stopping ED violence before it happens.* Retrieved November 14, 2007, from http://www.hhnmag.com/hhnmag_app/jsp/articledisplay.jsp?dcrpath=HHNMAG/PubsNewsArticle/data/2006September/0609HHN_FEA_Safety&domain=HHNMAG

9
Communication Strategies: Intra-Institutional

The most effective response policies and activities related to managing violence of any kind are those that never are called into play. While it is impossible to predict and develop contingencies for every potential threat to the Emergency Department (ED), hospital personnel, including managers and administrators, must have a variety of tools at their disposal to:

- Assist with understanding violence
- Manage groups that may instigate violence
- Mitigate the frequency and severity of violent episodes

Planning and communication also are fundamental to the successful outcome of a program to inform all stakeholders of the potential for violence in your ED. "Understanding and awareness can help thwart and avoid violent situations while saving the lives of staff, patients, and visitors alike. Training, protocols, and procedures can insure that safety measures are followed and that violence at the hands of street gangs can be greatly minimized" (L. Savelli, personal communication, August 20, 2008).

This chapter examines common approaches for the development and implementation of best practices and strategies to promote the culture of a violence-free environment, especially in the area of greatest violence potential, the Emergency Department. The goal is to communicate the potential for violence and to solicit the support and involvement of all stakeholders in the development of violence awareness and prevention initiatives.

BOTTOM-UP COMMUNICATION STRATEGIES

In clinical settings, communication via dashboards, trackers, and interpersonal communication is critical to achieving communication efficiency and continuity and to preventing delay in providing care for patients coming to the ED. Establishing methods for organizing and delivering information that work for your ED will improve your bottom line revenue by focusing on achieving quality outcomes and efficiency. The methods that you use to provide the rapid turnaround of data and consistent methods of information delivery are particularly important in the fast-paced, often-chaotic environment of the ED.

The same is true for interpersonal communications, within the ED, with other hospital departments, and with external customers within the community. The interpersonal communication methods that the ED selects to use should effectively share the message you wish to communicate and will be a particularly important tool to use when introducing education or training relative to violence-prevention initiatives. This holds true for both the internal customers (stakeholders) and the external marketplace. Your ultimate goal is to select a method that effectively influences others and establishes the Emergency Department as the authority with regard to the development of ED policy and practice of violence awareness and prevention. No Emergency Department is immune to violence. At some point, your ED will experience violence in one of its many forms. Everyone needs to be aware of this reality. Communicating awareness is an operating principle that can guide your actions to prevent serious consequences when violence does occur.

In today's competitive marketplace, hiring effective marketing and communication staff is a new necessity for hospitals. Marketing departments have the responsibility for continually keeping the hospital's health care message in front of customers. Hospitals are now business competitors, vying for patients and attempting to become the provider of choice by delivering hot-button products and services. The public relations (PR) or communication department's main functions are direct communication and relationship building with the public regarding the hospital, the promotion of the hospital's mission and goals, and the management of negative perceptions or communications about negative situations, such as ED violence.

Tip: Recruit marketing and PR employees who have a stake in enlarging the positive perception of the hospital and who will be incentivized to help create innovative programs to set the hospital apart from the competition.

VIOLENCE AWARENESS AND PREVENTION COMMUNICATIONS: DEVELOPING YOUR STRATEGY

Develop a communications strategy for the ED that will focus attention on violence awareness and prevention initiatives among external and internal customers. Begin your quest to proliferate the message of awareness of violence in the Emergency Department by starting with information that you already have. Utilize the results from the 12-question violence risk self-assessment questionnaire (see Chapter 8) to communicate the gaps in safety and security in your hospital and to establish the importance of the development of a successful violence awareness and prevention program for your ED and hospital. Sensing the specific vulnerabilities of *your* ED and the opportunities for improvement is one formula for focusing attention on the need for, and enlisting support for, the development of awareness and prevention strategies you will be proposing. Some recommended strategies include:

1. Customer service and communication skills training is a way to educate front-line ED personnel such as: receptionist, triage nurses, registrars, security officers, accounting personnel, and others who interact directly with ED patients, families, and visitors.
2. Train and educate hospital staff to identify the clues that indicate:
   - Anger or frustration in patients, families, and/or visitors that may lead to a violent episode
   - Drug or alcohol impairment in patient behavior that can make an individual prone to erratic or violent behavior.
3. Know local gang member colors and/or identifying tattoos (as described in Chapter 6) and alert personnel to take special precautions

if patients or others are suspected gang members; this patient cohort is capable of violence. Ask the gang expert from the local police department to help you learn and understand important information about local gangs and to communicate key indicators.

4. Keep patients and families informed of anticipated wait times and have ongoing communication with them during their wait. This is essential to keeping individuals calm during a time of increased stress and anxiety. Although the triage nurse will be evaluating patients while they are waiting in the waiting room, communication with patients and families is a critical strategy to meet patient needs and to prevent opportunities for an exacerbation of emotions.

The goal of a successful violence awareness and prevention program is for all employees to individually and collectively work together to communicate and practice safety and mitigation of violence in the Emergency Department and hospital. Encourage all stakeholders to embrace the necessity for violence awareness and prevention initiatives by providing opportunities to learn about violence. Some effective methods that can be used are:

- Sponsor focus groups and ED outreach meetings with other hospital departments to begin the discussion of violence in your workplace.
- Help participants identify your facility's SWOT analysis safety strengths, weaknesses, opportunities, and threats.[1] Hanging a large interactive poster or whiteboard in a visible, active hallway to encourage passersby to add their ideas and comments will encourage interactive communication and will generate a lot of interest in the process and in the outcome. An example of a SWOT analysis chart is displayed in Table 9.1.
- Identify each Emergency Department and hospital stakeholder and the impact that violence in the Emergency Department or hospital would have on each stakeholder. Who are some of your stakeholders? How might each stakeholder positively or negatively affect the occurrence and severity of violent events?
- Identify the gaps and opportunities that exist within your current safety environment. Does your hospital have a designated safety department? Is their role risk management, or is their role only to report statistics on violence or other events in your hospital?

Table 9.1

INTERACTIVE ED SWOT (STRENGTHS, WEAKNESSES, OPPORTUNITIES, THREATS) ANALYSIS: VIOLENCE IN THE ED TEMPLATE

STRENGTHS	WEAKNESSES
New ED will be complete in 3 months	Only regular staff trained in de-escalation procedures
ED lockdown capabilities	High nursing staff turnover

OPPORTUNITIES	THREATS
Enhance ED policies	Limited security officers in ED PRN or agency nursing staff and physicians not trained in de-escalation techniques

Add your thoughts—we value your input regarding the hospital and violence in the ED

Once you define the role of the safety department, you can decide if safety is a gap to be included in the plan you are developing to prevent violence in the ED. What is required to close any gaps to increase safety and to best leverage opportunities to reduce and eliminate violent episodes?

■ Workplace safety and the prevention of violence does not stop at the exits to your facility; beyond the ED doors lies the greatest threat to safety and violence—the customer walking through your ED entrance who has the potential for violence. Hospitals that are able to think beyond the confines of their campuses will find ample opportunity to affect the community in terms of education and awareness of the potential for violence in the ED and hospital.

A recent informal survey of Emergency Department personnel representing five hospitals revealed that no formal program to address violence awareness and/or mitigation had been made available to hospital employees (Allen, 2006). Several employees stated that they had received brief instruction regarding potential workplace violence during an employment orientation. Only a few employees indicated that they had received any communication, training, or program instruction beyond the initial employment orientation. Several ED personnel reported incidents of violence occurring in the emergency room but had no violence-prevention policies or initiatives to know how to respond or how to prevent a recurrence (Allen, 2006).

Many stakeholders or constituencies, including the communities served by the hospital, have a vested interest in maintaining a violence-free Emergency Department and hospital. Stakeholders include: the board of directors; owners; management/administrators; ED nurses, physicians, and staff; stockholders; unions; professional associations; customers/patients; families and visitors to the hospital; and the community as a whole. All stakeholders will benefit from process improvements that ensure a violence-free Emergency Department and hospital.

The majority of violence presenting to the ED tends to occur prior to hospital arrival (intimate partner violence, elder violence, etc.). Pre-hospital violence or violent events that begin away from the hospital can continue or escalate upon and after arrival in the ED.

The most dangerous violence is the violence that occurs within the Emergency Department and hospital because of the number of people (visitors, patients, and staff) and the potential impact to the operations of the hospital and to the environment of safety. Violence that occurs within the ED and hospital is the only type of violence over which employees have any control. Reducing the potential for violence is not only beneficial for all stakeholders, but is tantamount to ensuring a safe ED environment.

For employees, safety awareness and violence mitigation programs must be comprehensive, inclusive, evolutionary, and ongoing. Effective programs should recognize and acknowledge how violence affects each stakeholder and demonstrate how each stakeholder can benefit from and contribute to a safe environment. Stress that each stakeholder has the important responsibility to promote the culture of safety and reduce violence through the communication and reinforcement of program initiatives.

ACTION PLANS

Implementation of a violence awareness and prevention program starts with strategic communications designed to gather support for creation of a task force to develop the program and continues with the rollout of the strategies and tactics that are developed within the task force. The recommended approach is through five action plan activities.

Action Plan Step 1: Discussions Within the ED Personnel Group

The ED director and medical director together with the security chief should take responsibility for completing the violence risk self-assessment questionnaire. The answers that are derived from the questionnaire will not uncover all violence risk gaps that the ED may have, but it will point to some strategic deficiencies and gaps that can place EDs at risk for violence. Based on the information obtained from the questionnaire, edit the template letter provided in Exhibit 9.1 to customize critical information for the administration to be aware of relating to the potential for violence in the Emergency Department. Attach a copy of the questionnaire results and the ED responses to the letter.

The ED staff, including physicians and all PRN or agency staff, should meet to discuss the results. Meeting with all staff may require several sessions so that everyone is involved. Encourage the group to comment freely and ask if any of them feel unsafe at work. The goal is to expand the results of the questionnaire so that additional gaps and dangers can be identified. Engaging staff in creating solutions will ensure positive buy-in and may result in a plethora of suggestions for improvement. Share with the staff the letter that will be delivered to administration.

Action Plan Step 2: Educating the Administration About the Reality of Emergency Department Violence

Your goal, when communicating the necessity for implementing a violence awareness and prevention plan with the administration, is to make them aware of covert dangers in your ED. The ED normally reports to the chief nursing officer (CNO), so communicating the need for violence awareness and prevention should be an *easy sell* to the CNO. Solicit your CNO's assistance in communicating the need to the other members of the executive staff. Inform the CNO that you and the ED medical director will be meeting with the CEO and request your CNO's attendance at the meeting. Educating the CEO and the remainder of the executive team may be more difficult. The tips, listed in the following sections, regarding communication with the CEO apply to all members of the executive team.

Exhibit 9.1

TEMPLATE LETTER TO HOSPITAL ADMINISTRATION

To [Hospital Name] Administration and the Board of Directors:

The vulnerability of the Emergency Department and of the hospital for the potential of violence has been an increasing concern of ours. The concern is primarily for the safety of our Emergency Department nurses, physicians, and staff, but we must also take into account the potential danger to the patients, families, and visitors.

Recently, we completed a 12-question violence risk self-assessment questionnaire that confirmed our suspicions about the risk to the Emergency Department. We have determined that the Emergency Department is at significant risk for violence for the following reasons:

1. Nineteen percent of all patients coming to the Emergency Department come because they are in crisis from a serious exacerbation of their psychiatric illnesses. The state psychiatric hospital 6 miles from this hospital closed one year ago. The average length of stay for this type of patient is 15 hours because there are limited options for disposition. We have attempted to retrofit an existing treatment room for use as a safe room for patients who are frequently out of control, but we have been denied funding for this project. The short-term and long-term presence of this type of patient in our Emergency Department is putting our staff at risk, especially because of the fact that we have a security guard who is in the Emergency Department only between 12 midnight and 8 AM, Saturday and Sunday only. *[Use your statistics]*

2. Fifty-three percent of all patients coming to the Emergency Department are not emergency-level patients; most require primary care only. The low-acuity patient clogs the system for patients requiring true emergency care. On average, we have six patients *boarding* in the ED, waiting for inpatient beds, and the average time they must wait is 3.8 hours. The situation results in a great many patients waiting in the waiting room. Two days ago, one low-acuity patient verbally abused the triage nurse and the physician who both attempted to explain the reason for the extensive wait in the waiting room to him. Verbal abuse is a documented precursor to physical abuse. Aggression, violence, and abuse cannot and should not be tolerated by our staff. Mechanisms for reporting violent episodes need to be implemented. *[Use your statistics]*

We respectfully request your assistance to resolve the problem of security and safety in the Emergency Department.

Please attend a meeting tomorrow at 2 PM in the ED conference room so that we may discuss current issues and the safety measures that need to be implemented in the Emergency Department to benefit our staff and patients. Thank you.

Very sincerely yours,

[*Signature*]

RN, Director, Emergency Department

[*Signature*]

MD, Medical Director, Emergency Department

Action Plan Step 3: Buy in the CEO

Communicating a powerful *enterprise strategy* to prevent violence must start at the top. However, your Emergency Department staff, those on the front lines of potential violence, may need to educate the hospital administration and management about violence to get them on board and to gain their support for a violence-prevention campaign. It is critical for the CEO to be involved. Messages from the CEO will be listened to and taken seriously because everyone wants to do what the boss says! The Emergency Department may need to negotiate hospital leadership commitment to champion enduring strategies for the prevention of violence in the ED and hospital. While it would be unusual for the CEO/ administrator to be naïve about, or have no understanding of, violence as a problem in Emergency Departments, the CEO may not believe that violence can occur in your ED. Violence is a serious, bottom-line eroding problem that needs to be addressed.

Because CEOs understand numbers and costs, the best strategy to use when communicating with the CEO is to present statistics and evidence that violence can occur. Inform the CEO about violence in general and violence in your ED. Your goal is to have him/her communicate violence awareness and prevention in the ED (the program that you develop) from the CEO's office and to fill in the gaps in security that are missing—and that are essential for safety—in your ED.

The 10 tactics that are recommended for communication with the CEO are:

1. Hand-deliver the letter to the administration and board of directors. Ask the CEO to share the letter with other members of the executive team. Request a meeting date and time with the CEO in approximately 1 week to allow time for action from the CEO.
2. Prior to the meeting, obtain information from the local police department and provide the CEO with information regarding gang activity and intrusion into your hospital neighborhood. Cite statistics from the "Thirty-Six Compelling Reasons for ED Personnel and Administrators to Know and Understand Violence in the ED" located in Chapter 5.
3. Communicate the message that psychiatric hospitals have closed and that there are very limited community services. Psychiatric patients who live in the community and become uncontrollable have no place to go but to the Emergency Department. There is a high potential for violence from this group of patients.

4. The CEO will be aware of the crowding and boarding issues in the Emergency Department. Be certain that the ED medical director attends the meeting with you so that he can state specifics about your ED to the CEO. Crowding is a documented reason for violence in the Emergency Department. State the current level of security staffing in the ED. Include any problem that you have relative to safe levels of nurse staffing or the use of agency and staffing relative to physician and specialty physician issues—any situation that can threaten the safety of staff in the Emergency Department.

5. Describe any near-miss violence events that have occurred in the ED.

6. Share the results of the violence risk self-assessment questionnaire (Strategy 1 in Chapter 8) that point to the gaps in your ED safety.

7. Tie your requests for gap-fillers (24-hour security, metal detector, equipment for a secure room, etc.) to the actual costs for these items (pricing information is available in Exhibit 8.1). Prior to the meeting, ask your risk manager to provide the cost for disability due to stress of an employee and the cost for the death of an employee; share these costs with the CEO.

8. Give the CEO a copy of this book.

9. Inform the CEO that you are establishing a task force to identify additional gaps and to roll out a violence awareness and prevention program. As soon as the program details have been developed by the task force and the program is ready to deploy, request a second meeting with the CEO to share the specifics of the plan that the task force has developed.

10. Ask the CEO directly if his/her office will communicate the violence awareness and prevention plan rollout and the program details, including the reasons that he/she expects the staff to support the efforts to disseminate violence awareness and prevention.

Action Plan Step 4: Violence Awareness and Prevention Program Development

The way that any progressive program is developed and implemented varies by institution, facility, and location. Workplace cultures are unique, so there is no one standardized approach to implementing awareness or a program of operational change and improvement. Differing organizational structures, functions, organizational mission and vision, management styles, corporate histories, physical layouts, and communication systems contribute to your selection of the best method of communications for your specific environment.

Keep the two important components of program development in mind as you and the task force design the violence awareness and prevention program for your ED:

- *Awareness of the program,* including the reasons that the program is necessary
- *Implementation of the program components* to initiate change

Some of the suggestions to consider are:

1. Enlist buy-in and support from key corporate decision makers. Decision makers may vary by institution and could include one or more of the following: board of directors, CEO, CMO, senior management team, human resources management, loss prevention officer, security department, department heads, union representatives, and other key hospital individual or group decision makers. One imperative is that unconditional support for the program is communicated throughout the organization, starting in the CEO's office and expanding to include horizontal communication among the different levels of hierarchy, and vertically throughout all departments. Ensure that all clinical shifts are included in communications and that the program components, support, and rollout will be made available to all shifts. Violence can occur anytime and anywhere, so it is vital that all employees are aware, prepared, and know how to respond.

2. Select an individual or individuals whose main job will be to develop and deploy the program and to function as the program director. The ED director would be the ideal choice for program director, but the challenges that this individual faces every day may limit the success of the program. The program director should be selected from a group of involved employees who have been in the organization for at least 1 year, so that he/she understands the existing corporate culture and the type of effective communication methods that are successful and has a vested interest in protecting the Emergency Department.

3. Take advantage of what you know already works in your organization with regard to communication. The communication vehicles that are familiar to the employees, including existing newsletters,

bulletin boards, electronic message boards, orientation sessions, departmental and shift meetings, ongoing educational sessions, Internet and company Intranet sites, closed-circuit broadcasts, break- and lunch-room promotions, community service participations, and other methods unique to your organization, should be the communication methods of choice. There is no need to reinvent the wheel. Incorporating the functional and the familiar will ensure your success.

4. Informal organizational communication structures should not be overlooked when designing and implementing a program. One of the best informal methods is to select a champion within your organization to help communicate your message. Choose champions who are well-connected in your organization and who, as leaders, elicit respect from the majority of people; others will listen to people like this. Entice other champions who may interact with large numbers of people during the day: information desk clerks, cafeteria cashiers, security (of course!), evening supervisors, and so forth. The best champion of a violence prevention and awareness program may be the employee who has been a victim of violence or has witnessed aggression, violence, or abuse firsthand.

5. Implementing change takes time. Pay attention to the communication methods that work well over the long-term for your organization and continue to use them.

6. Involve all of the employees in communication of the program including the nonclinical areas of housekeeping, laboratory, account management, and so forth.

7. The employees in your organization are in a constant state of flux; employees depart and new employees enter. Communication of the violence awareness and prevention program is a critical component to include in hospital orientation sessions. If possible, schedule the program director to speak about violence awareness and prevention and the status of the program at every orientation session.

8. Reinforce and repeat the message continually.

9. Revise any program strategies, goals, and materials frequently to ensure relevance.

10. Continually assess and solicit feedback and information from all stakeholders. Ask the local police department, for example, to inform you about violence that has occurred at other hospitals,

businesses, schools, malls, or any site in your locale where large numbers of people gather and may have become a target for violence.

It is important to remember that no Emergency Department is immune to the possibility of violence, no matter how large or small the ED. Schools have learned many difficult lessons through their experiences and have implemented a range of violence-prevention barriers, including the installation of police or security personnel on site, limiting the access to school property, metal detectors to screen for weapons, training and drills for facility lockdowns, stun guns, instant message alert systems, and more. The same strategies are also appropriate for use in Emergency Departments (see the 10 strategies in Chapter 8).

Action Plan Step 5: Violence Awareness and Prevention Plan Rollout

The best program development tip that I can offer is this: keep it simple. There are eight simple steps in the implementation of a violence awareness and prevention program in your hospital and community.

1. Choose a program director. Use the simplified project plan and prepare an agenda for the first meeting. Keep meetings on time and no longer than 1 hour. Choose a meeting room with wallboard or chalkboard. Obtain a small allocation ($2,500–$5,000) from the ED budget or another source for expenses for a slogan contest, posters, signs, and other miscellaneous expenses.
2. Establish a task force of approximately 10 individuals from all segments of the hospital. Include marketing. Consider asking a board member. Share violence statistics and security gaps at the first meeting. Invite the CEO to the first meeting and introduce him/her to the group, even if they all know him/her.
3. Establish regular meeting dates and times that are no greater than 2 weeks apart.
4. Decide the community agencies to partner with (police, media, churches, other violence prevention groups, and hospital volunteers).
5. Roll out the slogan contest (internally and externally if desired) and set a date for selection of the slogan and announcement of the winner (minimum 2 weeks).

6. Decide how you will communicate your violence awareness and prevention message to internal and external stakeholders.
7. Decide on the wording of your message. Keep it simple (example: [Hospital Name] is Dead Set Against Violence).
8. Establish program goals: What do you want to accomplish? Set goals late in the meeting so that all participants have important information about the ED objectives to impart awareness about violence.

The process of implementing a program to benefit the community and all hospital employees offers great value for your employees and for the community. Activities that will connect your ED and hospital with the community and its vast resources will become an enduring asset. Because of the positive impact that a program such as violence awareness and prevention plan will have on the community, the ED and the hospital will attract more customers, which will boost profitability and place your hospital in the front of everyone's mind. The community will also benefit by recognizing your hospital as the leader in the health care community that has taken on the formidable task of preventing violence as a mechanism to protect its patients.

Reevaluate the progress of the program frequently, keeping your goal in mind. Revise the plan if there is a vital component of your program that is unsuccessful in its concept. Establish benchmarks and timelines that will force assessment of the program along the way through the accomplishment of measurable goals and objectives. Much can be learned from asking task force members for their candid opinions. If progress is slow, reevaluate and attempt to identify reasons. It may be necessary to rework one or more of the tactics.

While it is true that one size does not fit all when it comes to design and implementation of your plan to address emergency room violence, it is advisable to consider what other organizations have done or are doing to address the violence-related dilemma to which all hospitals are subject and vulnerable.

ED STAFF COMMUNICATION: DEBRIEFING FOLLOWING A VIOLENT INCIDENT

During the course of every day in the United States, emergency nurses and physicians are subjected to aggression, violence, and abuse from patients, families, and visitors in the Emergency Department, creating serious psychological trauma that does not necessarily result in death. Psychological trauma, short of death, is very serious and must be addressed to lessen the impact of stress and damage from violent episodes.

Anecdotal support and research evidence indicate that incidents of violence are unreported or underreported by professionals in the Emergency Department. One of the goals of this book is to establish an imperative for all Emergency Department nurses and physicians to report any incident of aggression, violence, or abuse that occurs. Erdos and Hughes, the authors of information about stress debriefing, advocate that "the best approach to staff assault in the medical workplace is prevention" (Erdos, 2001).

These experts suggest that to appropriately offer assistance to victims, you should develop a "response team" whose responsibility it is to assess the victim following a stressful incident, such as aggression, abuse, or violence. The response team should be led by a mental health professional trained in crisis intervention, stress, and posttraumatic stress disorder (PTSD), and the team may include a psychologist, a psychiatric nurse, a social worker or a psychiatrist, and individuals referred to as peer counselors. The most beneficial time to assess a victim is quickly after the event, optimally within 1 to 2 hours after the incident (Erdos, 2001).

Critical incident stress debriefing is referred to as an intervention to reduce distress and encourage the discussion and expression of emotions following an incident that has occurred, with a goal of alleviating the untoward effects of the incident (Erdos, 2001). Debriefing is indicated after major disaster, unusual violent events, serious injury, or other particularly difficult or stressful situations, according to psychiatryonline. com, such as the abuse delivered by a patient or another individual (Erdos, 2001).

Debriefing follows an established, six-step plan, implemented over a 3-hour period of time.

Step 1: Introduction. A facilitator explains the purpose of the session and ensures confidentiality to the victim.

Step 2: Facts. Individuals in the session introduce themselves and their roles. An overview of the incident is described.

Step 3: Feelings/emotions. Individuals discuss how they feel about the incident, and the emotional reactions are identified and shared.

Step 4: Symptoms. Individuals describe their physical and emotional symptoms, and the stress response is analyzed.

Step 5: Teaching. The facilitator describes the symptoms to be aware of, in themselves and in others. The response to stress and methods of recovery are discussed. Printed guides about stress are given to the individuals.

Step 6: Reentry. The facilitator repeats assurances and emphasizes that the dialogue will remain confidential. The facilitator answers any questions and establishes a follow-up plan. Referral to additional therapy may be provided (Erdos, 2001).

Using a debriefing session for all victims of violence has been shown to help reduce the long-term effects of stress. Distress from incidents of violence can be career ending and disability producing. Debriefing following any episode of violence can uncover important clues for providing additional resources to your staff and will be of immeasurable benefit in communicating to the staff that you care about their well-being (Erdos, 2001).

CASE STUDY

STRATEGIES FOR NO-BUDGET MARKETING AND COMMUNICATIONS

I had a limited budget dilemma a few years ago and had a need to market to a group of physicians who were typically treated to gourmet lunches supplied daily by pharmaceutical sales representatives. This group of physicians was critical to our success: quite simply, we needed their patients. We needed to get the attention of the physicians to show them the amazing patient outcomes that had been a benefit of our services. The problem was that we did not have a plan to compete—without a budget—to match the pharmaceutical reps. We came up with the idea to attend the Monday/ Wednesday/Friday mini-grand rounds and give the physicians the opportunity to meet and get to know us.

(Continued)

We arrived early for the first meeting and brought along a huge platter of cookies, purchased at low cost from our hospital cafeteria. I don't know if it was the cookies or our interest in learning about their patients during the meetings that convinced them to give us a try, but one by one the patients started arriving.

The challenge of a limited budget did not defeat our plan. Think outside your box and make the barriers, the ideas, and the changes your own.

CASE STUDY

DO YOU RECOGNIZE YOUR COWORKERS?

The scenario in this case study illustrates the importance of having face-to-face recognition among staff members and security staff and to have strict check-in procedures with PRN and agency staff. Ensure that your hospital has specific policies and procedures to address an employee—or alleged employee—who arrives at work without an official hospital photo identification badge. The following scenario is true:

An Emergency Department in Florida treated and discharged a patient one evening. The patient returned to the Emergency Department, claimed to be a nursing technician, but did not have the official hospital photo identification badge, as she claimed to have lost it.

The patient/alleged nursing tech was not challenged, and she worked for an entire shift, although the staff complained that she had very limited knowledge about the procedures that she would have been expected to know, had she been a real nursing technician. The next day the individual returned to the Emergency Department and asked to be readmitted—as a patient (Henry, 2007).

Fortunately, no patients were harmed, according to a risk management consultant/physician. The facility was extremely fortunate. "There is moral and ethical deception" (Henry, 2007), he says. The individual apparently did not ask for nor receive any

(Continued)

confidential personal information. Hospital patients including Emergency Department patients have a right to expect privacy, and they were at risk for having their personal information and confidence breached.

The incident clearly points to the value and necessity of having a check-in procedure for all nonemployee workers such as those coming from a nurse staffing agency. A policy to mandate the use and wearing of the official hospital photo identification badge is equally important. Emergency Departments and other nursing units in a hospital must think through policy requirements and ramifications. For example, if the policy states "no badge, no work," the loss of one employee for one shift could be astronomical in terms of patient care and safety. Having a process to manage the probabilities of each situation is difficult when writing policies, but it is a very important exercise.

It is commonplace for Emergency Departments to be chaotic and so intensely busy that staff rarely stop to take inventory or to ask questions. If a situation occurs that staff do not have time to address, it might be a reasonable suggestion to delegate the evaluation and resolution of a situation, such as the one described here, to security, or to an appropriate nonmedical individual.

Emergency Department management must communicate and stress the importance of wearing the photo identification badge and let staff know that it is OK to ask questions of individuals who are not recognized by regular ED employees. It is critical to avoid infringements of this kind, which could result in a much more serious outcome.

Often, a specialty physician is called in to evaluate a patient. The physician probably does not have a photo identification badge, and staff may not recognize the physician. Each specialty physician on staff or on the on-call roster must have and wear the official hospital photo identification badge. The Emergency Department physicians must make a serious effort to communicate to staff if they have called and requested a patient consultation from a physician who may not be on the hospital staff to evaluate a patient.

Staff, for some reason, seem hesitant to ask for credentials from someone they perceive to be a physician. Remember that it is as

(Continued)

*easy to falsely impersonate a physician as it is to falsely imperson-
ate a nursing technician. Don't hesitate: ask questions!
If staff are unsure of what to do, contact the director of the
Emergency Department for advice. The risk manager/physician in
this article recommends that staff take extra steps if and when you
believe that "something is amiss" (Henry, 2007).*

NOTE

1. Identification of strengths, weaknesses, opportunities, and threats is called a
SWOT analysis and can provide a method for participants to visualize opportunities for
improvement and the weaknesses that may lead to violence. Use a large conference
paper sheet; draw a large cross in the middle of the page using the entire page. In the
top left box, write "Strengths"; in the top right box write "Weaknesses"; write "Opportunities" in the box below "Strengths" and write "Threats" in the box below "Weaknesses."
Ask individuals to identify things about the ED and hospital that match each category:
for example, a strength is the CEO's support of a violence-protection program, but a
threat could be a large number of gang members as patients and no security guard. Get
the idea? It is very powerful and gets a lot of people involved in solutions!

REFERENCES

Allen, P. (2006). *Survey of hospital ED personnel.* Unpublished manuscript.

Erdos, B. H. (2001, September). *Emergency psychiatry: A review of assaults by patients
against staff at psychiatric emergency centers.* Retrieved October 20, 2007, from
http://psychservices.psychiatryonline.org

Henry, G. P. (2007, May 1). Patient comes back to ED in scrubs and works entire shift as
a temp. *ED Management, 19*(5), 49-51.

10 Community Communication Strategies

STRATEGY: PARTNER WITH THE COMMUNITY TO COMMUNICATE VIOLENCE AWARENESS AND PREVENTION

The rollout of the violence awareness and prevention program for both internal and external stakeholders has been outlined in the previous chapter. The focus of this chapter is to introduce information relative to communication with the community and provide additional strategies for a zero tolerance policy beyond the strategy presented in Chapter 8. Because the appropriate management of a crisis situation that occurs in the Emergency Department or hospital extends to the community, a comprehensive presentation of crisis management is included in this chapter.

External Stakeholders: The Community

Increasingly, marketing and advertising dollars are diverted into community service and philanthropic causes with an equal or greater return. Partnering with community agencies for assistance with fund-raising and program needs is a mutually beneficial arrangement for both your organization and the agency. For example, hospital sponsorship of a fund-raising event for an agency whose mission is to eliminate domestic violence within your community provides the agency with resources such as board leadership, volunteers, contributions, or other assets. In return the hospital receives media coverage, positive community relations, associate training and awareness, and resources for patients who are victims of domestic violence. In determining which agencies to support and partner with, consider the overall needs of your community as well as gaps in your violence awareness and prevention program. Do not hesitate to get input from your organization's associates who live in the community where your facility is located, staff social workers, community relations, and human resources staff.

Some ideas for community partnership events are to:

- Sponsor hospital and ED community forums or seminars
- Establish a speakers' bureau in partnership with police leaders to disseminate information about community gang activity and other critical violence issues
- Coordinate programs with appropriate city mayoral offices and the chamber of commerce
- Engage public relations (PR) and local media—become the mutual voice for violence awareness and prevention. The local media will be interested because they are competing intensely with other television and media for the next big story; together, the ED and the media can be a powerful communications tool.

STRATEGY: ZERO TOLERANCE FOR VIOLENCE

An important strategy for your hospital is the public communication of a zero tolerance policy to inform residents in the community that your hospital is serious about preventing violence in the Emergency Department and hospital. Zero tolerance means that your hospital will not permit or tolerate violence of any kind—and that there are consequences for any violent activity. A publicly communicated policy goes further to state your position and the consequences of any expression of violence. You mean business! Post signs, educate your staff, and communicate to the community via public service announcements that you will not tolerate violence on property surrounding your hospital or inside its walls at any time or in any form. See Exhibit 10.1 for a suggestion regarding zero tolerance signage. Let everyone know that

Exhibit 10.1

ZERO TOLERANCE SIGNAGE

[Hospital Name] has zero tolerance . . .

. . . for any individual who threatens or incites verbal or physical aggression, abuse, or violence against another individual, staff member, or patient.

There are serious consequences for aggression, abuse, or violence in this facility.

[Repeat in Spanish]

violence is forbidden and that any exhibition or threat of violence will be prosecuted.

Zero tolerance for violence has been implemented successfully and has helped airports control potential episodes of violence in aircraft and in terminals because they mean business. Any reference to aggression or threat of a violent act will have grave consequences. Emergency Departments and hospitals need to emulate the zero tolerance policies and activities of the Federal Aviation Administration and airports.

In 2006, the American Nurses Association (ANA) adopted a violence prevention resolution. The intent of the resolution was to censure violence against nurses and to protect nurses against prosecution for whistleblowing activities related to violence and abuse. The resolution and the ANA principles for the promotion of a healthy workplace are critical tenets for nurses in this volatile environment (Ray, 2007). Adopting and communicating policy and resolutions are a positive first step but need to include the consequences for violent behavior. See Exhibit 10.2 for the American Nurses Association principles for a healthy workplace.

Individual states are introducing or expanding legislation that would define an assault against a licensed health care practitioner as an *aggravated assault*. An aggravated assault is defined as a *reckless attack* with *intent* to *injure seriously*, as with a *deadly weapon*. Both California and Pennsylvania have passed legislation in the past 10 years that provides protection to licensed professionals in the form of a fine and/or imprisonment (Ray, 2007) of offenders, but neither the California nor

Exhibit 10.2

AMERICAN NURSES ASSOCIATION PRINCIPLES RELATED TO NURSING PRACTICE AND THE PROMOTION OF HEALTHY WORK ENVIRONMENTS FOR ALL NURSES

- "That all nursing personnel have the right to work in healthy work environments free of abusive behavior such as bullying, hostility, lateral abuse and violence, sexual harassment, intimidation, abuse of authority and position and reprisal for speaking out against abuses; and

- That the language of The Code of Ethics for Nurses with Interpretive Statements is nonnegotiable and the ethical precepts of the Code encompasses all nursing activities in all settings in which nurses practice, learn, teach, research, and lead, and may supersede specific policies of institutions, of employers, or of practice; and

- The registered nurse should report promptly incidents of abuse and advocate that no employee who experiences and reports workplace abuse faces reprisal; and

- Registered nurses should advocate for the implementation of policies that support abuse-free, harassment-free and violence-free workplaces through a comprehensive workplace security and violence prevention program; and

- The registered nurse should take appropriate action after an incident of abusive behavior to prevent recurrence of similar incidents."

From ANA Resolution, 2006, "Workplace Abuse and Harassment of Nurses," *Journal of Emergency Nursing, 33*(36), 257–261.

Pennsylvania legislation is enough to get the attention of the perpetrators or to have a positive impact on the occurrence of violence in the Emergency Department. It is going to take dedicated and committed advocacy by nurses and physicians to support and enact the type of legislation necessary to protect health care professionals and others against violence. We all know that the enactment of law is rarely the solution to a problem, but it may establish an essential first step in awareness of the problem. True change is created and begins to erode the foundation of problems such as violence when groups join to advocate policy and legislation and come together to say that they aren't going to take this anymore.

CASE STUDY

This case study illustrates the importance of communicating with the public who may be using your Emergency Department for primary care needs. One of the serious problems that EDs face is overcrowding (too many patients!), which can slow down the time it takes for providers to see and evaluate all patients. Patients having long waits in the Emergency Department can become frustrated and angry; pent-up emotions and situations beyond the control of the patient may lead to violence (frustration and anger are acknowledged reasons for violence). Educate the consumers in your hospital catchment area so that they understand the importance of using the Emergency Department for emergency care only! Much of this case study is from Birenbaum (2006, p. 1).

Medi-Cal is California's Medicaid health care insurance plan. Fifty percent of California health care consumers who are insured Medi-Cal public health care insurance are overusing the Emergency Department.

A recent study by the California HealthCare Foundation reports that Medi-Cal patients perceive the quality of care that they receive in one of California's Emergency Departments to be "superior" to the care that is available to them in the community. Medi-Cal holders say that they are likely to consider using the Emergency Department when a medical situation arises, such as a sudden illness or accident, according to the report.

Some of the reasons for consumers to use Emergency Departments, confirmed by the survey, are:

- *Community physicians are overloaded and cannot work patients into their overbooked schedules to allow for same-day appointments*
- *Community physicians do not provide care in the evening or on weekends*
- *Community physicians "do not communicate with their patients about urgent-care options"*

(Continued)

- *Patients say: [there is] lack of access to medical care outside the ED (e.g., same-day appointment with a primary care physician or evening and weekend appointments)*
- *Patients say: [there is] lack of advice on how to handle sudden medical problems*
- *Patients say: [there is] a lack of alternatives to the ED (e.g., nurse advice lines or urgent care clinics)*
- *Patients have positive attitudes about the ED as a site of care*
- *Seventy-six percent of the physicians say they have encouraged their patients to contact them before going to the ED*
- *But only 35% of patients say that their physicians encourage a telephone call before going to the ED*
- *Most of the (primary care) physicians say: I can accommodate same-day appointments .*
- *Greater than 50% of the patients say: I could not get an appointment the last time I needed urgent care*
- *Patients say:*
  - *I need to know why I should not use the ED for my chronic care needs*
  - *The ED provides easy access for diagnostic testing*
  - *The ED gives me a high quality of care*
  - *The ED allows me to see a specialist if I have a need to see one*
  - *The ED is convenient*
  - *The ED is affordable*
  - *The ED is overcrowded*
  - *All of the patients in the ED may result in less quality care for me*

The report reveals that 44% of patients who have used the Emergency Department have "one or more" chronic conditions. One in three patients in the survey say that their personal physician has encouraged patients to contact them prior to going to the ED, but more than half of those surveyed said that they "had difficulty reaching the physician after business hours."

(Continued)

California Emergency Departments are closing at rapid rates. The California Health Care Foundation is committed to ensuring that more appropriate—and reduced—use of EDs is achieved. The suggested improvements to reduce the Medi-Cal participants' inappropriate use of EDs for chronic care are derived from the problems that were identified in the survey:

- *Improve communication between physicians and patients*
- *Changing the processes in the ED to efficiently care for all patients*
- *Improve chronic care services*

CRISIS MANAGEMENT

Sonny Weide and Gayle Abbott, principles of the management consulting firm Hureco, Inc., in Virginia, offer compelling advice about hospital action following a crisis. The first moments following a crisis—such as a death from violence in the Emergency Department—are chaotic and confusing. The CEO of a hospital or the head of any organization must be decisive and take quick action to communicate and assure everyone that the situation (that created the crisis) is under control. Refer to Exhibit 10.3 for steps to take in developing a crisis management plan.

Crisis management is most effective when a plan is in place before a crisis has occurred. A *crisis management plan* must be an important part of the violence awareness and prevention plan for your hospital. Establish a plan, select tasks for specific members of the hospital staff, communicate the plan as soon as it has been written and frequently thereafter, reminding employees of the key tenets of the plan, and drill for perfection of crisis management strategy deployment. Knowing how to react before a crisis occurs will help diminish the impact of a crisis after it occurs.

Hureco, Inc. recommends that although each crisis will have unique circumstances, the following crisis management action plan can provide excellent guidelines:

- Engage counseling. The individuals who are closest to the situation and family members of the victims who have encountered trauma—psychological and perhaps physical—and need profes-

Exhibit 10.3

CRISIS MANAGEMENT ACTION PLAN

- Engage counseling for staff closest to violent crisis event
- Assemble a crisis management team (CMT) and deploy CMT activities
- Call victims' families
- Prepare media statement
- Arrange for clean-up of violence site
- Establish ongoing employee information/communication meetings
- Meet with hospital managers
- Respond to media
- Initiate internal and external investigations
- Establish employee committee to decide appropriate tribute for the victims of the violent event
- Establish employee reentry program
- Set up a rumor hotline (telephone)
- Manage insurance claims
- Set short-term and long-term goals

sional intervention so that recovery can begin. It is essential to provide counseling as quickly as possible. Hureco, Inc. reminds us that employees who have been in the vicinity of a crisis will not wish to stay in the area; the window of opportunity to provide immediate counseling is very narrow. Decide with the employee assistance program (EAP) or mental health professionals in advance how they can be contacted in the event of a crisis, especially if an event occurs after business hours. Small details are important, such as a location for the victims and/or eyewitnesses to go and who to call to arrange for comfort measures (food/drink, comfortable chairs, private areas, etc.). Arrange in advance for members of the EAP to be available and on site at the hospital 24 hours a day for up to 72 hours following the incident. Hureco, Inc. suggests having EAP professionals conduct walking rounds and be visible within the hospital. EAP counselors are professional mental health professionals and will be able to advise the crisis management team (CMT) if additional resources are required.

- Assemble a *CMT (Crisis management team)*. The CMT should include the following individuals: CEO, who functions as the CMT
leader; executive office representative; human resources executive; security executive; line manager; general counsel; and PR
executive. The CEO can turn leadership of the CMT over to another executive when the critical period of the crisis has passed,
after 72 hours or longer. Assign team members and specific tasks
and roles in advance of need. For example, in the event of a crisis, the CEO's assistant will contact the hospital internal security
department for details, to ensure contact with the local police department, and so forth. Hureco, Inc. recommends that each CMT
member operate with a sense of urgency. Following a crisis, the
facility will need a command or operations center located in a
convenient, central location. Plan in advance where the command
center will be located and have a schedule in place to staff the
command center 24 hours a day until the crisis has passed.
- The CMT has the following main obligations once a crisis has
occurred:

    - Gather and disseminate information as it develops. Open com-
    munication with the employees (first priority!) and with the
    public is essential to communicate that the leadership has
    taken action. Early communication goes far to help reestablish
    trust that will jumpstart recovery. Open communication will
    help dispel unnecessary rumors; great value and benefit results
    when employees hear credible accounts of events—told hon-
    estly and compassionately—from the CEO. Hureco, Inc. states
    that the longer the time between when you learn the facts and
    the time they are publicly disclosed, the less credible you (or
    you *and* your organization) become. Do not risk giving a stake-
    holder in your hospital or community a reason to distrust you
    or what is being said.
    - Take action to lessen the impact of the crisis. Part of the re-
    sponsibility of the CMT, by acting to lessen the impact of the
    event, is to dispel rumors that are naturally part of a crisis and
    have a life span of their own. Dispel rumors quickly so that
    the victims can begin the recovery process. The CMT can also
    make specific decisions about additional time off for certain
    employees or work reassignments if necessary. The other key
    task for the CMT is to coordinate the efforts of all groups or
    teams who are involved in the crisis.

- Create a plan to get beyond the crisis as quickly as possible. Some of the important functions of the CMT are to initiate future event planning such as establishing a committee for memorial events, initiating manager/employee meetings, establishing new or adapting current human resources policies, and providing ongoing EAP or professional counseling assistance for employees. See Exhibit 10.4 for a compendium of crisis management team activities.
- Call victims' families. The hospital has no legal obligation to call the victim's family, but the gesture communicates that the hospital cares about its employees and wishes to offer assistance during a time of significant stress. Families will consider the hospital as a partner that is helping to resolve details surrounding the event, and will be perceived by the victims and/or their families as compassionate, rather than being perceived as the wrongdoer that allowed the tragedy to occur. The individual who assumes the responsibility of calling the families must be very well-prepared prior to calling. Be cautious so as not to make any statement that could create a liability for the hospital. Ask legal counsel—in a precrisis management meeting—to discuss any situations or statements that could become legal liabilities for the hospital. The caller should be compassionate and is encouraged to not react negatively if the caller is berated or made to feel responsible for the event. The caller should provide the facts and offer the name and phone number of a hospital representative (CMT member) to call for additional information.
- Prepare a statement for the media. Write a statement of facts for the media and release it quickly following the event. A quick release to the press will present the facts as the hospital wishes them conveyed and will eliminate the chance of incorrect or haphazard statements. Hureco, Inc. recommends presenting the statement in a way that expresses grief at the occurrence of the event. Release updates with additional information as necessary.
- Clean up the site of the event. Coordinate the tasks that need to occur to conduct site cleanup with internal security and facilities engineering/maintenance. Professional services that provide clean-up services can be accessed or recommended by the local police department. If at all possible, redesign the

Exhibit 10.4

CRISIS MANAGEMENT TEAM ACTIVITIES
FOLLOWING A VIOLENCE CRISIS

EXECUTIVE OFFICE	HUMAN RESOURCES EXECUTIVE	SECURITY EXECUTIVE
Provide overall leadership	Coordinate counseling efforts and employee assistance program (EAP) interactions	Act as liaison between hospital and police
Provide regular updates to board, executive team	Schedule employee and manager meetings	Respond to security needs
Respond to media	Contact victims' families	Handle all details of worksite cleanup
	Manage insurance and OSHA issues	Conduct internal investigation
	Implement/adapt policies to assist employees through crisis	Respond to media
	Respond to media	
	Manage hotline responses	
	Act as liaison between crisis management team and employees	

LINE MANAGER	GENERAL COUNSEL	PUBLIC RELATIONS EXECUTIVE
Provide employee information programs	Manage workers' compensation issues	Prepare publicity/ media release
Update managers	Coordinate external investigation	Prepare publicity/ media updates
Coordinate communication between crisis management team and operations	Provide legal guidance for crisis management team	Coach executives with regard to press relations
Respond to media	Respond to media	
	Advise management in precrisis meetings with regard to preventing libelous statements following a crisis	

worksite before the employees return to work, to diminish the chance that employees will have posttraumatic reactions when returning to the site of the violence.

■ Establish employee information meetings. During the first few days following the crisis, management should hold meetings with employees every 2 to 3 hours to provide updated information and to encourage and answer questions. "Encourage employees to express their feelings," say Abbott and Weide. It is important to schedule the meetings as soon as the employees return to work, even though it is possible that not all of the facts will be available. Updates or additional information will benefit the employees and will help to reduce the proliferation of speculative rumors. Hureco, Inc. cautions that many negative comments and hostility will be communicated by the employees and directed at management; this type of reaction should be anticipated as a typical response. As time goes on, the frequency of the meetings can be reduced, based on attendance at the meetings or the diminished frequency of questions from employees. Hureco, Inc. advises that, generally speaking, meetings are no longer required within a week following the event. Suggest that the employees plan ways to honor the victims as an expression of an individual's typical response of wanting to help. Health care employees in particular will likely wish to reach out and offer assistance. The planning of memorial services or suggesting permanent installations are good and appropriate actions and will help control or manage activities that may create hospital liability.

■ Meet with hospital managers. Managers need to be consistently updated and kept informed so that they can respond to their employees. Specific instructional meetings for managers to train them in supporting the emotional needs of their employees and learning how to treat every employee in the same way will be especially important in the days following a violent event. Managers may require assistance to identify employees who would benefit from special care and additional counseling. Hureco, Inc. cautions that there is a "fine line between showing the extra measure of caring and the perception of favoritism." They recommend having manager meetings daily until the critical nature of the crisis has passed. Encourage managers to attend employee meetings as well. The key point is to recommend

that managers have direct involvement in the postcrisis phase so that the manager is perceived to be caring and involved with regard to the needs of the employees they manage.
- Respond to the media. Any individual who is a part of the hospital staff or management will be fair game for the media. The image of a cadre of reporters following an employee around and asking relentless questions that may put the individual on the spot is disconcerting. Stick to the facts and respond in the best way you know how. Generally, a hospital will designate a spokesperson who will interact with the media. Hureco, Inc. recommends the following:
  - Choose a spokesperson from the CMT.
  - Stick to concise responses, beginning with the critical facts and then fill in with details.
  - "Don't bluff; if you cannot answer the question, offer to find the answer." Follow up with the media once you have the answer.
  - Avoid "no comment" responses.
  - "Beware of hypothetical questions," say Abbott and Weide, and don't let the media suggest answers.
  - Tell the truth. Be completely truthful. "During a time of crisis, credibility is more important than ever," advise Abbott and Weide.
- Initiate internal and external investigations. Investigations are critical because litigation and accountability will be involved. The goal is to collect and document the facts. The earlier the facts of the crisis are determined, the sooner you can prepare your legal defense. Evaluate the necessity to establish or change hospital policy to prevent any recurrence. Internal investigations are to be conducted by the security department, and security will solicit assistance from the local police department. External investigations are managed by the legal department following the leadership of the hospital general legal counsel. Hureco, Inc. recommends the following:
  - Determine the relationship of the victims to the perpetrator(s)
  - Obtain the personnel file of the victims
  - Interview eyewitnesses
  - Obtain employment history, medical history, criminal history, red flag or documented change in behavior history of

the perpetrator(s) and obtain interviews with work friends or acquaintances of the perpetrator(s)

- Obtain information from the department manager regarding change in management, issues of production stress, and manager interactions
- Focus on prior documented hostile actions and prior documented violent activity between coworkers or with manager
- Establish an employee response committee. The purpose of the committee is to help employees learn to manage their feelings by encouraging and directing positive activities that will give each employee the feeling that he or she is doing something to help. Be aware that a crisis of this nature creates very real psychological trauma and reduces productivity. The grieving process that individuals experience is the same process that will impact a group of employees. The process of doing something is nearly as important as the event or permanent installation that is selected as a means to honor the victim(s).
- Establish an employee reentry support program. Following a crisis, policies of leave, sick time, or paid time off (PTO) approvals will need to be flexible and employee-focused. Individuals will have different needs and different responses and will require the opportunity for employees to communicate with one another. Anticipate that some employees will be unable to return to the worksite where the violence occurred; the most appropriate hospital response is to provide other career options within different departments or divisions. Some employees will not be able to return to work in the hospital no matter the length of time or support that is provided. The most appropriate response is for the hospital to assist with career transition via outplacement firms or direct assistance, attempting to find a position in another hospital if at all possible. Some employees will incur short-term or long-term disability related to posttraumatic stress.
- Set up a rumor hotline. Hotlines, staffed for specific hours during the day for as long a period of time as necessary, will help dispel rumors quickly. An additional purpose, advise Abbott and Weide, is that hotlines will disseminate accuracy and eliminate rumors. The hotline can be used to report incidents or new threats of violence in the postcrisis phase. The hotline can be staffed by counselors and/or employees. Employees will

need training to learn how to obtain the correct information from callers to the hotline. Each hotline operators will need to obtain a detailed description of the rumor, the department where the rumor is occurring, the day and time the rumor was heard, other witnesses to the rumor, and whether reports of the rumor have been communicated to management. Hotline operators should have a written statement of fact in response to the rumors that come in through the hotline and should offer a follow-up with the caller if additional information is required prior to making a response.

- Manage insurance/workers' compensation claims. Contact with all appropriate insurance carriers is to be done quickly following a crisis, including the completion and submission of all claim forms. Families of victims are prevented from suing employers in many states, based on the workers' compensation statutes of the state. Ask your risk manager or the insurance carrier for information regarding the law in your state. The possibility of negligence (negligent hiring, negligent supervision) may be levied at the employer or manager and could be the basis for a suit. In the case of an employee who kills other employees, the liability can be enormous because there is no insurance coverage for homicide, which is an illegal activity.
- Set goals for the future. For many days following a violent crisis the "activity level is high," but gradually, the environment will return to normal. It is paramount during this time that the ultimate six goals of crisis management are met:
  - Internal investigations are conducted quickly but methodically so as to capture all pertinent facts and are completed within 2 weeks.
  - External investigations are longer—often as much as 2 weeks—and are prepared with extreme care because the case will most likely involve litigation. External investigations should ideally begin very quickly following a crisis.
  - Limit liability by knowing what actions or activities—or the lack of actions—can create a potential for liability. By offering additional counseling, the hospital may be able to prevent disability claims of stress.
  - Employee response committee actions will be a key factor in helping employees return to routine work activities and helping employees cope. Abbott and Weide state that the

employees generally will have recommendations for ways to honor the victims within 7 to 10 days.

■ Recovery of productivity should be assessed by tracking improvement. Within 7 to 10 days, an improvement in productivity measures can be anticipated. Even in severe crisis events, normal productivity should be achieved within a few weeks.

■ An executive report summarizing the crisis and effecting a closure will need to be written and delivered within 30 to 45 days following the crisis. Statements of future policy and direction and assurances that similar events have been thwarted must be communicated (Weide & Abbott, 1994).

Crisis management, when handled efficiently and quickly, will be paramount to the credibility that the hospital will have following the crisis. Be very professional in approaches to the community and assure them that substantial procedures have been put in place with the goal of eliminating the possibility of any future violent incidents.

CASE STUDY

This case study illustrates the importance of communication with patients. The overall feeling of comfort of the patient and his family is enhanced as is the opportunity to diminish the chance that emotions can surge and potentially create a violent episode. The improved patient satisfaction scores clearly point to the benefit of strategic communication.

A survey of 1.5 million patients and 1,600 Emergency Departments revealed a surprising fact: patients claim they would feel much better—and give the ED better scores—if the ED would tell them how long they would have to wait to see a provider in the ED (Johnson, 2008). Patients want to be kept informed. Being informed about potential wait time ranked ahead of treating their chief complaint and controlling their pain as being highest on the patient's wish lists.

(Continued)

Consistent communication with the Emergency Department staff increased patient satisfaction because patients felt comfortable and cared for.

Patients who "waited four hours or more to see a provider but were kept well-informed regarding delays rewarded the ED with a high overall satisfaction scores giving them a ninety-six point six out of a possible one hundred points. Patients who were poorly informed gave patient satisfaction scores of forty-two point seven out of a possible one hundred points" (Johnson, 2008).

Communication is the key to keeping patients happy and at ease. Emergency Department nurses and management have known the immense benefit of communication with patients and families for a long time. A response of "I don't know but I will find out" is better than no information at all. Keeping patients comfortable, content, and feeling cared for is essential to the prevention of mounting frustration that has the potential to develop into violent incidents (Johnson, 2008).

CASE STUDY

Scottsdale Healthcare in Scottsdale, Arizona, has added a beneficial service for its potential Emergency Department patients, and it is the first—or at least one of the first in the United States—to do so. The three Emergency Departments in each of Scottsdale's three local hospitals post the real-time Emergency Department waiting room time on their Web site (www.shc.org) so that patients can anticipate knowing how long they may be expected to wait from the time they walk in the ED until they are escorted to a treatment room. Posting wait times on the Web site is Scottsdale Healthcare's answer to the 60-minute or no-wait guarantees that some hospitals offer to their Emergency Department patients and probably represents a better approach. Guarantees are "very difficult to live up to," says the director of emergency services Nancy Hicks-Arsenault (Jones, Keith [Public Relations], 2008).

(Continued)

Scottsdale Healthcare, as with every hospital in the U.S., continues to make positive changes for its patients. Scottsdale Healthcare is making strides to reduce the Emergency Department wait times, having beaten both the state's and the nation's wait time average. Two of the Emergency Departments have 100,000 patients annually, and the third ED, which opened in late 2007, is on pace to see nearly 15,000 patients this year.

Various sources, such as Press Ganey and the CDC, quote different times for the U.S. national average Emergency Department wait times (Nawar, Niska, & Xu, 2007; Press Ganey, 2008). Often, the time is measured from the time the patient enters the Emergency Department until the patient is seen by a provider. However, the Press Ganey report uses the total ED length of stay (LOS), which measures the time a patient enters the ED until the patient has received a disposition, or discharge, from ED care. Press Ganey quotes the national average ED wait time (LOS) as 4 hours; Scottsdale Healthcare LOS is 3 hours (Press Ganey, 2008).

There are a few considerations to posting ED wait times on the Web site.

- Posting wait times caters more to the population of non-emergency or primary care patients. Nonemergency/low-acuity (primary care) patients are the patient population that EDs all over the U.S. have been trying to discourage from using Emergency Department services. Low-acuity patients clog the system for those needing true emergency care.
- Patients needing true emergency care may not have time to access the Web site to evaluate which Emergency Department has the lowest wait time.
- Not everyone has access to the Internet.
- The Web-posted wait times are one more innovative service for patients/customers of Scottsdale Healthcare.

Emergency Department waiting room times are one of the more important measures that EDs continuously work to improve, to be sure that patient satisfaction scores stay high and to ensure that

(Continued)

reasons for patient frustration and anger stay low. One of the most-reported and documented reasons for patient violence in the Emergency Department is the patient frustration and anger due to the extended times patients must wait in the ED waiting room before they can see a provider.

CASE STUDY

In 2006, a small suburban hospital came face to face with its vulnerabilities related to Emergency Department violence. It is rare to read about this type of incident occurring in hospitals or Emergency Rooms, and I give the CEO and leaders of the hospital a great deal of recognition, congratulations, and credit for having the courage to share their experiences with the news media. I know that the lessons they have learned and have communicated will be extremely beneficial to all of the hospitals and Emergency Departments in the U.S. who believe that "it can't happen here."

"Today, every hospital is at the same risk of exposure to drug and alcohol abuse, domestic violence and psychiatric patients. All of it shows up in your Emergency Room, and your security officer at the front door has to have a better level of training than being told to say, 'Good morning. How are you?'" says Roger Sheets, the president of International Association for Healthcare Security and Safety, following the altercation that occurred in the Howard County General Hospital, a suburban hospital in Maryland, in 2006 (Harris, 2006).

One quiet Saturday night in early summer, a crowd of angry individuals showed up at the ambulatory entrance to the Emergency Department, trying to overpower the security guards, and attempting to climb over the reception desk to see a friend who had been fatally shot. It is obvious from studies that have been done about gangs that this was a gang intrusion, doing everything that they could to gather around their dead gang member and

(Continued)

possibly take up residence in the waiting room, in case a rival gang would show up. Fortunately, the situation was controlled before that happened.

The hospital and Emergency Department lost a great deal more than their naiveté that night. Emergency Department patients were diverted away from the hospital for a number of hours (loss of revenue), but maybe even worse, the hospital had to face the fact that it was vulnerable to violence. Hospital administration had been providing a level of security that was appropriate to the level of risk that had been typical at Howard County General Hospital. Until that night, the security officers, who were not police officers, did not have weapons of any kind, and only the security supervisor had access to a chemical deterrent spray. Only a few of the doors in the hospital could be locked electronically. Additionally, the publicity to which the hospital was exposed was not glowing or beneficial. Hospitals are now exposed to situations that put the hospital, the Emergency Department, and the staff at risk for violence that can lead to injury and death.

Security experts for health care institutions explain that "concerns have escalated at virtually every institution—urban and suburban"—since 9/11 (Harris, 2006). There are huge gaps in the levels of security that hospitals provide, which is the reason that Emergency Departments need to evaluate their own risk. Most large facilities have come to terms with the fact that they need a high level of security, including security guards who carry weapons, metal detectors, security cameras and a staff to monitor the real-time videos, and doors that can be locked electronically.

In Maryland, state or local police officers stay with a patient they have brought into the Emergency Department if they anticipate that the patient will be charged with a violent crime. In other cases, the police must determine if they have the personnel to continuously guard the patient.

One hospital tells about the patient who was involved in a violent altercation and came into the Emergency Department on life support. The decision was made to not post a guard because of the fact that the patient was unconscious and on life support systems. The patient's girlfriend, who was carrying a butcher knife, was

(Continued)

able to gain access to the Emergency Department, "cut all of the lines and wheeled him out" (Harris, 2006). The impact of violence on the community is substantial. It is critical to communicate the true prevalence of violence and any potential outcomes to get full permission and support from all community stakeholders to implement focused violence-mitigation activities. As in my community, many of the residents of a community are most likely not aware of the proliferation of gangs and violent gang activities. It is, in my opinion, our job to let them know. Through the creation of innovative programs that will provide information and opportunities for community involvement and participation, we will equip individuals and communities with the tools to understand and thwart violence.

REFERENCES

Birenbaum, S. (2006). *Nowhere else to go: Why California's emergency rooms are filled with insured patients.* Retrieved July 22, 2008, from http://www.chcf.org/press/view.cfm?itemID=126090&printFormat=true

Harris, M. (2006). *Hospitals face intrusion of violent world into facilities.* Retrieved July 18, 2007, from http://www.baltimoresun.com/news/health/bal-m.o.hospital17jul06,4286517.story?

Johnson, B. (2008). *The doctor will see you . . . in a while.* Retrieved August 22, 2008, from http://www.washingtonpost.com/wp-dyn/content/article/2009/06/13/AR200806130 3435_pdf

Ray, M. M. (2007). The dark side of the job: Violence in the Emergency Department. *Journal of Emergency Nursing, 33*(3), 257–261.

Sonny Weide, G. A. (1994). Murder at work: Managing the crisis. *Employment Relations Today,* 139–150.

Outcomes and Future Directions

You must be the change you wish to see in the world.
                                                    —*Mohandas Gandhi*

11 The Benefits of Implementing Violence Prevention Strategies

Janet R. Cooper (2005), assistant professor of nursing at the University of Mississippi, has validated many of the assumptions that were made in this book. Professor Cooper, in her March 2005 letter to the editor of the *Online Journal of Issues in Nursing*, confirmed the growing incidence of Emergency Department violence and went as far as quoting societal costs and proposing some of the same general solutions that are recommended herein. Professor Cooper agrees that violence in the emergency room is a serious, significant, and a recurring theme for U.S. hospitals. Nothing in the research for this book has indicated that the trend will reverse any time soon. The opportunity to confront the challenge and make significant, important changes must not go unanswered.

This book attempts to bring together all pertinent facts about violence in the Emergency Department into one compelling book for health care professionals and for the general public alike. For hospitals and Emergency Departments, the intention of this book is to create a red alert so that the all-too-real potential for violence won't become buried in the myriad of other issues occurring right now in the ED. The issue of Emergency Department violence needs to be highlighted, shouted from the rafters, run up the flag pole, made a priority, and addressed—today.

Hospitals and health care facilities are hesitant to act when it comes to addressing violence and implementing violence prevention. As we have explored, part of the reason is that the administration or other decision makers may be doubtful that investments of this nature yield a good return on money invested, or they may have difficulty committing to a problem that they do not perceive—or understand. Educating the administration and the decision makers is an essential task in helping the hospital leaders recognize and understand what Emergency Departments are dealing with relative to violence. Suggest that the administrator-on-call (AOC) be called to the Emergency Department whenever a dangerous or potentially violent patient arrives for care—day or night. The administration may need visual explanations of the seriousness of the problems and the reality of violence.

Communicating a commitment to safety for the Emergency Department and hospital is an important message for any health care facility to convey—and it is a valuable insurance policy. If employees do not have the commitment, support, or insight of the hospital leaders, there is a serious problem, and those employees may want to consider reevaluating a commitment to the hospital. The administration needs to take a leadership position and an active, visible role relative to violence, leading focus groups and task force meetings to combat violence and to achieve workable solutions. Once administrators understand the concerns, they will be supportive.

Violence prevention strategies and tactics have long-term benefits for hospitals. Employee retention, in particular, is a tangible and cost-saving benefit for any company. Employees will stay with a company when they are given opportunities to learn and grow, when they are paid what they believe is a fair wage, when they are provided with life-enhancing benefits that allow them to care for themselves and their families, and when they have a supportive and safe work environment and culture. Developing a culture that is safe and violence free is growing in importance as a necessary benefit for hospital and other health care employers. Health care leaders must work hard to put controls in place against patient, family, and visitor violence and must also become aware and knowledgeable about lateral violence and the extent of it in your hospital or facility. Learning to recognize lateral violence and to champion training and policies against lateral violence will be a key retention strategy in the future. A case study was presented in Chapter 6 illustrating the effects of lateral violence in a large hospital system. The hospital had a culture that propagated lateral violence but was not aware of the rampant nature of lateral violence or the impact that it had in the facility. The hospital was also struggling with a very low 50%

registered nurse (RN) retention rate. One of the nursing leaders identified the problem of lateral violence as the reason that so many of the hospital's nurses were leaving hospital employment so soon after orientation. The hospital implemented an educational program and policy support against lateral violence, communicating a zero tolerance policy for all violence—including lateral violence. Within a short period of time, the retention rate rose dramatically. In another case study in Chapter 3, department managers regularly discouraged staff from reporting violent episodes—even the reporting of physical injuries. The staff in the latter case study most likely did not feel cared for, and this may have led to a culture of distrust and underlying dissatisfaction. Nursing leaders can have a significant impact on keeping their staff feeling valued and important to their mission. Sincere expressions of caring will translate to long-term job satisfaction and positive retention efforts.

The cost to recruit and retain one RN for 1 year is in excess of $60,000. The cost projection is based on expenses for training and orientation, perks, and salary and benefit costs but does not include any sign-on, retention, or performance bonus. Trained, experienced, professional nurses are at a premium because of the very limited supply and the dwindling pool of RNs.

Employee satisfaction is a key quality measure for most hospitals. Hospitals ask their employees to assess the hospital performance in terms of their ability to take care of the employee and to ask if the employee would recommend the hospital as a first-class place to work. Employees are the most important asset that any hospital—any company—has. The smart hospitals let their employees know how much they are valued! Informing employees that they are a large factor in the success of a company is an immense benefit to a hospital or to any company. Happy and satisfied employees typically stay employed for the long term, thereby improving retention rates, lowering costs of recruitment and training, and accelerating operational continuity.

Hospitals and all companies can significantly and positively affect their institutional risk by having long-term and satisfied employees who will help drive down the risk incurred by an institution and reduce insurance premiums. Long-term employees—versus dayworkers or agency staff—reduce patient errors and lower the risk of liability for the facility. The risk incurred by a hospital for disability claims, liability, and Occupational Safety and Health Administration (OSHA) fines relative to violent injury or death could potentially be very high, possibly rendering the hospital insolvent.

Happy employees are a hospital's best source of advertising. If a customer or employee is satisfied, he will tell one person about his good experience; if he is dissatisfied, he will tell two people about his bad experience! Excellent customer service—starting in the Emergency Department waiting room by communicating, offering small tokens of comfort, adding amenities, and generally taking excellent care of patients—can boost trust and generate an influx of new patients. Remember that hospital profits are derived from inpatient revenue, and a majority of these patients are from the Emergency Department. Not all patients are uninsured or charity care.

Employees—most especially hospital and Emergency Department employees—should feel protected and safe at work and should be backed by a supportive administration that listens to their concerns. But this is not always the case. In recent years, companies seem to be doing a better job taking care of their employees and making the employees a part of problem-solving processes and improvement projects. Recognizing employees during a Nurses' Week or Physician Appreciation Day are methods that hospitals have been using to promote their hardest-working employees and to let individuals know they are appreciated. The one mistake that employers make is to give inexpensive tokens to their employees. The token gift may be perceived by the recipient as insincere or cheap. A better idea—and easier to administer—is to provide a free lunch or a few extra paid hours off—gifts that employees really appreciate and that let them know they are valued.

Keeping employees happy is a benefit to all employers but is an especially effective tool for hospitals. Happy employees will naturally generate customers. Customers want to know that the employer—especially in service industries, such as health care—takes care of its employees and will take care of its patients in the same manner. Unions or the threat of union activity for nurses can produce a negative message to the community. Nurses, in particular, have always been known as the caring profession, and the integration of a nursing union in a hospital environment may leave many customers confused and thinking that either overwork, too few staff, or low pay may be responsible for union activity or entrance. Of course, neither of these situations may be the actual cause, but the perception in the community may be that the hospital is not taking care of its employees and the employees were forced to bring in a third party to help defend and protect their rights or their working environment.

THE CORE COMPETENCY OF CUSTOMER SERVICE

A core competency is a service or a product that companies do or make well—better than most of their competitors. The best explanation for core competency for the Emergency Department is that of a deep proficiency that enables a company to deliver unique value to customers and creates a sustainable competitive advantage (Rigby, 2008). The Emergency Department can become a core competency for hospitals and would create nonstop patients and revenues for the hospital. The current circumstances of Emergency Departments are that of chaos and patients boarded everywhere waiting for inpatient beds, transfers (often, to chock-full psychiatric hospitals), waiting for specialist physician evaluations, and patients and families waiting for hours in the waiting room to see a provider. Why would the ED want or need more patients?

The problems that hospitals are facing are vast, and they are not and will not be easy to correct. For years to come, the ED will be dealing with a large majority of the problems that affect it today. But hospitals and particularly nurses are amazing magicians and will probably have developed work-around solutions or will have created ways to lessen the impact of all of the problems. Hopefully, legislation will help things along by addressing the immense problem of the uninsured.

It is important to continue to attract patients who will become loyal customers—in good times and in bad—and will use and support the other services and programs provided by the hospital. Sometimes, revenues and profits from other products (CT scans, adult day care, diabetes care, etc.) are the only way that hospitals have to survive and to retain a small chance to counterbalance the losses they are incurring in the Emergency Department.

Services in the Emergency Department can become a core competency for your hospital. Even in the face of numerous patient visits and many inappropriate visits, the services that you provide to take good care of your patients—your customers—can yield benefits. Subscribing to a hospitality strategy and adding small comforts will go a long way to making your waiting patients and families happier. Providing consistent communication is critical to adding to the comfort level and decreasing stress. Employing some ideas that have been presented in this book, such as posting ED waiting room wait times on the front page of the hospital Web site as Scottsdale Hospital has done, can give patients a sense of more control. There are many ideas that can be used, and hopefully this book has helped you find the one idea that will work for your ED.

Violence prevention can also become a core competency for your hospital. The prevention of violence is a customer service strategy that will go one step further to comforting and caring for your patients because they know they are in a safe environment. Violence prevention is critical to protect the hospital and employees from harm delivered by violent patients or violent street gangs. The communication strategies that were introduced in Chapter 9, for implementing a violence awareness and prevention program in the ED will provide a benefit to the Emergency Department, to the hospital, and to the community. The core competency of violence prevention can be used to market the hospital and the ED; just be certain that all gaps in security and safety have been plugged and that violence-prevention strategies have been implemented. It would be a devastating blow if the hospital were to communicate violence prevention as a core competency and to then have a violent episode occur in the ED.

A violence-prevention strategy is an essential platform in a hospitality strategy. Simply put, customers will not choose your hospital if there is the reality *or* the perception that it is a dangerous place to be. Do whatever is necessary to communicate the tactics your hospital is using to combat violence at the front door and to let patients know that they are safe and that their business is valued.

Making the Emergency Department your hospital's core competency—the reason that your patient/customers choose you—can pay off handsomely. The key is to continuously provide the best services in the way that you promise you will. Communicate your plans and successes often so that the community will be aware of your measures toward efficiency and safety and the fact that you want them to continue to choose your hospital for their care.

CASE STUDY

The following case study is a partial story reporting the murder of a devoted psychiatrist by one of her own patients. The story not only depicts the horrendous death of a health care physician by violence, which is the focus of this book, but it tells the bigger story that the

(Continued)

employees have been asking for additional security protection for years. Because the hospital faces a $25 million shortfall this year, they could not afford to provide additional security. In addition, the hospital will incur another $30,000 fine from OSHA and untold liability costs.

There must have been an awful commotion, although no one heard a thing. It was a busy county psychiatric hospital, after all, and the Unit C exam room door was closed. But inside, a terrible story was unfolding. During a routine afternoon checkup this past November, Dr. Erlinda Ursua was slain by one of her own patients, a severely mentally ill woman who had been brought to John George Psychiatric Pavilion that morning. The doctor was beaten savagely, according to sheriff's department records, her head and face smashed again and again into a solid object. She also was strangled, according to a not-yet-released autopsy report. Outside the door and just up the hall, nurses, mental health specialists, and doctors went about their work completely unaware of what was happening inside the room. Although the examination room had a panic button, the sixty-year-old MD, who stood only four-foot-eleven, couldn't get to it during the attack.

A hospital janitor made the ghastly discovery later that afternoon. [The janitor] opened the exam room door so he could empty the trash and found the doctor's lifeless body on the floor. Her physician's coat was open and her shoes sat next to her feet. An earring, a piece of a jade bracelet, and paperwork were strewn around. No one else was in the room.

Alameda County Sheriff's Department detectives told [the husband] that his wife probably didn't die during the beating. She lay there undiscovered for an hour and a half, they estimated, and was most likely alive for at least some of that time.

The suspected killer, thirty-seven year-old [female patient] whose hands were scratched and swollen when she was questioned by detectives later that day, said she became upset when the doctor tried to take her pulse. "I punched her in the neck and her blue wallet and keys went up in the air," she reportedly said. Then, according to a sheriff's department report, [the patient] began to ramble unintelligibly.

While staffers at the eighty-eight-bed psychiatric hospital were deeply saddened by their colleague's murder, hardly anyone was shocked. For years, they have complained of assaults by patients, many of whom are severely mentally ill and are brought to the San

(Continued)

Leandro facility against their will by the cops. Some are homeless; others are transferred from area jails. Many [patients] show up after going off their psychiatric medications and arrive in frightening states: They are brought in unkempt and reeking, covered in feces, barking like dogs, or dressed up in costumes. Patients also have been admitted with knives and other weapons stashed in their pockets.

"I've seen so many of my co-workers taken out on stretchers. It's terrible," says [employee] a mental health specialist at John George who is out on stress leave after saving a colleague's life during a Christmas Day stabbing in 2002.

Stretchers for wounded staff members were all too common in the twelve months prior to Erlinda Ursua's death. One nurse was stabbed twice in the back. Another was punched in the face and had his nose broken. A staff member's head was slammed into a wall so hard she suffered a concussion, and another nearly lost an eye to a pencil-wielding patient. A doctor's jaw was dislocated, and one aide's knee was injured so severely that it required surgery and now has to be re-placed. These, according to Dr. Harold Cottman, a hospital psychiatrist, are in addition to numerous less-serious assaults. In 2003 alone, at least six hospital employees went out on workers' compensation leave following patient attacks. But because of poor record-keeping, a top hospital administrator was unable to say just how many other employees went on leave in prior years. Only one thing was certain, the administrator said: "I can tell you there were others."

Despite the repeated attacks and a growing chorus of employee complaints, hospital administrators made few real improvements. By last April, safety had become such a concern at John George that five staffers approached the California division of Occupational Safety and Health, the state's workplace safety agency, to complain.

In June, following an investigation, Cal-OSHA cited the hospital and fined it $30,000 for failing to report two of the attacks as required by law. The state agency also issued a citation for the hospital's failure to maintain an adequate worker safety program. "On a regular basis," one of the citations reads, "employees are suffering injuries from violent patients who assault the employees." (Goldsmith, 2004)

A NOTE OF CAUTION

Emergency Departments are generally cost centers; that is, they perform few functions that create revenue for the hospital, so it is essential that Emergency Departments are operated at maximum efficiency. Reimbursement rates for a majority of the patients who need and use the ED for primary care or low-acuity needs are very low. Hospitals are willing to make investments in the Emergency Department because the ED is the new front door to hospitals and can generate business through inpatient admissions. For these reasons, solving the problems of crowding and boarding are very important initiatives for hospitals and Emergency Departments.

Hopefully within a few years, providing health care services through either a national insurance program or some other solution, in tandem with fewer unwise government regulations, and the initiation of improved funding methods and sources will be in place to benefit Emergency Departments, rather than holding them responsible for all of the problems of society. The Emergency Department needs to be supported in its enormous task of caring for the community in the best way that it can and to help generate revenue for the hospital via the rapid and efficient admission of inpatients.

A word of caution is required. The process of off-loading or decompressing the Emergency Department can have untoward and unexpected effects. While we should not expect that we will wake up in 3 years and all of the inappropriate and uninsured patients will be gone from emergency services, the dramatic decrease in the number of patients coming to the Emergency Department is a reality. It wasn't too many years ago that hospitals closed entire inpatient floors and laid off cadres of nurses because the hospitals did not have enough inpatients to support the services.

It is important to continue to provide customer value through services that best serve the community and respond to its needs. Offering unique programs, educational courses, or delivering a high-quality (and highly reimbursable) service in more efficient ways can improve the chances that customers in your community will continue to choose your hospital and Emergency Department when they need care. Provide ways to connect with your customers, and they will be your customers for the long run.

A hospitality strategy for the Emergency Department is a relatively new concept. Attracting and retaining customers wasn't necessary before for-profit health care—your customers came because you had the only hospital in town. However, a hospitality strategy—to make your customers/patients feel valued and happy that they chose your Emergency Department and hospital—is one of the most important strategies that can be implemented. Refer to Chapter 8 for tactics and ideas to develop a hospitality strategy.

Today, generally, every hospital provides the same services and each hospital attempts to provide a better service than its competitors. In Nashville, one particular physician group regularly moves back and forth between two hospitals, depending on which hospital gives them the best deal: the marketing and the resources to be able to provide the very best medical care, better pay, more patients, more perks, all wrapped up with a big bow of clever marketing slogans and valet parking. By changing hospitals, the physicians are afforded the opportunity to provide the best care for their patients in a very competitive market.

PUBLIC RELATIONS

According to Clarke L. Caywood, PhD, the integrated marketing and communications chair at Northwestern University, public relations brings together an organization's stakeholder relationships, old and new, via a communication strategy to develop and manage messages coming from the organization. The goal, of course, is to cleverly brand the organization while developing a positive reputation that will result in profits (Caywood, 1997). Dr. Caywood believes that the leaders in an organization must take on the role of public relations (PR) and learn to integrate all internal and external relationships. This new leadership role will help the organization achieve its overarching marketing goal. There are four levels of integration that are recommended:

1. Relationship-building with stakeholders. PR focuses not on the concentrated activity and sphere of marketing to customers, but, rather, manages an "outside-in perspective" with those stakeholders who are familiar with your organization. For a hospital, this might be positive feedback and the reputation of an innovative program teaching child development to new parents.
2. Management function relationships. This is the integration of all jobs within the organization with the message the organization wishes to deliver. In other words, the organization brings together all functions within the organization and communicates the organization's public message as interpreted by each department. This type of integration strategy is a mini-MBA for hospitals. The "financial perspective of violence" can be communicated by them in terms of the huge cost of violence. In my view, this integration tactic gets all employees involved in the message you are trying to communicate.

3. Corporate structure integration. Corporate structure integration is very different for large organizations than it is for small organizations and would necessitate different methods—perhaps even different messages—for each size of organization. For hospitals, learning how to communicate with the various departments and integrating their involvement into the organization's message is a key. As a simple example, at the hospital level, involving all levels of the organization in developing the message is to involve all employees—all stakeholders—in the message by sponsoring a slogan contest as was suggested in Chapter 8.

4. Societal integration. This is the easy part. Create and communicate your message to the public to inform them that you have the interest of the community and its needs in mind: Violence is dangerous to our community; this hospital has implemented a zero-tolerance policy against violence. Your message to benefit the community will integrate the public's interest (no violence) into a marketing message (zero tolerance at this hospital), and will deliver your message to the public (Caywood, 1997).

The purpose of a violence prevention program is to protect patients and staff from violence. Preventing violence will also create the perception of a shield of safety for your customers. Negative public relations in the event of a violent episode that occurs at your hospital can rapidly undermine and eradicate the positive forward progress that an organization has made in providing great health care services and establishing outstanding customer-focused service and communication.

REFERENCES

Caywood, C. (1997). Advanced public relations practice in key industries. In C. Caywood (Ed.), *The handbook of strategic public relations & integrated communications* (pp. 436–439). New York: McGraw-Hill.

Cooper, J. (2005, March 15). *Online Journal of Issues in Nursing.* Retrieved May 19, 2008, from http://www.nursingworld.org/MainMenuCategories/ANAMarketplace/ANAPeriodicals/

Goldsmith, S. (2004). *The lunatics have taken over the asylum.* Retrieved July 2, 2008, from http://www.eastbayexpress.com/news/the_lunatics_have_taken_over_the_asylum/Content?oid=286560

Rigby, D. (2008). *Management tools.* Retrieved August 18, 2008, from www.bain.com/management_tools/tools_competencies.sap?groupCode=2

12 Future Directions

Health care delivery in the Emergency Department is at crisis point and is at imminent risk of breakdown. Violence occurring in the waiting room and treatment areas is a very serious—and very real—problem. But violence, as critical and dangerous as it is, is only one of the many serious predicaments for Emergency Departments in the United States today.

Street gangs infiltrate EDs seeking drugs or vengeance against rival gang members who have been brought to the Emergency Department with gunshot or stab wounds or as victims of beatings. Typically, calm patients wait for hours in the waiting room to see a provider and can often lash out in frustration at caregivers. There are not enough nurses to care for the patients in Emergency Departments or in hospital inpatient units. The result is an inconsistent workforce that lacks—through no fault of its own—methods to provide excellent health care afforded through continuity of care. A lack of nurses also produces limited numbers of caregivers for patients in hospitals, resulting in an equally limited number of available staffed inpatient beds.

Patients who cannot be moved out of the Emergency Department to an inpatient bed must remain *boarded* in the ED, which results in a backlog of patients waiting in ED beds in the hallway or outside emergency treatment rooms. These waiting patients require the same level of care as those emergency patients who continue to arrive for care via EMS or ambulatory entrances. But, because of the boarded patients waiting for inpatient beds or the psychiatric patients who cannot be referred to appropriate psychiatric treatment facilities—because there is a significant lack of psychiatric resources—there are often no beds in the ED available to treat emergency patients. Newly arriving EMS patients are diverted from one Emergency Department to another in the attempt to locate an ED that can accommodate and care adequately for the patient.

The Emergency Medical Treatment and Active Labor Act (EMTALA) regulations enacted by Centers for Medicare and Medicaid Services (CMS) require that all patients who arrive in the Emergency Department must be evaluated and treated. EMTALA was created to ensure that patients could not be unceremoniously dumped or transferred to other facilities because the patient lacked the ability to pay. Today, Emergency Department physicians struggle to see and treat all of the patients who arrive in the Emergency Department. The uninsured populations who do not typically have a primary care physician often wait until their medical condition is a bona fide emergency before arriving in the ED for care. The cost for treating an emergency is much higher and more long-term than the cost to prevent or manage a less-serious medical problem, or to intervene in the problem before it becomes an emergency. A hospital receives approximately 30% reimbursement for the care of an uninsured patient or $0.30 out of a $1.00. Who pays the remainder? The hospital and the Emergency Department physicians who provide hours of free care to patients every week do. A recent report reveals that all physicians provide an average of $4 billion annually in uncompensated care (Blum, 2005). Additionally, hospitals provide thousands of dollars every month in charity and bad debt care.

To add to the dilemma, there is a shortage of primary care physicians across the U.S. Insured patients who may not be able to arrange a timely appointment with their own primary care physician utilize the emergency room for primary care problems, which further exacerbates the crowding in Emergency Departments. Physician specialists—surgeons, gastroenterologists, and others—have been enticed with huge financial incentives to provide on-call services in the Emergency Room. Specialty physicians are in very limited supply so that providing on-call services to all hospitals is becoming a problem without a solution. Emergency Departments are required by CMS to have specialty physicians on-call for ED patient consultations, yet they may be unavailable, even when on-call, because of an emergency surgery or office visits with their own patients. Specialty physicians and surgeons are typically in high demand. There is growing evidence that these physicians have begun to value their infrequent time off and prefer not to cover Emergency Department services. Patients who cannot be seen in a timely manner in the ED must wait—often for hours—until a specialist can arrive to evaluate the patient, adding to further crowding in the Emergency Department.

And through all of this, psychiatric patients who are not controlled with essential medication because of the limited psychiatric services in the community and very low insurance coverage and reimbursement have nowhere else to go, and disgruntled patients and families, who have waited for hours and have escalating stress, strike out at the Emergency Department nurses and physicians, often causing serious injuries to the staff. These amazing caregivers erroneously think that aggression, violence, and abuse are part of the job.

And so the sequence continues...

ED violence and violence against ED nurses and physicians is frequently unreported and severely underreported, causing a continuance in the acceptance of aggression, violence, and abuse, leaving vulnerable staff at risk for injury and death. The first step that needs to be taken is that every stakeholder needs to understand that Emergency Departments were designed to assess and treat only life-threatening medical emergencies.

SUGGESTED TOPICS FOR FUTURE HOSPITAL-SPONSORED AND GOVERNMENT RESEARCH

The U.S. has a lot of work to do. The current health care system is seriously flawed, and there is clear evidence that our nation's leaders do not have the essential information they need to initiate reform or to halt the breakdown of U.S. health care—especially in the Emergency Department.

The election of a new administration is the ideal time to implement change. The new U.S. government will have the opportunity to prioritize health care change. Nursing and physician leaders must help the new administration recognize factors affecting the crisis in health care—especially in the Emergency Department.

The staid, ineffectual approach to change in health care is not working, and the attempts to create innovation through governmental channels result in delays from the red tape of government process. As a new administration, the leaders have the attention of the U.S. citizens, who will be anticipating and demanding new ideas and new methods to improve health care delivery for all U. S. citizens. The administration, with the help of health care and Emergency Department leaders, can and must take prompt, proactive steps toward revolutionary solutions and real transformation.

Emergency Departments are in crisis; violence in the Emergency Department is only part of the problem adding to the crisis. Understanding the issues that are creating the crisis is the first step toward understanding the bigger problems impacting the ED. It will help explain why violence is the serious problem for the U.S. that it is.

THINKING OUTSIDE THE BOX

The total reform of the health care system in the U.S. cannot be accomplished quickly. The facets and components that feed into the whole of the U.S. health care system create a complex web of cause and effect that need to be carefully evaluated to achieve optimal outcomes.

The incoming administration needs to focus on immediate changes that can be made to resolve the issues creating chaos in health care delivery systems, especially in the Emergency Department today. To accomplish change as rapidly as possible, a consortium of health care leaders from U.S. hospitals and Emergency Departments, consultant leaders from the Canadian National Health Service (NHS), members of key economic and health care think tanks, research organizations (such as the Centers for Disease Control), the secretary of the Department of Health and Human Services, and nonpartisan congressional champions for change need to join forces to strategize and create a proactive but realistic plan for the next 5 years. Periodic outcomes from the discussions and recommendations need to be delivered directly to Congress and to the president.

I have identified seven critical topics that can serve as action items and a potential starting point for government focus in the next 5 years:

1. Violence in the Emergency Department
2. Emergency Department crowding and boarding
3. The uninsured
4. Psychiatric and mental health resources (inpatient and outpatient)
5. Dwindling availability of nurses and physicians
6. Emergency preparedness
7. Electronic health records (EHR) (see Exhibit 12.1)

STRATEGY: SEVEN IN FIVE

TOP 7 HEALTH CARE FOCUS TOPICS FOR THE NEXT 5 YEARS

1. Violence in the Emergency Department
2. Emergency Department crowding and boarding
3. The uninsured
4. Psychiatric and mental health resources
5. Declining numbers of nurses and physicians
6. Emergency preparedness in the Emergency Department and for EMS
7. Electronic health records (EHR)

    The beginning of *total health care reform* starts here.

ACTION ITEMS FOR GOVERNMENT

Action Item 1: Violence in the Emergency Department

Key deliverables: Understand the drivers of violence in the ED. Support legislative models to increase criminal penalties for assaults against nurses. Carve out funding to support and initiate measures to shield Emergency Departments from violent intrusions. Initiate a national campaign against violence in the Emergency Department.

Several states have increased penalties for assaults against nurses (Ray, 2007). The legal definition of assault is "a crime that occurs when one person tries to physically harm another in a way that makes the person under attack feel immediately threatened. Actual physical contact is not necessary; threatening gestures that would alarm any reasonable person can constitute an assault" ("Assault: Legal Definition," 2009). California has updated its penal code to include assaults specifically carried out against nurses or physicians who are involved in the care of persons needing emergency care. Any Emergency Department perpetrator of violence now faces up to a $2,000 fine, a year in the county jail, or both.

Pennsylvania, too, has introduced and expanded legislation to enforce justice for acts of violence against licensed professionals. The term *licensed professional* is defined as an individual in a state who holds a professional or occupational license. The bill would expand the meaning of acts of violence against professionals to aggravated assault (Jost, 2007).

Legislative bills and legal remedies for nurses represent a beneficial, positive step forward. Finally, states are beginning to implement legal protection for the nurses who have been vulnerable to Emergency Department aggression, violence, or abuse for many years. Nurses often have no support from their employers to report or prosecute against the violence of patients, leaving nurses faced with tolerating aggression, violence, and abuse or leaving their jobs.

Apply for easy-to-obtain annual federal grants that Emergency Department leaders can use to establish violence protection plans and to install necessary security barriers such as metal detectors, security staff, and other protective measures that may not be affordable in current ED budgets.

To draw attention to the national problem of violence in the Emergency Department, the Emergency Nurses Association (ENA) and the American College of Emergency Physicians (ACEP) need to join forces, as they routinely do. The groups must launch a national campaign against violence in the Emergency Department. A nationally focused campaign would accomplish three objectives:

1. Launching of a national awareness platform regarding the problem of violence in the ED and of the aggression, violence, and abuse that Emergency Department personnel are enduring. ED violence must stop.
2. Communication to all Emergency Department nurses and physicians that violence is not just part of the job and that all episodes of aggression, violence, and abuse must be reported.
3. Providing the initial opportunity for all hospitals and Emergency Departments to establish and communicate a zero tolerance policy against violence for their facilities, including the initiation of a written policy and procedure, including a mechanism for reporting violence. A zero tolerance initiative must include consistent and frequent communication to the public about violence and violence controls, including education for all staff, signage, and administrative support.

For Consideration

The enactment or expansion of laws to prosecute individuals for violence against nurses may inadvertently function to keep patients who really need emergency care away from the Emergency Department. Some patients, by the very nature of their disease, may have episodes of out-of-control or psychotic behavior. Will laws such as these de-incentivize a certain population of patients from even going to the Emergency Department to get care that they need? Will the psychosis spill into the streets because they or their caregivers realize that there is a possibility of prosecution if they go to the ED for care, and injure a nurse? There are so few specialized psychiatric Emergency Departments that the possibility of having a psychiatric Emergency Department in close proximity to everyone needing this service is, at best, remote.

Options for legislative protection for nurses and physicians (and for all emergency personnel) need to be explored to provide legal remedies in the event of injuries that individuals incur as the result of aggression, violence, and abuse in the Emergency Department and in all areas of health care.

Action Item 2: Emergency Department Crowding and Boarding

Key deliverables: Continue the joint work of Congress and the ACEP to further understand the drivers of ED crowding and boarding. Work with the ED leaders to implement current strategies and solutions (Kaplan, 2007) that have been recommended and proposed by ACEP. Establish low-cost or no-cost community resources for 24/7 primary care and psychiatric needs to reduce the inappropriate use of the Emergency Department as a stop-gap measure in the national problem of the uninsured. Look to other nations (Canada, Europe, and Australia) for solutions. Start pilot programs for house calls, medical home concepts, and the expanded use of Nurse Practitioners (NPs). Develop a pool of resources for psychiatric and psychological issues and primary care options, implement nurse advice lines, and pilot 24-hour low-acuity care clinics attached to EDs (Rosenthal, 2008).

The problems of crowding in the Emergency Department are due in part to the excessive numbers of patients visiting the Emergency Department. EMTALA requires Emergency Departments to see and stabilize every patient who arrives. ACEP has been educating Congress and the federal government over the past few years to help frame the problems and to strategize solutions regarding Emergency Department crowding and boarding and to evaluate the unintended consequences of the EMTALA regulation. ACEP has developed several generic strategies, and the hope is that Congress will become enlightened about the seriousness of the problem and the underlying causes and will move quickly to enact change.

We cannot assume that all Emergency Department physicians are members of ACEP. It would be extremely beneficial to establish a government grant that provides low-cost membership to ACEP so that all Emergency Departments and physicians will have access to the leaders for ED change and to visionary solutions.

Communication of the strategies alone is not the answer. The way that the federal government can help create realistic and enduring solutions, is to:

- Understand the problem and the drivers of ED crowding and the necessity for boarding due to crowding.
- Reexamine the programs and funding options that are currently available to communities for primary care and psychiatric services and understand the deficiencies that exist.
- Establish a *model community* clinic as a learning lab, funded by federal government grants and private foundation funding. Establish a fund-raising team to generate revenue (grant writing, etc.) for operating expenses. Implement community or regional plans to develop services for communities with the goal of alleviating the numbers of patients visiting the Emergency Department. Learn from the clinic and roll out duplicate models in other communities if the clinic resolves some of the Emergency Department problems and provides improved care at a lower cost. Evaluate the deficiencies and the successes biannually and evaluate outcomes after 5 years.

The model community clinic services could include:

- Establishment of multiple locations of community-based 24/7 clinics that are staffed by nurse practitioners and provide low-cost, no-cost, or sliding-scale payment for primary care, obstetric care, pediatric care, and psychiatric care services for the safety-net population. Position the clinics in close proximity to Emergency Departments whose populations have the need for the services. Partner with local community hospitals and medical and nursing schools.
- Partnering with pharmaceutical manufacturers and durable medical equipment suppliers to provide previously used and sterilized goods at low or no cost.

- Implementing house calls and outreach teams to establish communication with the homeless and the population atrisk for visiting the Emergency Department. The concept has been successfully implemented on a small scale and needs to be tested on a large scale (based on the Camden, New Jersey, model; Addis, 2008).
- Establishing 24/7 nurse advice lines based at the community clinics or in the nurses' homes for registered nurses to provide advice to callers from evidence-based protocols for primary, pediatric, and psychiatric care.
- Establishing multilingual communication methods to inform the public about appropriate utilization of the ED and of the availability of the community clinic to be used for after-hours primary care needs in order to prevent unsuitable utilization of the Emergency Department.
- Decisions must be made about access to the services for undocumented /illegal individuals and children.
- Be aware that shifting the population to a secondary care site will create some of the same problems that are currently experienced by EDs.

The crowding and boarding problem in U.S. Emergency Departments is a situation that has developed over time and is the result of many factors. The factors include limited primary care and psychiatric resources in the community, which drives low-acuity patients to the only place they can receive 24-hour care: the Emergency Department. The increase in community resources and the 24/7 availability of ancillary medical and health care resources will create partial solutions. A large percentage of inappropriate patients—those *not* requiring emergency care—will be automatically redirected by the triage nurse, without having to come through the Emergency Department. However, relying on in-hospital resources to direct patients to appropriate care will continue to consume the limited resources of Emergency Departments.

ED crowding and the necessity to board patients in the Emergency Department negatively affects patient safety. The reasons that crowding occurs in the ED are varied and may be unique to each Emergency Department and hospital. Administrations must take a leadership role and proactively approach the problem as a hospital problem and not assume that ED crowding and boarding are strictly ED problems. Enhancing communications and launching opportunities for improvements via an interdepartmental team to work toward operational solutions will be a good first start. ACEP has developed several excellent generic strategies that are useful for all Emergency Departments.

Action Item 3: The Uninsured

Key deliverables: Is the answer to provide free health care services for the uninsured? Could a very low-cost insurance solution for all U.S. citizens provide enough revenue to enhance services at 24-hour primary care and psychiatric clinics? Are there enough educated and trained medical and psychological providers to even consider this option?

The uninsured population presents a serious challenge. All people—even those who are not citizens and those who cannot afford to purchase health insurance—get ill and need health care and emergency services. Hospitals cannot be expected to carry the entire cost burden of uninsured patients via a dwindling state-funded charity care or bad-debt write-offs.

One short-term solution may be to provide around-the-clock care clinics to reduce the strain on Emergency Departments. There are several charity care models that offer quality care for individuals who have no insurance or are of low-income means. For example, one pediatric provider—Mercy Children's Clinic in Franklin, Tennessee—offers free or low-cost services through its own foundation, supporting it through donations, fund-raisers, and grants.

Until health reform or Medicaid enhancement can be accomplished, government grants could be established to provide capital to open clinics providing quality care services for the poor. An important component in the success of this measure would be to decrease the timeline for grant approval and to simplify bureaucratic requirements and streamline grant approval and payout.

Action Item 4: Psychiatric and Mental Health Resources

Key deliverables: Add community psychiatric resources and build psychiatric EDs and crisis inpatient facilities in each hospital, improve reimbursement for psychiatric services and safety-net services, establish financial incentives to entice medical students to consider psychiatry as a career, and legislate for health insurers to cover more mental health services. Mental health parity was signed into law in October 2008 as part of the $700 billion economic bail-out package, thanks primarily to Patrick Kennedy who, as a consumer of mental health services, recognized the serious gap in mental health insurance benefits and attached his name and focus to legislating necessary change!

Psychiatric resources are extremely lacking. There is a severe scarcity of child and adult psychiatrists and the dramatic drop in available inpatient psychiatric beds. Often, psychiatric hospitals lack resources and operate on very limited budgets that do not support appropriate staffing of health care professionals or security officers. Additionally, reimbursement for psychiatric services is very low.

Many medical students are not interested in pursuing psychiatry. Establishing financial incentives for residents to pursue psychiatry would introduce needed talent into the workforce. The passage of legislation giving psychologists prescriptive authority to prescribe stabilizing and therapeutic medication would eliminate the necessity for psychiatrists to see patients who have already been diagnosed by a psychologist. Currently, patients must also visit a psychiatrist to have medication prescribed.

Action Item 5: Reverse the Trend of Diminishing Numbers of Nurses and Physicians

Key deliverables: Integrate federal government and community resources to address the declining numbers of Emergency Department nurses and physicians and enhance educational resources to train new nurses and physicians.

Workable strategies that would add more nurses and physicians into the marketplace are going to require specific measures and new ways to train new physicians and nurses in the most rapid method possible. It is critical to increase the numbers of physicians and nurses but to do so in a way that preserves the quality of the education so as to have a didactically trained and functional workforce that is also grounded in theory.

There are five strategies for consideration to provide a surge of new health care talent into health care systems to fill current gaps. The suggested strategies are:

1. Establish an advanced level of nurse practitioner education nurses by recruiting advanced-degree nursing personnel—those who are registered nurses and have advanced degrees such as MS, MSN, MBA, or MEd—to establish different and accelerated training methods for nurses that would fill the gap of primary care physicians and certain other specialties. The barriers will be training locations, professors/educators, and the cost of the education.

2. Physician training methods need to be reevaluated so as to accelerate training, especially for primary care physicians and gerontologists. The provision of free medical school tuition for all qualified medical school students to eliminate the enormous debt that must be repaid when medical students complete education and training would ensure the addition of talented physicians into the pool. When students face huge debt repayment, the circumstance may force physicians to obtain highly compensated specialty training. However, if students exit medical school debt-free, new physicians may be enticed toward primary care, emergency medicine, and gerontology because there will be no burden to repay thousands of dollars in tuition costs. Adding strategic business courses for physicians in training will aid in helping new physicians establish practices and offices and make prudent decisions about large capital expenditures for necessities such as EHR and health care information technology.

3. Establish new practice models for registered nurses, nurse practitioners, physician assistants, and advanced-degreed experienced registered nurses. Evaluate new practice models for certain physician groups.

4. Work with the federal government to revamp health care–related regulations and establish new hospital- and physician-friendly regulations that remove barriers to excellent patient care and access to health care.

5. What health care models are working in other countries? Many countries have national health care, so the comparisons may not be equal. An educated task force can seek out innovation in other countries that may be worth a trial in the U.S.

Action Item 6: Energize Emergency Preparedness

The U.S. would sustain a great many deaths if an enemy successfully violated our borders and attacked us today; we simply aren't prepared for a mass casualty. EMS is too fragmented to be useful, much as was the case in New York City during 9/11. U.S. Emergency Departments are already bursting at the seams and are not equipped with either capacity, manpower, or the ability to manage a surge in the event that a pandemic or a national disaster occurs. Recently, Vanderbilt University Medical Center adult Emergency Department had 88 patients boarding, each waiting for an inpatient room. What would occur if suddenly 3,000 additional people had serious, life-threatening injuries or had experienced an exposure to a potentially life-threatening virus or bacterium and required care? There is no easy solution for a problem of this magnitude, but the U.S. needs to have a proactive plan for an event of this nature and this scale.

One suggestion that should be initiated is to have a progressive task force composed of EMS and congressional leaders working toward an emergency solution. Currently regional planning groups are in place, but their plans and resources are generally unknown to their communities. Integration of the planning should be pushed down to the local level to allow for communication, fund management, and innovation.

The implementation of a visual learning lab/model Emergency Department to try out best practices and training that would be located in five central locations in the U.S. in upstate New York, in southern Georgia, in western Arizona, in Utah, and in central Texas could help practitioners determine the best methods for managing surges in demand and for establishing essential local and national communications. Taking this idea a step further, a paperless or all-electronic hospital would be an exciting trial-and-error opportunity to see which methods are workable and which systems need to be developed further (Osterweil, 2008).

Action Item 7: Nationalize Electronic Health Records

The possibility of a *national electronic health record* plan that would include all health care entities—hospitals, physician offices, clinics—utilizing the same technology platform would be a remarkable accomplishment and would control, diminish, or eliminate the problems of interoperability of information technology systems. Establishing the platform and foundation for one system today would eliminate having to redo the system at some point in the future and would accomplish the simplicity and consistency of one system for all.

It would be a valuable exercise for the government to explore the possibility with an EHR supplier. The EHR system would not be nationalized but would, preferably, be privately run and managed. Start-up costs could be financed and supported by federal government grants and other interested entities. Current U.S. investments in pharmaceuticals and research are massive, as would be the investment in a national EHR project. Although a national EHR project of this magnitude and initial complexity would be an enormous task, the long-term benefits are worth considering. Business intelligence and capital would be necessary to ensure success.

Health care entities could be incentivized to use the national EHR system through tax credits or by rewarding the hospital's participation via guarantees of investments of only small amounts of time and money.

OTHER ISSUES FOR CONSIDERATION

- A short-term solution for the uninsured. One possible immediate solution for the uninsured population in the U.S. is to offer a very low-cost insurance for all U.S. citizens that would cover routine health, dental, and emergency care and would provide coverage for catastrophic events. The revenue derived from even a tiny contribution from families could finance less-expensive care in 24-hour clinics and would allow savings of state charity care funds.
- Wellness pays. It costs less to provide care for healthy individuals than it does for ill individuals. Trends are moving in this direction, although the insurance companies could do more to incentivize participation.
- Pay for performance and other incentives. Physicians are reimbursed based on the volume of patients that they evaluate and treat. The only incentive that physicians have is to see as many patients as possible during the course of a day as a means of increasing their reimbursement, allowing for a viable practice. Many complex patients who are elderly and have multiple comorbidities frequently must choose to visit the Emergency Department because the primary care physician does not have the time to work up the patient or to diagnose and/or treat time-consuming problems. The pay-for-performance model has had positive results, although it has been tested only in small-scale studies. CMS needs to consider pay-for-performance incentives for Medicare.
- Charity care. Some states have begun to retract charity care payments to hospitals in their states. Because of the large number of uninsured patients in many states, the withdrawal of payments has created the dissolution of many hospitals, especially in New Jersey. The only solution is to increase taxes to reimburse hospitals and to increase the funds available for charity care so that hospitals are provided with cash for operations in those states that cannot fund hospitals, expenses for charity care (Rosenthal, 2008).

■ Rethink EMTALA. Although the involvement of *government* in health care usually involves the addition of new, cumbersome, and difficult regulations, a change in the way that government supports the Emergency Department may be beneficial. The EMTALA requirement establishes an unfunded mandate to accept and treat uninsured—and all—patients. The result of regulation without a method to fund it is a rapid deterioration of profit or surplus revenue. The EMTALA regulation has inadvertently created a financial fiasco for hospital and Emergency Department budgets and needs to be reevaluated (*ACEP Task Force Report*, n.d.; Blum, 2005).

There is encouraging change that could positively affect Emergency Departments. The Centers for Medicare and Medicaid has proposed allowing hospitals to share on-call physician coverage in what is being termed a regional or community plan. In April of 2008, CMS suggested changing its current on-call physician regulation to allow hospitals within a designated region to essentially share their specialty physician on-call responsibility that is now mandated by CMS through EMTALA. This change is in response to the difficulty that hospital Emergency Departments are having in complying with the portion of the regulation requiring a full complement of specialty physicians on the on-call list, to be able to respond to the needs of Emergency Department patients who may require a particular specialty service. But, because of the limited supply and availability of specialty physicians, Emergency Departments found themselves lacking in specialty coverage, and Emergency Department physicians were spending a great deal of time trying to find a specialty physician to provide a specific service (*CMS Proposes Changes*, 2008).

In 2004, 67% of Emergency Department physician-directors and other hospital physicians reported to ACEP that they were having difficulty supplying on-call specialty physicians. By 2005, in a re-survey to the same population of physicians, the figure had risen to 73% (Vanlandingham, 2006).

The dilemma, aside from the particulars of sharing the on-call physician and the logistics that the plan may entail, is that CMS does not know how to ensure that the same financially risky patients will not be dumped at the community call–plan hospital. The original tenets of EMTALA were designed to protect and prevent patients who represented a financial risk to the hospital or Emergency Department from being dumped at other hospitals.

CMS will issue a final ruling soon. It would be welcomed if CMS would rethink the entire EMTALA act to evaluate and measure the financial affect on hospitals and Emergency Departments (Glendinning, 2008).

ACCESS TO EMERGENCY MEDICAL SERVICES ACT OF 2007

Senate Bill 1003, introduced on March 28, 2007, an amendment to title XVIII of the Social Security Act sponsored by Senator Debbie Ann Stabenow (D-Michigan), would:

- Improve access to emergency services and the quality and efficiency of the care provided in EDs, hospitals, and critical access hospitals
- Establish a bipartisan commission to examine the factors that affect the efficient delivery of ED services
- Provide additional payments for certain physician services
- Establish a CMS working group (ostensibly to work on EMTALA provisions)

Clearly, Congress is reticent in its responsibility to learn the details of the peril in which Emergency Departments find themselves. The last reported action on the bill was March 28, 2007, the day it was introduced, according to www.GovTrack.us, a Web site that tracks the activities of the current congressional sessions. If patients and issues in the ED were handled in a similar slow and inefficient manner, Emergency Departments would implode. The health care industry needs an uncompromising health care–educated advocate who will get this type of bill introduced and passed *quickly*. Similar iterations of this bill have been introduced on 11 previous occasions since the 104th Congress. Each time, the bill has been killed (S. 1003: Access to Emergency Medical Services Act, 2007).

Surely our government can help us out better than this. It is difficult to understand how such a significant problem that has been addressed with Congress by ACEP can be abruptly forgotten or pushed aside for allegedly more important discussions. How can we get this issue in front of the individual or committee who will understand and promote the issue until change can be enacted?

Many hospitals and EDs are closing every week in the U.S. because of the financial complexity that hospitals and EDs have encountered—largely due to the overwhelming number of patients who do not have health insurance. State charity care funds have been re-allocated to support other critical needs. EDs and hospitals are struggling to comply with requirements that dig into their profit base, and many hospitals can no longer afford to operate and are forced to close, leaving patients to crowd into the remaining hospital EDs. Several encouraging solutions in operation now include:

- Medical home. The medical home concept may have some merit, but at this point, there is little data to understand if financial benefits can be derived from the concept.
- Malpractice reform. Texas may become the model for malpractice reform. Costs for malpractice insurance coverage have dropped significantly. The result is that Texas is benefiting from an influx of physicians into the state. Malpractice liabilities need to be reduced or eliminated for specialty physicians who are on-call for hospitals. Currently, specialty physicians have greater costs, exposure, and liability for patients that are seen in the Emergency Department. The current method of assessing specialty physicians is counterproductive and needs immediate reform to either limit or eliminate physician liability for providing on-call services in the ED (Blumenthal, 2008).

CASE STUDY

In a recent article in Investor's Business Daily, *Mike Leavitt, the former secretary of the U.S. Department of Health and Human Services, provides a compelling argument for the U.S. to develop—as a starting point—"package deals" for health care. Mr. Leavitt points out that if we purchased cars the way that we currently purchase health care, no automobile manufacturer would ever sell a car. Why?*

To begin with, the automobile manufacturers would not know the final price the consumer would be paying. It is doubtful any of us would be satisfied with a guess as to the final price of the

(Continued)

car. But we are forced to be satisfied purchasing our health care in this manner. For health care purchases, we never really know the final price we will be paying. What we pay for doctors, facilities (hospital rooms or outpatient service centers), and other services (anesthesiology, for example), is a moving target and cannot be absolutely quoted in advance.

Mr. Leavitt's department was adamant in his suggestion that Congress join with Medicare officials to recreate the U.S. health care delivery system. His goal is to initiate a reform of the current health care system and begin providing high-quality, low-cost health care, based on "four cornerstones [that] are standard quality measurements, cost comparisons, EHR (electronic health records) and value-based incentives" for physicians (Leavitt, 2008).

PAY-FOR-PERFORMANCE (P4P)

The current trend in physician incentives is termed pay for performance (P4P). Pay-for-performance is the method that was introduced early in the 21st century to incentivize physicians to meet certain quality targets and is currently being used as a trial to evaluate the process that health plans and government programs use to pay physicians for their services. The underlying premise is based on the accomplishment of quality target outcomes within specific disease groups for patients. For example, a physician would be paid the full scheduled reimbursement fee for a diabetic patient if the physician scheduled periodic patient Hemoglobin A1C testing.[1] The goal of pay-for-performance was to remove disincentives of quantity of patients and to "align financial reward with improved [patient] outcomes" (Baker, 2003, p. 3). A recent program evaluation has concluded that "not all P4P continue to evolve" because "several programs have stalled in their development." "Provider participation levels, having achieved modest goals without strong impetus from employers or providers for continued expansion or refinement" (Baker, 2003, p. 6).

Physicians are reimbursed for caring for Medicare patients via a fee-for-service plan that pays the physician for each office visit and each hospitalization day. This fee-for-service arrangement forces physicians to think in terms of quantity—the actual numbers of patients seen and treated—rather than focusing on the quality of the health care services provided. Despite encouraging progress toward positive incentives for physicians, pay-for-performance has not yet been adopted by CMS for Medicare reimbursement. Pay-for-performance methods were used by approximately eighty percent of commercial health care maintenance organizations in 2006 (Rosenthal, 2008). Currently, the pay-for-performance trial has less than 10 years of experience. Much remains to be evaluated to ensure that quality is indeed being improved and achieved. "Health plans talk about shifting to outcomes-based payment models, putting more demand on doctors to meet standards of care by developing 'best practices' approaches, while at the same time providing no additional reimbursement to do so," laments internist Jordon Lovy, MD (as quoted in Baker, 2003, p. 5).

EVIDENCE-BASED VIOLENCE PREVENTION PRACTICE IN THE EMERGENCY DEPARTMENT

Efforts similar to those proposed by Congressman Randy Forbes to champion the cause of controlling gang activity in the U.S. are a positive step forward in legislating actions that ultimately may help diminish violence that spills over into Emergency Department waiting rooms. Although Mr. Forbes's 2005 bill proposal (reintroduced in 2007), referred to as the Gangbuster Bill (Gang Deterrence and Community Protection Act of 2005), has not yet passed in the Senate, we can hope that one knowledgeable champion for change will recognize the value of this bill and of other similar bills to diminish violence in society.

Mr. Forbes's bill has a two-pronged objective:

1. Teenage gang members will be tried as adults in a court of law.
2. A minimum jail sentence of 10 years would be imposed on teenage gang members for involvement in violent, gang-related criminal activities.

Additionally, the bill would:

1. Authorize funding for the investigation and prosecution of gang crimes
2. Create a statute to prosecute any enterprise that is supported and run by gangs and to fund gang investigational technology and database creation

The bill is explained on Mr. Forbes's downloadable pamphlet about the proposed Gangbuster Bill (*It Stops Now: The Gangbuster Bill*, 2005).

CASE STUDY

PREVENTION AS A STRATEGY FOR REDUCING HEALTH CARE COST

Wishard Health Services whose health care–system participants' are diverse, has the following population distribution: 28% of the population is covered by Medicaid, 34% is uninsured, and only 10% owns commercial health insurance. The system knew that the chance for serious financial risk was high.

To manage this risk, the executives of the hospital/health care system focus on providing preventive and primary care, to keep patients from becoming ill. The improvements they have made have kept ED utilization low. The preventive care has limited the risk and number of premature births and has kept people healthy and out of the hospital. The efforts have paid off. The hospital projects they will have a $5.5 million surplus at the end of the year (Lee, 2008).

Perhaps similar wellness and primary care–centered programs could also reduce the risk of violence in the Emergency Department. By controlling overcrowding in Emergency Departments, facilities would have the necessary resources to treat life-threatening emergencies within efficient timeframes, thus reducing the opportunity for laborious ED waits that can lead to frustration, anger, and violence.

CASE STUDY

ROBOTIC TRIAGE

A robotic triage system is being developed for use by battlefield medics, allowing them to assess an injured soldier from afar, up to

(Continued)

several miles away. The triage robot serves to prevent additional injuries and trauma to the medics in charge of caring for injured troops.

While this particular triage system is not the same type of triage used in Emergency Departments, there may be an application for using a similar apparatus down the road, *and to perhaps assess and reassess patients in the ED waiting room and additionally for use in mass casualties. The company says that the robot could also be use for mine disasters or building collapses, or any situation that requires an emergency response that would risk human life.*

PERL, the company developing the system, won the contract from the Army Medical Research and Materiel Command following a tough competition with 35 other manufacturers and will have the robot ready for testing in approximately 2 years.

Some of the features of the robot are thermographic sensors to measure vital signs without touching the patient. The robot extracts the measurements, and software gathers the data and evaluates it. A video camera and communication device allows the remote medic to evaluate the injured soldier via visualization and communication (Accardi, 2008).

The expansion of the science of robotics offers the opportunity for the U.S. to capitalize on its domination in research and to create applications for health care. In addition to being a valuable battlefield tool, robotics may have utility in the areas of EMS, telemedicine, and Emergency Department trauma.

CONCLUSION

Nurses in the ED are on the front lines of violence, and hospitals need enact safety, security, and training to be certain that each and every nurse is protected and feels safe when he/she arrives to work in the Emergency Department. One hospital encouraged nurses to return to work after a particularly bad altercation with a violent patient, and there are other EDs that have discouraged the reporting of injury-producing aggression. Nurses are entitled—and you must know that it is essential—to report all episodes of aggression, violence, and abuse to help diminish the influence of violence for all nurses.

Exhibit 12.2

FIVE PROPOSALS TO REPAIR A BROKEN HEALTH CARE SYSTEM

MANDATE COVERAGE POSSIBLE REFORM	EXPAND MEDICARE	END TAX BENEFITS FOR EMPLOYER-PROVIDER COVERAGE	REWARD EFFICIENCY	ENCOURAGE PREVENTIVE-HEALTH INITIATIVES
Create a system requiring all Americans to have health insurance, just as all drivers are required to have auto insurance. Premiums could be adjusted to keep coverage affordable. Businesses would be required to provide health coverage or pay into a fund.	Broaden Medicare to include the entire population. This proposal has support among those who believe it would take wasteful administrative cost—and profits—out of the system. An interim step could be to allow people aged 50–64 to buy into Medicare.	Treat employee health benefits as ordinary income. Americans would become more aware of the total cost of health insurance and care. This would push prices down.	Offer incentives to make the system more efficient. Financially reward physicians for providing high-quality care at lower cost. Require that all providers use a common computerized medical record system.	Financially reward or penalize the habits of individual policyholders—to encourage people to quit smoking or to lose weight, and so forth. Government would play a role through education or even through tax incentives.

PROS

Everybody would have health insurance. Eliminating the costs of uncompensated care for the uninsured would lower prices for everyone. The health of those now uninsured would improve.	Insurance companies pocketed billions in profits last year—money that could instead be used to offset basic health care costs. Medicare spends much less on administrative costs.	If patients were able to shop for coverage, they might be able to negotiate lower rates, as they have done on electronics and airline tickets. Or they might demand government intervention.	Efficiency rewards would boost quality, make the system work leaner, and trim costs. Electronic record keeping would eliminate needless duplication and would improve patient safety.	If Americans adopted a healthier lifestyle it could greatly reduce the number of people diagnosed with chronic illnesses and the costs to treat these diseases and lead to longer life span.

CONS				
Some people might be forced to buy insurance they think they can't afford or don't need. This proposal would be politically difficult to enact.	Medicare expansion puts providers—doctors, hospitals and others—at the mercy of the government and leaves them little choice but to accept whatever prices Medicare choose to pay.	The sick and the injured—especially in an emergency—will most likely have neither the time or the ability to hunt for a bargain.	Electronic records could jeopardize patient privacy. Hospitals and providers making the capital investment won't benefit financially.	Some believe that these are strictly personal matters and should not involve government mandates or tax incentives. Longer life spans could cost the system more in the long run.
OUTLOOK				
Massachusetts is moving in this direction, and a similar attempt in California failed. There may be reluctance to mandate coverage until more states prove that this is a workable approach.	Some countries already use this single-payer system; U.S. analysts are watching carefully. But in the U.S., there is widespread resistance to the idea, so it may be difficult to pass.	There is growing awareness that employer-provided coverage is shrinking, necessitating an alternative. But this is a radical proposal for a system that tends to adopt incremental changes.	Electronic records alone would yield only a modest reward. Electronic records are not a comprehensive solution but would likely be included in broader reforms.	In the past, it has been difficult to launch and coordinate large-scale and sustained preventive-health campaigns.

Note: From "Five Proposals to Repair a Broken [Healthcare] System," by J. Jaffe, July/August 2008. *AARP*, p. 56.

Physicians also are in harms' way of dangerous and violent patients. The hazards that are inherent to the Emergency Department have evolved because of the large numbers of patients who visit Emergency Departments: uninsured patients, psychiatric patients, low-acuity patients, and those needing actual emergency care. The inefficiency of inpatient operations and the sheer numbers of patients in the waiting room and in the hallways can produce violent reactions from minor irritations and place the nurses and physicians in peril.

Violence affects our patients. The unconscionable act of abuse to a child or to an elderly person or another human being is discussed in Chapter 6 so that Emergency Department nurses and physicians can be alert to situations and help ED personnel recognize violence against these vulnerable individuals.

Lateral abuse is violence against coworkers. And, unfortunately, lateral violence is extremely prevalent in nursing. Dr. Barry Stein, a psychologist in British Columbia, believes that nurses abusing other nurses is because of the high levels of stress that they encounter every day at work. Lateral abuse is violence and needs to be reported (Thomson, 2004).

This book presents the impetus for change for hospitals and Emergency Departments. Violence exists: hospitals must implement barriers to protect their EDs from the occurrences and the impact of violence. The federal government needs to step in and assist Emergency Departments and hospitals with reform and change to current regulations that are placing financial burdens and unconquerable barriers on health care institutions. Together, perhaps we can generate innovative short-term and long-term solutions for U.S. health care—especially in the Emergency Department (Jaffe, 2008; see Exhibit 12.2 for suggestions to repair the U.S. health care system).

NOTE

1. Hemoglobin A1C is a blood test that measures the level of blood glucose (sugar) control over a specified length of time, usually 4 months. HA1C levels of 7% or less indicates excellent blood sugar control whereas 9%–12% reflects a less-than-optimum control. HA1C levels greater than 12% indicate very poor blood sugar control.

REFERENCES

Accardi, M. (2008, August 29). *Robotic triage system aims to keep combat medics safe.* Retrieved September 30, 2008, from www.emsresponder.com/online/printer.jsp?id-8191

ACEP Task Force report on boarding and emergency department crowding; ACEP's suggested boarding solutions generate national support. (n.d.). Retrieved August 13, 2008, from http://acep.org/advocacy.aspx?id=33074

Addis, N. (2008, July 13). Super users are swamping the ED. *Star-Ledger* (Camden, NJ).

Assault: Legal definition. (2009). Retrieved April 29, 2009, from http://www.nolo.com/definition.cfm/term/22542b6f-fedb-450a-889a82a49ea50ceb/alpha/a/

Baker, G. W. (2003). *Pay for performance incentive programs in healthcare: Market dynamics and business process (executive briefing)*. Retrieved April 29, 2009, from http://www.leapfroggroup.org/media/file/Leapfrog-Pay_for_Performance_Briefing.pdf

Blum, F. M. (2005, November 21). *Recommendations to the EMTALA tag*. Retrieved December 31, 2008, from www.acep.org/workarea/showcontent.aspx?id=5166

Blumenthal, R. (2008, October 5). *More doctors in Texas after malpractice caps*. Retrieved December 31, 2008, from http://www.nytimes.com/2007/10/05/us/05doctors.html

CMS proposes changes to EMTALA requirements. (2008). Retrieved December 31, 2008, from http://www.mwe.com/index.cfm/fuseaction/publications.nldetail/object_id/c0eb083c-ea55-4e4a-b9c5-6479b25193a1.cfm

Glendinning, D. (June, 16 2008). *EMTALA flexibility proposed to relieve on-call shortages*. Retrieved July 22, 2008, from http://www.ama-assn.org/amednews/2008/06/16/gvl20616.htm

It stops now: The Gangbuster Bill. (2005). Retrieved July 22, 2008, from www.streetgangs.com/laws/gangflyer.pdf

Jaffe, J. (2008, July/August). Five proposals to repair a broken [health care] system. *AARP*, p. 56.

Jost, T. (2007). *Health care at risk: A critique of the consumer-driven movement*. Durham, NC: Duke University Press.

Kaplan, J. C. (2007, October 9). *Tackling emergency department crowding from the inside out*. Retrieved July 22, 2008, from http://meetings.acep.org/NR/rdonlyres/0A32CA38-1365-4534-90CF-117861515E20/0/TU141.pdf

Leavitt, M. F. (2008, June 24). *Time to adopt a value-driven health system*. Retrieved June 25, 2008, from http://www.hhs.gov/secretary/opeds/valuedrive.html

Lee, D. (2008). *Wishard says early action aids patients, bottom line*. Retrieved August 4, 2009, from http://www.indystar.com/apps/pbcs.dll/article?AID=2008807270395&template=printart

Osterweil, N. (2008). *US emergency preparedness found wanting*. Retrieved December 31, 2008, from http://www.medscape.com/viewarticle/585862?src=mp&spon=21&uac=123131J

Ray, M. M. (2007). The dark side of the job: Violence in the Emergency Department. *Journal of Emergency Nursing, 33*(3), 257–261.

Rosenthal, T. (2008, December 22). *The medical home: Growing evidence to support a new approach to primary care*. Retrieved December 31, 2008, from http://www.medscape.com/viewarticle/585208_1

S. 1003: Access to Emergency Medical Services Act of 2007. (2007, March 28). Retrieved August 12, 2008, from http://www.govtrack.us/congress/bill.xpd?bill=s110-1003

Thomson, H. (2004). *Study shows nurses are regular target of violence but 70% of incidents go unreported*. Vancouver: University of British Columbia.

Vanlandingham, B. M. (2006). *On-call specialty coverage in U.S. emergency departments*. Retrieved April 29, 2009, from http://www.acep.org/workarea/downloadasset.aspx?id=33266

Appendices

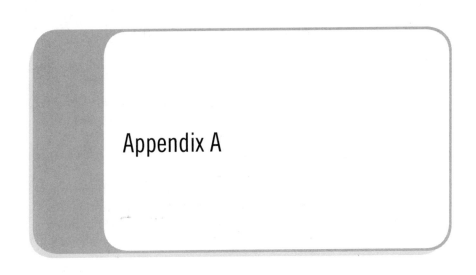

Appendix A

RECOMMENDED WEB SITES FOR VIOLENCE REDUCTION
RESOURCES

http://www.EDViolence.com—Violence in the Emergency Department

http://www.JenniferAnn.org—Dating violence resources

http://www.chooserespect.org—Centers for Disease Control dating violence site

http://www.loveisrespect.org—Dating violence Web site presented by Liz Claiborne

http://www.loveisnotabuse.com—Dating violence Web site presented by Liz Claiborne

http://www.Homefrontprotect.com—Gang information and consultation

http://www.YouthAlive.org—Preventing (street and youth) violence, developing youth leaders

http://www.ENA.org—Emergency Nurses Association

http://www.ACEP.org—American College of Emergency Physicians

http://www.Texashealthresoureces.com—

http://www.texashealth.org/body.cfm?id=1848—Family/Intimate partner violence cost calculator estimates the cost impact of IPV on businesses.

http://www.youtube.com/watch?v=mBCRBaLHR1k—Lateral violence scenarios

http://www.youtube.com/watch?v=4MT8Wnb9ZY8&feature=related —Lateral violence scenarios

http://www.Capindex.com—Crime forecasting and geographic risk

http://www.access.gpo.gov/nara/cfr/waisidx_04/42cfr482_04.html— Web site guidance for restraint policy and restraint use

http://www.GovTrack.us—Nongovernmental Web site to track progress of congressional bills

http://www.streetgangs.com/laws/gangflyer.pdf—Gang Busters bill

https://www.ena.org/government/Advocacy/Violence/PositionStatement.pdf—Emergency Nurses Association Position Statement: Violence in the Emergency Care Setting

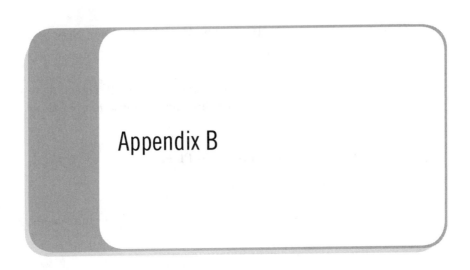

Appendix B

RECOMMENDED POLICIES FOR EMERGENCY DEPARTMENT VIOLENCE REDUCTION

- Zero tolerance for possession of weapons in the Emergency Department; scanning for weapons (ambulatory and EMS patients) including zero tolerance signage policy
- Zero tolerance for aggression, violence, or abuse; reporting of violence or abuse or threats of violence or abuse, including lateral violence
- Staff debriefing and counseling following a violent incident
- Possession of illicit substances forbidden; confiscation/surrender required
- Identification of potentially violent individuals or individuals with a history of violent behavior; flagging of records
- Triage reassessment policy; identification of patients who have increasing stress
- Assessment policies: intimate partner violence, dating violence, elder abuse, child abuse, suicide potential
- Employee and visitor access to ED including EMS entrance
- Hostage policy
- Forensic reporting policy

- Code V, Dr. Duress, Dr. Tough, Dr. Alert, Dr. Red, Dr. Now
  - Whichever paging moniker is used, be certain it is not similar to the name of a current physician.
  - Be certain that you communicate the name and the meaning to everyone in the hospital, including any in-house telephone or Telex operators and receptionists.

Policies That Should Already Be in Place

- Restraint policy
- Use of secure-room policy
- Bomb threats or other threat response (tornadoes, hurricanes, child abduction, etc.)
- Emergency preparedness/surge response
- Human resources dress policy to include no visible tattoos, no sports team clothing
- Human resources background check on all employees

Downloadable Policies That Are Available on the Web Site www.EDViolence.com

- Street gang policy
- Duress alarm policy (Strategy 4 in Chapter 8 of this book)
- Security assessment timing to ensure duress alarms, door access controls, and lockdown mechanisms are in working order
- Extra security in ED when prisoner brought to ED for evaluation
- Customer service policy
- De-escalation training
- Code V policy

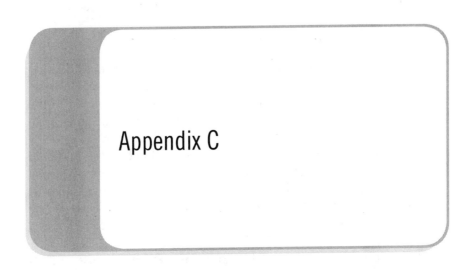

Appendix C

AMERICAN COLLEGE OF EMERGENCY PHYSICIANS:
EMERGENCY DEPARTMENT CROWDING AND BOARDING
STRATEGIES WHITE PAPER

SHORT-TERM SOLUTIONS/MODEL PRACTICES

Short-term solutions to the crowding problem involve cooperative efforts between the ED and other stakeholders, including the various hospital inpatient units, ancillary and support services, the hospital medical staff, administration and EMS providers. Simply expanding ED facility space and increasing hospital bed capacity are two approaches that alone are unlikely to be successful in relieving ED crowding. Likewise, any strategies that do not have the enthusiastic support of senior hospital management are doomed to failure. Most of *the strategies that have been found to be successful* were those that *addressed primary factors external to the ED*.

This list of model practices can be viewed as short-term solutions, and can be grouped under several health care domains having individual and shared responsibilities for alleviating crowding. These domains are EMS, ED, hospital and regional services.

EMS MODEL PRACTICES

- **Medical direction.** The EMS medical director should develop policies and protocols for the delivery of patients to appropriate hospitals, based on knowledge of the specialty capabilities of the system's facilities. The medical director also should be involved in the development of system-wide diversion protocols.
- **Diversion protocols.** Each ambulance within the system should carry a written protocol that defines explicit criteria for diverting patients, and includes contingency plans for alternative transport destinations. Familiarity with such diversion protocols should be part of the knowledge base for all paramedics and EMTs working in the system.
- **Regional information management system.** The use of EM-System™ software is one example of an Internet-based tool that can help manage hospital diversion status and collect real-time information for current and future planning by EMS agencies. The ED Alert network, used in Massachusetts, is another example. The goal is to be able to direct ambulances to the nearest open and appropriate facility prior to initiation of patient transport. Information collected from these tools must also be made available to local health authorities with responsibility for planning and disaster management.
- **Regional diversion saturation override.** A process must be in place to account for times when there is saturation of all hospitals in a region, so as to not leave EMS providers without an appropriate hospital destination. In Boston and Denver, for example, at the point when the last available hospital is poised to go on diversion, all hospitals are automatically taken off diversion and re-opened to incoming ambulances.
- **Documentation.** Diversions (number, length of time, hospitals involved, reasons) and EMS turnaround times (the time intervals spent by EMS waiting at hospitals) should be tracked, tallied monthly and reported to ED medical directors, hospital administrators, and regional public health authorities.
- **State Public Health Authorities.** All of the above activities should be coordinated with those agencies responsible for hospital oversight, EMS systems, disaster response, and current preparations for bioterrorism preparedness.

EMERGENCY DEPARTMENT MODEL PRACTICES

Although the major characteristics of ED patient flow—random arrival of patients having varying degrees of acuity—is beyond the direct control of the ED staff, the ED does have the ability to influence the throughput process. The following are some recommendations:

- **Real-time monitoring of ED crowding metrics.** Through weekly measurement of Key Performance Indicators, such as ED patient volume, hospital census, boarders, staffing levels, critical care bed capacity, throughput times and ED waiting times, EDs may be able to predict in advance when diversion is imminent. The goal, of course, is to identify and correct problems *before* they get out of control and lead to hospital diversion. One example of this functionality is the "Emergency Department Demand/Capacity Management System" used at Overlook Hospital in Summit, New Jersey, which uses a color-coded matrix to define the level of ED activity. This is said to have reduced the admission cycle time from 129 minutes to 78 minutes in 2001, with a 13-month hiatus in the incidence of diversions.
- **Best Demonstrated Processes.** A detailed analysis of ED patient lengths of stay (LOS) in a large multihospital system leads to the identification of "best demonstrated processes" (BDP) that distinguish top-performing from bottom-performing EDs. The BDP methodology can then be applied to the slowest EDs in the system to improve their patient throughput times and reduce their LOS. Examples of BDPs include clear identification of a person responsible for a task, clear transfer of responsibility from one step in a process to the next, and explicit process performance expectations with a designated individual charged with monitoring each process.
- **ED automation.** The ED is amenable to multiple automated processes. Examples include patient tracking software, template charting and check-box systems, automated discharge instructions and prescriptions, on-line ordering of lab tests and imaging studies, point-of-care bedside testing, pneumatic transfer of drugs and supplies, bedside computer registration and the use of fax machines to receive stat radiology reports.

THREE SYSTEM-WIDE SOLUTIONS TO DECOMPRESSING VOLUME IN ED

The American College of Emergency Physicians (ACEP) has identified **three system-wide tactics** that provide immediate solutions for decompression of patient volume in the Emergency Department (crowding) and may eliminate the need for patients to board in the ED:

1. **Full-capacity protocol (FCP).** Implement Full-capacity protocol when ED is nearing, or at capacity. Full-capacity protocol is the moving of boarded ED patients to the hallways or other open areas of the inpatient units where they will be admitted. Precautions must include professionals to care for these patients and there are certain patient type exclusions.[1]
2. **Discharge all inpatients by 12:00 noon.** Prior to discharge, and especially if the patient will be delayed beyond noon, patients should be moved to an ambulatory discharge unit to free up inpatient bed space.
3. **Smooth the surgery schedule.** Schedule planned surgeries from Monday–Friday instead of clumping surgery procedures on Monday, Tuesday, and Wednesday.[2]

NOTES

From *ACEP Task Force Report on Boarding and Emergency Department Crowding; ACEP's Suggested Boarding Solutions Generate National Support.* (n.d.). Retrieved August 13, 2008, from http://acep.org/advocacy.aspx?id=33074

1. S. Kershaw, "City Hospitals Reinvent Role of Emergency." *New York Times*, February 12, 2008.
2. (Corporate author); Emergency Department Crowding and Boarding Strategies White Paper: Short-term Solutions/Model Practices; ACEP (American College of Emergency Physicians) Web page.

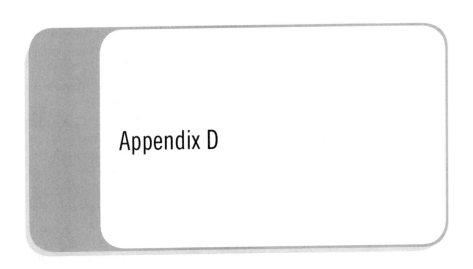

Appendix D

THE AMERICAN COLLEGE OF EMERGENCY PHYSICIANS:
THE NATIONAL REPORT CARD ON THE STATE OF
EMERGENCY MEDICINE FOR 2009
(THE NATIONAL GRADE: C−)

EXECUTIVE SUMMARY

Emergency medicine needs to be there, "where you need it, when you need it." It's something that few people think about until the moment an emergency occurs—and then their lives may depend on it. The recent Hurricane Katrina disaster shows just how important it is to have effective emergency medicine systems in place at all times. An effective system, however, requires more than the dedicated work of highly trained medical professionals—it needs the support of government to function.

The National Report Card on the State of Emergency Medicine is an assessment of the support that each state provides for its emergency medicine system.

The American College of Emergency Physicians (ACEP) prepared this report to underscore the challenges facing patients who need emergency care, as well as to recognize efforts being made to address these needs. The objective of this report is to motivate state and national policy support for improving emergency care. This effort is the first in a series of report cards, which will serve as a baseline to show progress in the future.[1]

ACEP began this intensive effort more than a year ago, with the appointment of a task force with research and policy expertise to oversee the project. The task force developed 50 objective and quantifiable criteria that were used to measure the performance of each state and the District of Columbia. These measurements were weighted and aggregated, and grades were assigned based on a comparison to the best state's performance.

Each state has an overall grade, plus grades in four categories— Access to Emergency Care, Quality and Patient Safety, Public Health and Injury Prevention, and Medical Liability Environment. These grades are not evaluations of physicians or hospital emergency departments, but they show the overall effort of states to support effective emergency medicine systems.

The results are sobering. The national emergency health care system is in serious condition, with many states in a critical situation. While no state receives an overall failing grade, many have serious deficiencies, and almost all have areas in which there is substantial room for improvement. State and national policymakers should take the results to heart and support efforts to improve emergency care.

NATIONAL GRADE

The emergency medicine system of the United States as a whole has earned a grade of C—barely above a D. This represents an average of the overall grades for all states and the District of Columbia, as well as data received from ACEP's Government Services and Puerto Rico chapters. No state scored either an A or F for its overall grade.

California, Massachusetts, Connecticut, and the District of Columbia led the nation with overall grades of B. Rating worst in the nation with overall grades of D+ or D were Alabama, Arizona, Arkansas, Idaho, Indiana, New Mexico, Oklahoma, South Dakota, Utah, Virginia, Washington, and Wyoming. More than 80 % of states earned poor or near-failing overall grades (C+ to D).

FACTS BEHIND THE NATIONAL GRADE

Despite the life-saving importance of emergency care, the emergency medicine systems in many states are under extreme stress. The number of people coming to Emergency Departments continues to increase, with nearly 114 million patient visits in 2003, the highest number ever, according to the Centers for Disease Control and Prevention (CDC). At the same time, the overall capacity of the nation's emergency systems has decreased, with hundreds of emergency departments closing in the past 10 years. The number of Emergency Departments has decreased by 14 % since 1993, according to the CDC, and hospitals are operating far fewer inpatient beds than they did a decade ago. During the 1990s, hospitals lost 103,000 staffed inpatient medical-surgical beds and 7,800 intensive care unit beds nationwide.

In addition, hospital Emergency Departments have a federal mandate to medically screen and stabilize all patients, regardless of their ability to pay. As a result, increasing numbers of uninsured patients with nowhere else to go for medical care are coming to Emergency Departments. Thus, a large number of people pay nothing for their care.

Soaring amounts of uncompensated care means fewer resources for everyone. At the same time, all health insurance payers, including private insurance companies, Medicare, and Medicaid, are paying less for services, and state governments are cutting health budgets.

Local Emergency Departments are at the front line of this national health care crisis. They are increasingly crowded, often to the point that ambulances must be diverted to another hospital. A key cause is the lack of staffed inpatient beds. Often, when emergency patients need to be moved into hospital beds, they must wait in Emergency Department hallways for hours and sometimes days. Another cause is the high cost of medical liability insurance, which has led some specialty doctors to leave medicine or to be less willing to be "on-call" for emergency situations, aggravating hospitals' ability to provide emergency care.

Federal medical liability reform would help states prevent medical specialists from leaving the practice of medicine and end the on-going battles against the reforms in place. For example, Wisconsin last year lost its battle and rescinded its reforms. Federal policymakers also could increase the number of physicians available in Emergency Departments by supporting liability protections for physicians who provide EMTALA(Emergency Medical Treatment and Labor Act)-related care.

AMBULANCE DIVERSION SURVEY

The report cards include the first-ever national survey of state government emergency medicine services officials on ambulance diversion. The Quality and Patient Safety category included the question, "Does the state require hospitals to submit data on diversions?" The survey sought to determine which states, on a statewide basis, require reporting on the frequency of diversions. State government emergency medical services (EMS) offices were contacted by telephone to obtain this information.

The survey found that only 10 states currently collect this data. Only with adequate data about the extent of the diversion problem will the country begin to confront this serious problem. ACEP is calling on all states, as well as the federal government, to begin systematic monitoring of ambulance diversion. Gathering this data will allow the nation to know the true dimensions of this rapidly growing symptom of the gridlock in emergency departments. Understanding the scope of the issue is the logical first step in confronting a complex and critical issue.

HURRICANE KATRINA

The Hurricane Katrina disaster demonstrated the critical role of emergency medicine in times of natural or man-made disasters. It also showed the need for "surge capacity" in the critical time between when a disaster occurs and when state or federal resources can be mobilized to respond.

The report card statistics from Louisiana and Mississippi are effective as of September 1, 2005, prior to the hurricane. Clearly, the loss of additional resources, particularly in New Orleans and the Gulf Coast areas, indicates even greater need for infrastructure, capacity, and local resources. At the same time, the report card offers some insights into how these areas can be rebuilt effectively.

UNDERSTANDING THE FOUR CATEGORIES

The states' overall grades are an average of their grades in four categories.

Access to Emergency Care

Evaluating patients' access to care is fundamental to evaluating the overall delivery of emergency care. Emergency departments play a vital role in providing care and access to the health care system in every community; however, their ability is limited by the system's capacity and the number of trained professionals in the state. Hospital emergency departments also play a key role in the health care safety net, treating patients regardless of whether they can pay or have health insurance.

The access category measures the availability of emergency care resources in the state, as well as certain kinds of state health care spending, including public funding of health insurance. This category also measures what percentage of a state's population is uninsured. It also measures the number of hospital-staffed beds, because a larger bed capacity reduces overcrowding and preserves everyone's access to emergency care. This category was weighted most heavily because patient access is a critical measure of how a state is meeting the emergency care needs of its residents.

Quality and Patient Safety

This category measures state support for training emergency physicians and EMS personnel, patient access to ambulances and 911 services, and state commitment to measure the extent of ambulance diversion.

Research shows emergency medicine residents usually stay to practice in the states where they trained, or nearby. This suggests that support for emergency medicine residency programs will help increase the number of qualified emergency physicians in an area.

Public Health and Injury Prevention

This category measures state support for health and safety programs, such as seat belt, helmet, and drunk driving laws. Emergency physicians see firsthand the tragic consequences of traumatic injuries in states where injury prevention laws are weak or nonexistent. Nearly 40 % of all emergency visits are attributable to traumatic injuries. Trauma is the leading cause of death for persons younger than age 34.

This category also examines the percentage of the population that is immunized, the availability of emergency preparedness programs, and the presence of public health programs that promote safer environments. These are programs through which governments help reduce preventable injuries and diseases. This is relevant to emergency medicine because emergency physicians and nurses are on the "frontlines" of caring for patients with preventable injuries and diseases.

Medical Liability Environment

This category assesses increases in state medical liability rates and support for medical liability reforms, including caps on noneconomic damages and legal protections for physicians who provide emergency care. A problem with a state's medical liability climate can lead to physician shortages, delays in patient care, and increased patient transfers, all of which have a direct bearing on the emergency medical care system.

In some areas of the country, Emergency Departments have closed because medical specialists, such as neurosurgeons, obstetricians, and orthopedists, could not obtain medical liability insurance. In almost all states, some areas do not have critical on-call specialists. Many of these specialists no longer provide services because they fear lawsuits. The problem could worsen as liability concerns drive medical students away from high-risk specialties, such as emergency medicine, surgery, neurosurgery, orthopedics, and obstetrics.

States that have addressed the problem by enacting caps on noneconomic damages—often at $250,000—have protected patients and maintained an environment in which good physicians are not forced out of practice. In the absence of federal legislation, states must act to preserve access to life-saving medical care, while also protecting patients from malpractice.

METHODOLOGY

The report card was assembled in four steps. First, a task force of experts carefully considered the available data and developed 50 appropriate evaluation criteria. The most difficult constraint was finding data collected consistently in all the states.

In some cases, important measurements were available in some states, but not all, which would not allow for comparison. Preparing this report makes it clear that federal and state governments could help improve emergency care through better, more frequent, and more consistent data collection. Overall, there were fewer than 20 pieces of data missing in the final document, out of a total of thousands of pieces of data, a gap that did not have a significant effect on the final grades.

Second, the task force divided the criteria into the four broad categories. The task force recognized that not all categories or criteria were equal, and assigned percentage weightings to reflect this. The four categories and their percentages of the final grade are as follows:

- access—40 %;
- quality and patient safety—25 %;
- public health and injury prevention—10 %;
- and medical liability environment—25 %.

The grades then were allocated as follows:

- States that reached at least 80% of the top state score received an A
- States that reached at least 70% of the top state score received a B
- States that reached at least 50% of the top state score received a C
- States that reached at least 30% of the top state score received a D
- States that fell below 30% of the top state score received an F

The task force also assigned each of the 50 criteria percentage weightings that were used to develop a score within each category. These percentages are shown in the list of criteria in the next section.

Third, the performance of each state in each of the 50 criteria was compared and points awarded. In most cases, the states and the District of Columbia were ranked from top to bottom, with the top state receiving 51 points. For criteria requiring a yes or no answer, 51 points were awarded for a "yes" answer. The points for each criterion were then multiplied by the weighting factors. Those totals were added to determine each state's point total for each of the four categories.

Fourth, the states' point totals were compared using a modified-curve scoring system. Each state's total was compared with the total of the state with the highest grade in that category. This means that no state has been judged on the basis of an abstract "ideal," but rather on the basis of what has been achieved by the best state.

This scale, which was applied across all four categories, offered a generous range in which states could earn a good grade. For example, a state that scored at least 50 % of the highest state score still received a C, both overall and within each category. States in the top or bottom third of each letter-grade range received a "+" or "–" grade accordingly. A state's overall grade is the average of its grades in the four categories.

In summary, the report card methodology is an objective evaluation using data collected consistently in all states from governments and major medical associations. The grades are based strictly on how a state's support compares to the highest scoring state. All the data used in the evaluation are included in the state's report card, and all sources for this data are listed in the table at the end of this report.

ACEP gathered the best data available, but there were shortcomings. In a few cases, the most recent data were several years old. To maintain consistency, the report cards use data published in official government reports, even though a state-by-state review might have generated some updated data points.

Finally, all states have unique circumstances worthy of consideration when grading the four categories. The narrative sections of the report cards discuss the most significant of these circumstances.

The results of the 2009 Report Card present a picture of an emergency care system fraught with significant challenges and under more stress than ever before. *The overall grade for the nation across all five categories is a C–*. This low grade is particularly reflective of the poor score in *Access to Emergency Care* (D–). Because of its direct impact on emergency services and capacity for patient care, this category of indicators accounts for 30% of the Report Card grade, so the poor score is especially relevant. This category also incorporates many of the issues that states have identified as their top areas of concern. These include:

- Boarding of patients in Emergency Departments and hospital crowding
- Lack of adequate access to on-call specialists
- Limited access to primary care services
- Shortages of emergency physicians and nurses
- Ambulance diversion
- Inadequate reimbursement from public and private insurers
- High rates of uninsured individuals

Table AppD 1

TOP RANKED STATES (HIGHEST TO LOWEST)	BOTTOM RANKED STATES (LOWEST TO HIGHEST)
1. Massachusetts	51. Arkansas
2. District of Columbia	50. Oklahoma
2. Rhode Island	49. New Mexico
4. Maryland	48. Nevada
5. Nebraska	47. Oregon
6. Minnesota	46. Idaho
7. Maine	45. Arizona
8. Kansas	44. Kentucky
8. Pennsylvania	43. Michigan
10. Delaware	42. Wyoming
10. North Dakota	
10. Utah	

The grades for the other categories are slightly better, but not strong enough to pull up the full national average. Both *Disaster Preparedness* and *Quality and Patient Safety Environment* receive a C+, *Public Health and Injury Prevention* receives a grade of C, and the *Medical Liability Environment* receives a grade of C−.

Note: For further information, interactive state-by-state results, and access to the complete Report Card document please refer to: http://www.emreportcard.org/uploadedFiles/ACEP-ReportCard-10-22-08.pdf.pdf.

ADDITIONAL LINKS

Individual state reports: http://www.emreportcard.org/statereports.sap
Summary statistics for state comparisons: http://www.emreportcard.org/uploadedFiles/
    SummaryStatsForStateComp.pdf

NOTE

1. This report is posted on the ACEP Web site (www.acep.org), and significant developments will be added to the site as they become available.

Index

AAMC. *See* Association of American
    Medical Colleges
Abbott, Gayle, 279
Abuse, child. *See also* Dating
    violence
  adult manifestations of, 204
  case study on, 209–210
  categories of, 205
  checklist tool for, 208
  cost of, 124
  description of, 204–205
  MSBP and, 210, 211
  as prehospital violent condition, 186
  signs of, 207–208
  statistics on, 206
Abuse, elder. *See also* Elderly
  case study on, 203–204
  checklist tools for, 200, 202
  description of, 197–198
  financial abuse and, 201–202
  neglect as, 200–202
  as prehospital violent condition,
    186
  psychological abuse and, 201
  risk factors of, 198
  screening for, 203
  signs of, 199–200
Abuse, financial, 201–202
Abuse, psychological, 201
Abuse, substance
  aggressor types and, 144
  inpatient facilities for, 67–69
  LOS and, 59
  prior diagnosis regarding, 68
  violence regarding, 134, 135, 144,
    172, 174
Access
  Bush regarding, 180
  controlling, 217–218, 231–235

cost/training regarding, 235
door policies for, 234
efficiency and, 33–34
government regarding, 324
ID badges and, 232
ID technologies and, 233–234
as quality measure, 32–33
report card on, 349
trust and, 233
visitor policies for, 234–235
Access to Emergency Medical Services
  Act (2007), 324
ACEP. *See* American College of
  Emergency Physicians
Acuity, 64, 107, 215
Advise nurse, 104–105
Aetna, 35
Aggression
  biology of, 14–15, 16
  cognitive dissonance creating,
    18–19
  collective, 12
  de-escalation management for, 237
  delayed, 18
  economy and, 13
  genetics and, 14
  humiliation producing, 17–18
  hypothalamus and, 14–15
  magical thinking and, 19–20
  mechanism of, 8, 12–13, 14, 19
  psychology of, 16–17
  relative deprivation and, 19
  risk assessment and, 143–144
  socialization influencing, 16
  social norms and, 12–13
  substance abuse and, 144
  testosterone regarding, 15, 16
  theories of, 14–17
Alabama, 346